A MANUAL OF PRACTICAL ORTHODONTICS

BY

W. J. TULLEY

Ph.D., B.D.S., F.D.S. R.C.S., D.Orth. R.C.S.

Professor of Orthodontics, University of London, Head of Department of Orthodontics, Guy's Hospital, London. Extra Mural Lecturer, Eastman Dental Hospital, Institute of Dental Surgery, London

AND

A. C. CAMPBELL

B.D.S., F.D.S. R.C.S., M.R.C.S., L.R.C.P., D.Orth. R.C.S.

Consultant Orthodontist to Guy's Hospital and Hammersmith Hospital, London

WITH A FOREWORD BY

R. E. RIX

F.D.S. R.C.S., M.R.C.S., L.R.C.P., D.Orth. R.C.S.

Dental Surgeon Emeritus, Dental Department for Children, Guy's Hospital, London

THIRD EDITION

BRISTOL: JOHN WRIGHT & SONS LTD.

1970

First Edition, August, 1960
Second Edition, September, 1965
Third Edition, October, 1970

Distribution by Sole Agents:
United States of America: The Williams & Wilkins Company, Baltimore
Canada: The Macmillan Company of Canada, Ltd., Toronto

ISBN 0 7236 0265 4

PRINTED IN GREAT BRITAIN BY JOHN WRIGHT & SONS LTD.
AT THE STONEBRIDGE PRESS, BRISTOL BS4 5NU

TO

EILEEN AND MARGARET

PREFACE TO THE THIRD EDITION

In this third edition the authors have attempted to correct a number of points where research has established certain facts having a practical bearing on treatment. The first important point arises from a paper by Ballard (1967), 'A Morphological Basis of Prognosis Determination and Treatment Planning' (*Trans. Br. Soc. Study Orthod.*, **11**, 95). In this paper Ballard describes how to estimate the possibilities of producing a stable position of the upper labial segment. Secondly, comment is made on the effect of extractions on the lower labial segment with particular reference to Mills (1968) (*Dent. Practnr dent. Rec.*, **18**, 293). Thirdly, with regard to the extraction of the second molars, information from the paper by Cryer (1967), 'Third Molar Eruption and the Effect of Extraction of Adjacent Teeth', has been included. This treatment is rarely advocated in the light of Cryer's findings.

Apart from further attention to detail, the book maintains its original form. The bibliography has been widened to give further guidance on reading for postgraduate students. The chapter dealing with extraction of teeth has been completely revised.

There are several additional illustrations and others have been replaced to give greater clarity.

No attempt has been made to cover the use of multibanded appliances as there are many texts available in this field for the graduate student.

We would again like to express our thanks to the many colleagues who have helped us with constructive criticism and those who have given us permission to use their material. Due recognition is given in the text. We would especially like to thank Mrs. Rawlins and Mrs. Howell for their patient secretarial assistance and our publishers for their constant help and attention to detail.

W. J. T.
A. C. C.

Guy's Hospital,
*London, S.E.*1.
1970

FROM THE PREFACE TO THE FIRST EDITION

THIS book is designed to meet the requirements of undergraduates and to act as a basis for general reading for postgraduates.

The chapters dealing with the practical aspects of treatment are designed to be of assistance to the general practitioner. With this in mind we have tried to show treated cases with serial models, where possible, illustrating progress and the final result.

In a volume of this size it is impossible to cover all aspects of the subject and the reader is referred to the bibliography for more detailed studies. The book may be criticized for oversimplification and dogmatic statements, but these are essential for clarity. The literature on the subject shows the breadth of individual views and the prejudices which still exist.

In the chapters on treatment the accent is almost entirely on removable appliances as we believe that with very few exceptions a satisfactory result can be obtained in this way. Emphasis is placed on simplicity of appliance design and only one or two ways of effecting various tooth movements are described, although in fact there may be many alternative methods.

A scientific approach to the subject of orthodontics is beginning to appear with further research in the field of genetics, facial growth and development, and oral function. However, so complex are the individual variations of facial form that it is most unlikely that any method of scientific appraisal will supplant clinical judgement acquired by experience. Some orthodontic procedures are still practised quite empirically because they have been successful.

W. J. T.
A. C. C.

Dental Department for Children,
Guy's Hospital,
London, S.E.1.
1960

CONTENTS

FOREWORD TO THE FIRST EDITION

By R. E. Rix, F.D.S. R.C.S., M.R.C.S., L.R.C.P., D.Orth. R.C.S

Most derangements of the dentition are genetic in origin. They are not the effect of relative disuse of the jaws nor are they the effect of environmental influences in the Lamarckian sense, though there are some postnatal factors which can adversely affect a potentially poor dentition but which do not affect a potentially good one. Preventive orthodontics in the literal sense is extremely limited. Interceptive orthodontics (that is, early interference to improve incipient derangements) is a more fruitful field of endeavour. Orthodontic practice, however, deals mainly with derangements of the dentition which are already established.

The adjective 'abnormal' is frequently used in orthodontic literature and reveals an unconscious attachment to a morphologically ideal 'normal' which comparatively few children possess. Derangements, even those which are severe, do not have a harmful effect upon nutrition as there is such diversity and plenty of food in the modern diet. In the old edentulous patient one seldom hears of authenticated nutritional disorders.

Orthodontic treatment is seldom able to produce a complete and morphologically ideal dentition. In general terms it aims at making a compromise with Nature in order to improve appearances and to create stable conditions which favour the long survival of a healthy dentition.

Cephalometric teleradiography has demonstrated clearly the wide variations in the skeletal structure of the face and has shown that only the dento-alveolar structures are susceptible to modification by orthodontic treatment. This statement excludes mandibular displacements which form but a small part of occlusal derangements.

Cephalometric analysis with its geometrical allusions comes as a surprise to a student whose training has had a strong biological background. It does, however, demonstrate clearly the many skeletal characteristics associated with dental derangements. The value of such an analysis is not reduced by the admission that it cannot form a precise yardstick for treatment of a particular individual.

Having once grasped in principle the associations between the teeth and the facial skeleton, the student is best served by cultivating his clinical acumen. His examination of the patient must extend, in any case, beyond the hard tissues and include an appraisal of the soft-tissue environment of the dentition.

Orthodontic treatment can help to foster conditions for the survival of a healthy dentition but the proper shape of the dentition is not enough. There are certain factors of a general rather than a local nature, which can protect the dentition, despite local conditions which are not theoretically correct. Recognition of these factors helps the orthodontist to preserve moderation in his outlook. This is important when deciding whether treatment is desirable for those cases which are on the fringe of generally accepted standards.

The more derangements of the dentition hinder natural self-cleansing of the mouth, and the more unusual stresses are concentrated on one or two teeth, the more beneficial is orthodontic treatment. The relationship between occlusal stresses and periodontal disease is a continuing source of inquiry and controversy, but there are differences in the reaction of individuals. As for the relationship of incisors, unless they are actually traumatizing the gum margins, a deep overbite *per se* is of little significance.

The application of orthodontic treatment depends upon the cultivation of several skills, some of which are quite remote from the patient. The impact of treatment on a child and indeed on the whole domestic scene needs sympathetic consideration. The authors have endeavoured to point the way to obtaining satisfactory results with the minimum of interference by appliances.

Although aesthetic standards are subjective, in a sophisticated society such as ours they tend to be too rigid for the orthodontist to be able to satisfy or for him to wish to satisfy. With our population becoming increasingly cosmopolitan, rigid standards of aesthetics are obviously unrealistic.

It is sometimes difficult to convince parents of the limitations of treatment and the orthodontist himself may hope for too much by using appliances with high mechanical efficiency.

Medical practitioners also tend to hope for too much when advising orthodontic treatment to improve the nasal airway or to correct mouth-breathing. The airway cannot be enlarged by any change in position of the teeth and their alveolar process. Mouth-breathing is not automatically overcome when an incisor overjet is reduced to the point where the teeth themselves form no hindrance to closure of the lips.

Orthodontic treatment to improve speech defects is disappointing, as they rarely stem primarily from a dental derangement.

I welcome the opportunity of commending this book by two men whose orthodontic training and experience was gained at Guy's Hospital, where the amount and variety of clinical material has helped to evolve a sound approach to the speciality.

A MANUAL OF PRACTICAL ORTHODONTICS

CHAPTER I

INTRODUCTION

Definition of Orthodontics.—The definition published by the British Society for the Study of Orthodontics in 1922 is as follows:—

'Orthodontics includes the study of the growth and development of the jaws and face particularly, and the body generally, as influencing the position of the teeth; the study of action and reaction of internal and external influences on the development and the prevention and correction of arrested and perverted development.'

Very few dental irregularities are due to pathological lesions and to include these as a prominent factor in the definition would be to high-light this aspect unduly.

The authors would prefer this definition:—

'Orthodontics is the dental science which is concerned with the study of the growth, development, and infinite variations of the face, jaws, and teeth and particularly with the treatment of dentofacial abnormalities within the limits set by certain biological factors.'

History.—Although reference to some simple forms of orthodontic treatment can be traced in early civilizations it was not until the eighteenth century that Pierre Fauchard, John Hunter, and others published extensive works on the subject and they must be considered as the fathers of modern orthodontic thought. The middle of the nine-teenth century saw an increasing interest in the aetiology and treatment of irregularities of the teeth.

There were many men who were responsible for the forward look at the end of the last century. Certainly Edward Hartley Angle deserves mention as the first man to found a postgraduate school for the study of this subject. In the British Isles, Northcroft, Badcock, and Chapman were amongst those responsible for founding the British Society for the Study of Orthodontics in 1907.

The men who have made a major contribution to the study of aetiology of dental irregularities will be referred to specifically in Chapter V.

Aims and Objects.—The term 'malocclusion' suggests that all deviations from the ideal occlusion are deserving of treatment. It would be quite wrong to suggest to the lay public that some of the variations are really defects; many are quite functionally and aesthetically acceptable for the individual. It is unrealistic to state a great number of reasons for orthodontic treatment. The primary reasons are listed here:—

a. To Improve Facial Aesthetics within Certain Limits.—The fact that orthodontic treatment is often considered necessary purely for aesthetic reasons should not detract from its value. A severe dentofacial abnormality may give rise to psychological disturbances in sensitive children if they are teased. A severe malocclusion may be a social embarrassment in later life. It is also important for children to take an interest and pride in their teeth if they are to look after them.

Orthodontic treatment which eliminates an excessive overjet may also assist natural lip seal, but only when the teeth are a primary cause of separation of the lips. This will give the gingivae natural protection. However, it must be remembered that many lips which fail to seal at rest are anatomically too short and incompetent to effect a seal.

b. To Improve the Function of the Dentition.—Many malocclusions are quite functional and in no way impair the efficiency of mastication. A deep overbite, *per se*, is not an indication for treatment. This only becomes necessary when there is direct trauma to the gingival tissues.

It has been said that certain irregularities, e.g., unilateral cross-bite, by causing mandibular deviation, disturb the muscular co-ordination and may give rise to symptoms related to the temporomandibular joint in later life. However, orthodontic treatment which allows teeth to tilt and causes abnormal premature contacts of teeth is far more likely to produce symptoms of this nature.

Function can be improved in a number of instances, e.g., anterior cross-bite where the upper incisors are inside the bite.

c. Elimination of Crowding.—

i. Apart from the elimination of anterior crowding for aesthetic reasons, crowding in less visible areas may not allow the teeth and gingivae to be naturally or artificially cleaned. In subjects susceptible to periodontal disease or caries, elimination of areas of stagnation may help to reduce the problem.

However, many crowded mouths remain quite healthy so that crowding should not be considered a primary cause of dental or periodontal disease.

ii. In certain circumstances, orthodontic treatment eliminates or prevents impaction of second premolars and third molars owing to interception of crowding by judicious extraction.

d. As an Adjunct to other Forms of Dental Treatment.—

i. Preparation of the mouth for prosthetic apparatus. In cases where teeth are lost through trauma or are naturally missing, orthodontic treatment can so dispose the teeth to make the preparation of dentures, bridges, or crowns more satisfactory.

ii. Late orthodontic treatment may be a useful adjunct in the treatment of periodontal disease, prior to splinting. Surgical treatment by osteotomy may require minor tooth movements to improve the position of the standing teeth both aesthetically and functionally when the jaw segments are to be re-positioned.

iii. To assist the movement of aberrant unerupted teeth in certain situations in conjunction with surgical exposure.

Terminology.—The authors believe that terminology used in orthodontics should be as simple as possible and generally follow accepted anatomical, physiological, and medical terms. This leaves remarkably few terms which need to be specifically defined and these will be explained as they appear in the text.

CHAPTER II

THE GROWTH OF THE JAWS AND THE DEVELOPMENT OF THE DENTITION

In this chapter a brief description will be given of the postnatal growth of the face and jaws. The development of a 'normal' or average dentition will be discussed in relation to this. It must be emphasized that there are infinite variations in the human dentition which make it as individual as a finger-print.

The Gum Pads at Birth.—At birth the gum pads contain the developing deciduous teeth in their bony crypts. For a short time these

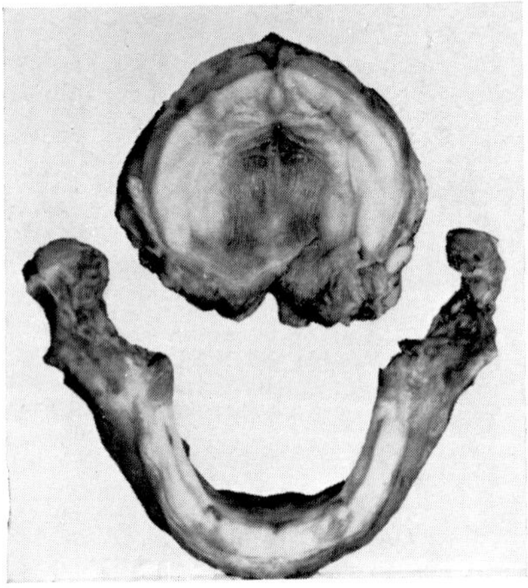

Fig. 1.—Occlusal view of gum pads showing their shape and segmentation. (*By courtesy of Professor B. E. D. Cooke.*)

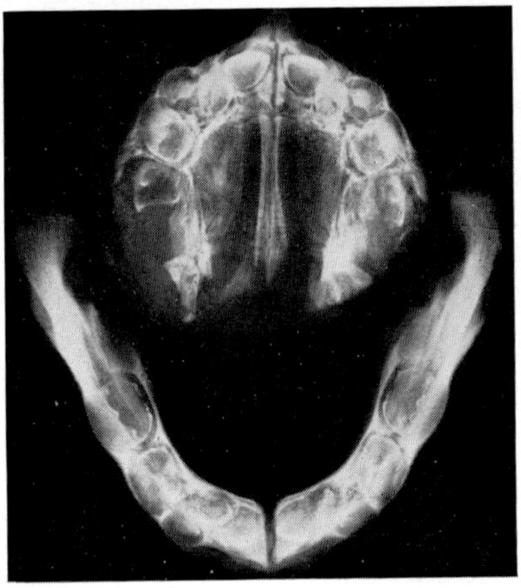

Fig. 2.—Occlusal X-ray of gum pads at birth showing position of teeth in their crypts.

crypts are not completely covered with bone. The upper gum pad is horseshoe-shaped and the lower U-shaped and somewhat flattened anteriorly (*Fig.* 1).

They are divided into segments which indicate the positions of the underlying teeth with the exception of the second deciduous molar area, which is not well defined for the first few months. *Fig.* 2 illustrates the typical position of the teeth in their crypts at this time.

The arch of the upper gum pad is both wider and longer than the lower and the palate is flat. The gum pads are probably not brought together in function and their anteroposterior relationship is difficult to assess. Sillman describes this relationship by reference to the relative position of the lateral sulci distal to the developing canine. The lateral sulcus in the lower arch is well distal to that in the upper. *Fig.* 3 illustrates a typical relationship of the gum pads. Clinch has shown that there are many variations even at this stage.

At rest the gum pads are widely separated. The tongue is blunt and large relative to the size of the jaws, resting between the gum pads in contact with the lower lip and the cheeks. The upper lip is

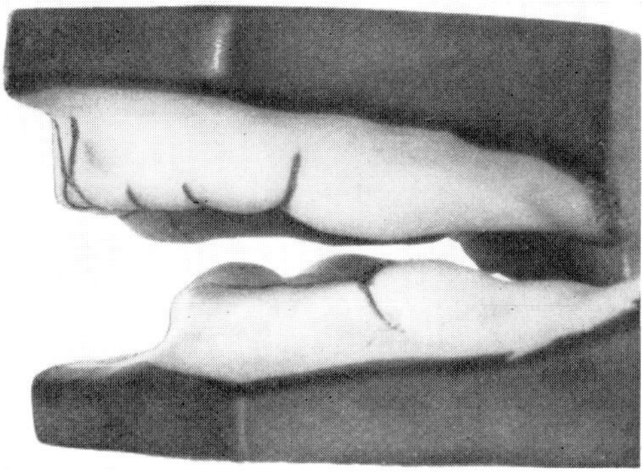

Fig. 3.—The gum pads at birth. (Note relation of lateral sulci distal to canine segment.)

rather flaccid and everted, with its fraenum attached to the crest of the upper gum pad. The lower lip is dimpled and recedes under the upper.

The Jaws at Birth.—At birth the small facial skeleton constitutes about one-eighth of the total skull size, whereas in the adult it constitutes nearly one-half. The maxillary complex is a small replica of the adult, without the alveolar process. The maxillae have overgrown the premaxillary element on the facial aspect.

The body of the mandible is a gutter of bone containing the developing teeth. The condylar and coronoid processes are small and the condyle is in almost the same plane as the body (*Fig.* 4). During the first year of life there is fibrous union between the two halves of the mandible and this fibrous tissue may contain small mental ossicles. There is no real mental eminence and in profile the mandible appears retrusive. The temporomandibular joint has a very shallow glenoid cavity and no well-defined articular eminence. The condyle itself is rather flat, so that there is lack of definition of the articular surfaces.

The Growth of the Facial Skeleton.—John Hunter probably made the first really serious contribution to the study of jaw growth.

By comparing many skulls at different ages he showed the three-dimensional changes in the facial skeleton. Many of his observations were extremely astute and are still the basis of modern views. Animal experimentation by Brash and others, using vital staining methods, helped in an appreciation of areas of bone deposition in the jaws. Although this technique showed up areas in which bone deposition was extremely active at the time the animals were sacrificed, it did not

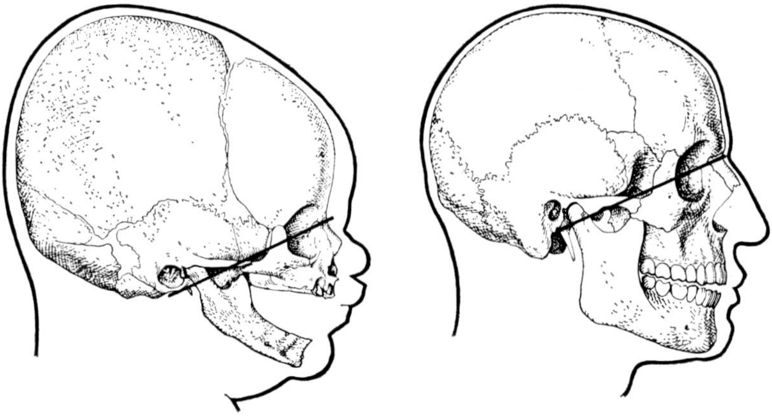

Fig. 4.—The jaws at birth compared to the adult. (Note relative size of facial skeleton.)

take into account the fact that bone is constantly being remodelled and did not highlight the main growth centres.

It was not until the introduction of a serial cephalometric X-ray technique by Broadbent that it was possible to make an appraisal of the growth pattern in the same individual using human material. This work in the Bolton Study was a great step forward, and among the other major contributions to cephalometric studies was that of Brodie. At the present time, there are many serial studies of facial growth with particular reference to ethnic groups which have been modelled on Broadbent's original work.

Sicher, Rushton, Scott, Symons, and others have added to our knowledge of the mechanisms of growth by studying the histology of the growing tissues. Björk has made the most recent contribution to the subject using a group of metallic implants in each jaw. Serial radiographs can be superimposed using the implants as reference points as they appear to remain in a stable position relative to each other. This has overcome one of the difficulties of having a stable point and plane of reference for superimposition.

From these serial studies it is obvious that there is an overall pattern of growth which evolves along predetermined lines. This growth pattern has individual characteristics and no two faces are alike, with the exception of identical twins. For the sake of convenience it is customary to describe growth in the cranial base, maxillary complex, and the mandible separately, but these are closely interrelated.

Recent work by Moss stresses that the overall genetic pattern is not merely related to the skeletal growth but is embodied in the mesoderm of the embryonic facial processes. His concept of a 'functional matrix' which determines the skeletal development is perfectly consistent with previous views but there is a danger of interpreting Moss's theories to support the contention that environment plays a major part in influencing the development of facial skeletal structures which is not consistent with clinical findings.

The Growth of the Cranial Base.—The cranial base consists fundamentally of basi-occiput, basi-sphenoid, and the ethmoid, all of which have lateral connexions. At birth they are separated by areas of cartilage, the most important of which is a synchondrosis connecting the basi-sphenoid to the basi-occiput. The age at which active growth at this synchondrosis ceases is extremely variable. Brodie has shown evidence of bony fusion in some subjects as early as 8 years. In most cases it can be seen by puberty.

As the mandible is attached to the posterolateral aspect of the cranial base and the maxillary complex attached anteriorly, this is a most important area of growth, allowing an increase in length of the cranial base which needs corresponding adjustments in growth of the maxillary complex and mandible to maintain the anteroposterior relationship of the growing jaws. In achondroplasia, where interstitial growth of cartilage fails, the maxillary complex is not projected forward.

The Growth of the Maxilla (*Fig.* 5 A).—The maxilla enlarges in all dimensions mainly by surface apposition of bone. Its vertical height increases with the building up of alveolar bone supporting the teeth. It is buttressed against the neighbouring bones (principally frontal, zygomatic, and sphenoid) and joined to them by obliquely placed sutures containing connective tissue. In the early years of life the cells of this connective tissue are proliferating rapidly. Cellular activity at these suture sites with new-bone formation at their margins makes an early contribution to the downward and forward projection of the maxilla. As the maxilla increases in size, the antra, which at birth were mere depressions on the lateral wall of the nose, become established by internal resorption and they reach half adult size by 7 years. The palate descends with the downward growth of the maxilla coincident with surface apposition on the oral aspect and resorption on the nasal floor. The palatal vault deepens as the alveolar process develops. Growth at the median palatal suture is probably not a primary factor in the increase of palatal width. It has been noted that where there is a cleft of the hard and soft palate posterior to the incisive canal which has not been closed surgically, there is no interference with normal dental arch width.

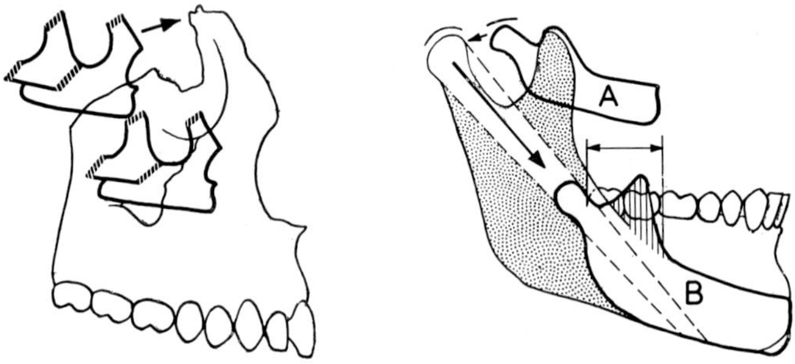

A B

Fig. 5.—A, Diagram of maxillary growth illustrating: (1) Forward growth of the cranial base carrying the maxilla forwards (indicated by arrow). (2) Sutural growth making some contribution to the downward and forward projection (indicated by cross-hatching). (3) Overall enlargement by surface apposition with internal remodelling. (4) Development of the alveolar process.

B, Diagram of mandibular growth illustrating: (1) Change in position of cranial attachment due to growth of cranial base (small arrow). (2) Main growth site in condylar cartilage projecting the mandible downwards and forwards (large arrow). (3) Marked enlargement of muscular processes (indicated by dotted stipple). (4) Building up of alveolar process.

Scott states that the nasal septum acts as a primary growth site in the maxilla, being a cartilaginous structure capable of interstitial growth of its cellular elements. The evidence that it is a primary growth site comparable to that of the condylar cartilage in the mandible is far from conclusive, but there is no doubt that growth of the cartilage in the nasal septum occurs to keep up with the general growth of the maxillary complex. Early submucous resection of the septum appears to have no adverse effect on the growth of the middle face. On the other hand, the unrestricted growth of the nasal septum in bilateral clefts of the lip and palate indicates the importance of this septal growth.

The Growth of the Mandible (*Fig.* 5 B).—Rushton, Symons, and others have made it clear that each half of the mandible must be considered as a long bone with two muscular processes and a dental process.

The active growth site on each side is an area of cartilage beneath the fibrous covering of the condyle. Interstitial and appositional growth of cartilage at this site propels the body of the mandible downwards and forwards. Owing to the divergence of the rami, the condyles become increasingly separated, keeping pace with the widening of the cranial base (*Fig.* 6). The two main muscular processes increase in size coincidentally with the growth of the muscles of mastication.

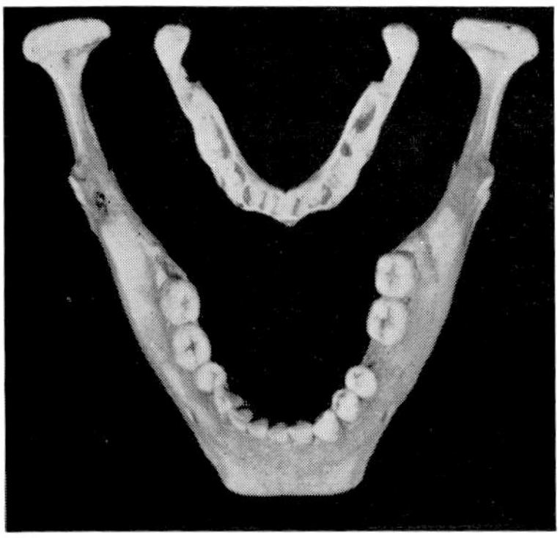

Fig. 6.—Diagram of infant and adult mandibles showing increasing condylar separation.

The bone increases in thickness by surface apposition, but there is surprisingly little addition of bone to the lower border. The increase in height of the so-called mandibular body is due mainly to the alveolar growth as the vertical height between the jaws increases. The chin becomes more prominent as the mandible elongates. There is little surface apposition of bone at the chin point, but it does occur after puberty in some cases, as indicated in *Fig.* 7. Remodelling at the anterior border of the ramus and the rising level of the alveolus meeting with the sloping ramus provide space for the eruption of the teeth, as shown in *Fig.* 5 B. The contour of the gonial region does not usually change, but the angle between a tangent to the lower border and the posterior border of the mandible (described as the 'condylar angle' by Sicher) becomes less obtuse (*Fig.* 8). In some cases, however, there is a postpubertal apposition of bone, changing the contour of the gonial region coincident with increase in size of the mental eminence and supra-orbital ridges (*Fig.* 7). There is bony union at the symphysis at the end of the first year and the connective tissue here makes no contribution to growth.

The 'Dental Bases'.—The parts of the mandible and maxilla on which the alveolar processes and the teeth are superimposed may be described as the 'dental bases' or the 'apical bases'. There is no anatomical dividing line between this area and the alveolar process, particularly at the age of 6–7 years, when both jaws are literally full of

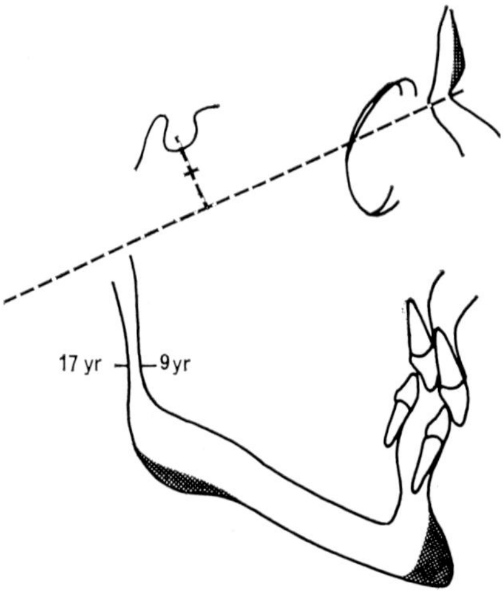

Fig. 7.—Tracing from serial study by cephalometric X-rays showing an instance where there was postpubertal apposition of bone at the chin, supra-orbital ridges, and angle of mandible. Tracings at 9 yr., and 17 yr. 7 mth. (*By courtesy of Dr. Broadbent.*)

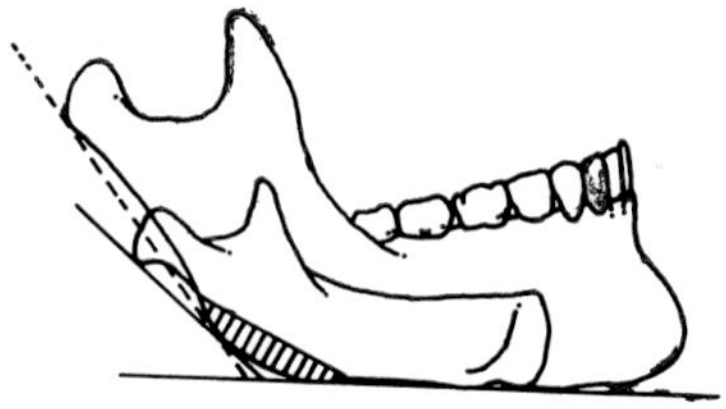

Fig. 8.—Diagram of mandible at birth superimposed on adult mandible to show changing condylar angle but relatively constant gonial contour (indicated by cross-hatching). (*After Sicher.*)

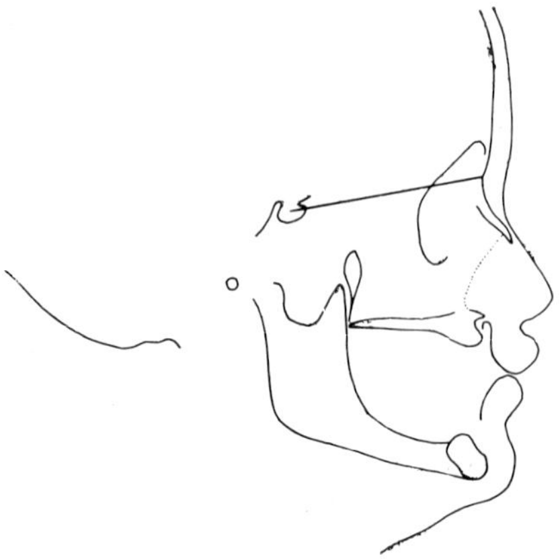

Fig. 9.—Tracing from case of anodontia showing that part of the jaws which represents the 'dental bases'.

teeth. It is convenient to think of the so-called 'dental base' of the mandible and maxilla as that part of the bone which is present in a case of anodontia where there is no alveolar process supporting teeth (*Fig.* 9). Serial radiographic studies of growth have shown that where all the teeth are missing the downward and forward translations of the anterior nasal spine and the chin point are within the limits of 'normal'.

Facial Height.—The height of the face at rest is not dependent on the presence of the teeth and alveolar process. The posture of the mandible in relation to the maxilla is determined early in infancy and is maintained with remarkable constancy by the supporting musculature.

The gum pads of the infant are widely separated in the resting position, and as the jaws grow downwards and forwards the increasing vertical space is taken up by the development of the alveolar process and the teeth. This vertical development establishes a level of the upper and lower teeth with an interocclusal clearance (freeway space) of approximately 2–3 mm. at rest (Thompson). The occlusal level is established in such a way that the elevator muscles reciprocally relax on contact in the reflex manner described by Sherington. The clinical significance of the rest position of the mandible and the maintenance of occlusal height will be discussed in Chapter V.

The Environment of the Developing Dentition.—The dental arches develop on the main scaffold of the jaws which have been described as the 'dental bases'. There are certain factors which are

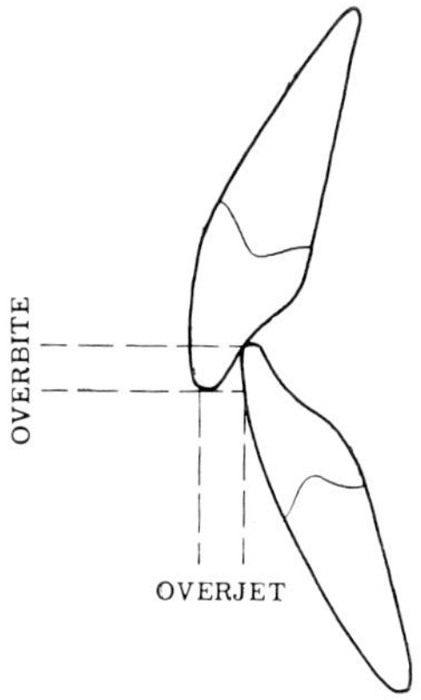

Fig. 10.—Diagram to illustrate the terms 'overbite' and 'overjet'.

necessary for the development of a 'normal' acceptable dentition with the 'normal' incisor overbite and overjet illustrated in *Fig.* 10.

First, and by far the most important factor, is that the bony bases grow to an adequate size to accommodate all the teeth and they must be correctly related both anteroposteriorly and laterally. Secondly, the perimeter of the dental arches will be influenced by the size, shape, and consequent function of the lips, cheeks, and tongue. These soft tissues act rather like a rubber mould which influences the position of the teeth and adaptive alveolar process. It is the posture of the soft tissues rather than their functional activities which has the dominant effect. As the facial skeleton grows, the attached musculature will change in its relationship and will have a modifying effect on the dental arches. This will be discussed at some length in Chapter III.

Too much stress has been placed on the integrity of the dental arches influencing the position of the labial segments. There is very little evidence to support the idea that extractions or absence of teeth in one or both arches will affect the incisor relationship. The relevance of this problem will be discussed in Chapter V.

The upper and lower teeth should be so placed that a simple hinge movement of the mandible can occur from the position of rest (centric jaw relationship) into the position of maximum cuspal interdigitation. Under these circumstances this can be the true 'centric occlusion'. Occlusal forces will assist in directing the teeth as they erupt and establish the occlusal level of the cheek teeth.

The Development of the Dentition (*Figs.* 11–13).—Studies of the developing dentition have been made by Friel, Sillman, Bonnar, Moorrees, and others. Leighton has made an important contribution to the study of occlusal development and emphasizes the variations which can occur within the range of normal. His findings have also influenced the timing of orthodontic treatment, which will be discussed later. During the first 6 months of life the gum pads enlarge and their arches widen. The anteroposterior relationship of the gum pads changes so that the mandibular arch is no longer distal to the maxillary arch. The deciduous incisors can then erupt in their correct relationship and this usually takes place between 6 months and 1 year of age but is subject to extreme variability. The deciduous dentition may not be completed until $2\frac{1}{2}$–$3\frac{1}{2}$ years of age. In some instances the incisors erupt with spaces between them which close with the completion of the deciduous dentition, leaving a fairly constant space mesial to the upper canine and distal to the lower canine. Occasionally the deciduous incisors erupt spaced and stay spaced. Most clinicians would agree that they like to see the deciduous incisors becoming more spaced prior to being shed. Baume has shown that 40 per cent of cases that did not exhibit incisor spacing prior to their loss developed crowding in the permanent dentition.

The anteroposterior relationship of the deciduous arches cannot be fairly assessed until the first deciduous molars are in occlusion. Friel describes the 'normal' dentition at 3 years of age as having the distal edges of upper and lower second deciduous molars flush. The incisors are upright and the overbite is fairly deep. The lower deciduous canines, although mesial to the upper canines, are to some extent covered by them. There is no appreciable lateral growth of the arches during the period 3 to $5\frac{1}{2}$ years, but there is an adjustment in the anteroposterior relationship, the lower teeth migrating forward in relation to the upper. Bonnar has shown that these occlusal adjustments vary considerably in their timing.

Occlusion in the Mixed Dentition.—The phase of the mixed dentition commences with the eruption of the first molars at the age of $5\frac{1}{2}$ to 6 years. The lower second deciduous molars are at this time farther forward than their upper counterparts, so that the newly erupted first permanent molars have their distal edges flush. The 'normal' cuspal relationship described by Angle may not be established at this time (*Fig.* 11 *d*, e). The deciduous incisors have usually suffered considerable attrition and are becoming loose.

The phase of eruption of the permanent incisors may be spread over 2–3 years. Normally the lower incisors erupt before their upper counterparts. They may appear instanding, as they develop on the lingual side of the deciduous incisors and move labially as the latter are shed. The upper central incisors develop on the palatal side of their predecessors. As the roots of the deciduous incisors are resorbed, the permanent incisors move downwards and forwards into a wider arc. This movement and their increased proclination compared with the deciduous incisors enable the larger teeth to be accommodated. There is a little increase in arch width in the canine region between 5 and 8 years of age. It is of the order of 3 mm., being slightly greater in the upper than in the lower arch.

It is normal for a space to be present between the newly erupted upper central incisors (*Fig.* 12 e). The labial fraenum does not grow down with the alveolar development, so that it is no longer attached to the alveolar crest. Before they erupt, the upper lateral incisors are palatal to the centrals. As the upper central incisors erupt, space should become available for the lateral incisors to disengage themselves from their palatal position and to erupt downwards and forwards into the line of the arch, but the apices remain slightly palatally placed in relation to the central incisors. The lateral incisor crowns may have a slight distal inclination and overlap the deciduous canines giving the appearance of mild crowding. This position is associated with the proximity of the crowns of the unerupted canines to the roots of the laterals. Broadbent has described this as the 'ugly duckling' stage

(*Fig.* 12 e). As the permanent canines erupt the lateral incisors assume a more upright position.

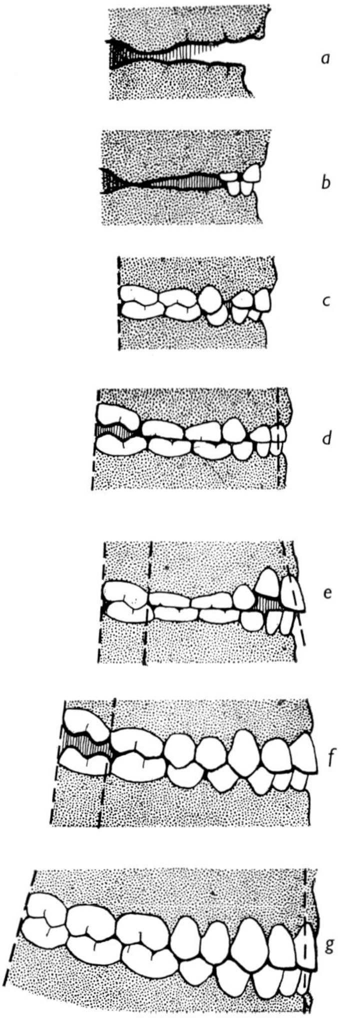

Fig. 11.—Diagram showing development of the dentition. Lateral view. (For details *see* text.)

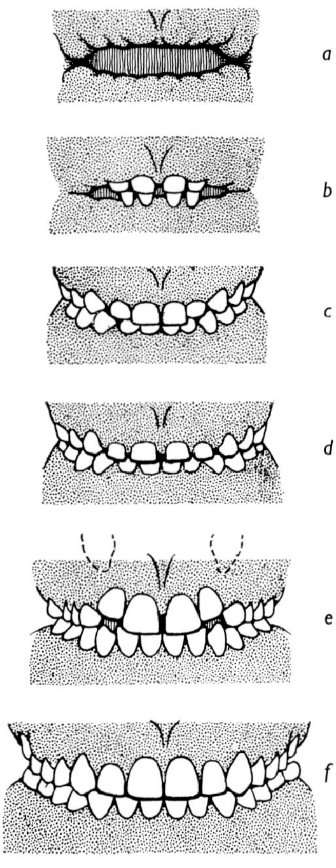

Fig. 12.—Diagram showing development of the dentition. Frontal view.

The natural spacing between the upper central incisors begins to close with the eruption of the laterals and should disappear completely with the eruption of the canines.

The phase of permanent incisor eruption with its minor irregularities is a common source of concern to parents, as crowding which may have been present but not obvious in the deciduous dentition becomes more apparent with the eruption of the larger permanent incisors.

Replacement of Deciduous Cheek Teeth.—The replacement of deciduous cheek teeth by their successors may begin as early as 7–8 years of age and may not be completed until 13–14 years. The deciduous molars, particularly the lowers, are larger mesiodistally than their

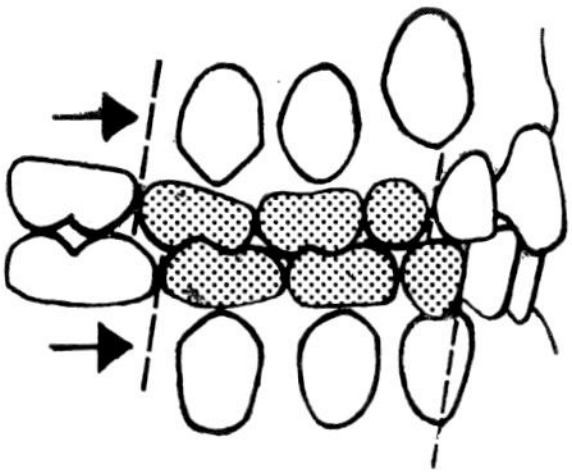

Fig. 13.—Diagram showing discrepancy in size of successional teeth and deciduous predecessors.

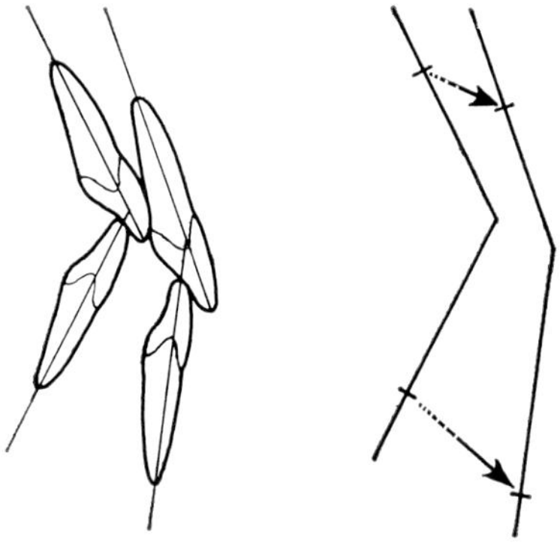

Fig. 14.—Diagram of growth trends showing tendency of incisors to move upright in late growth stages. (*After Björk.*)

successors. The upper deciduous canine does not in itself maintain enough space for its successor and the lower deciduous canine maintains barely enough space. However, like the incisors, the permanent canines erupt into a wider arch and utilize any space remaining in the incisor region.

The discrepancy in size between the deciduous cheek teeth and their successors is greater in the lower jaw than in the upper. The upper first molar moves forward to a lesser extent than the lower when the dentition changes, to take up the cuspal relationship described by Angle (*Fig.* 13), if this has not occurred at an earlier stage. Any early loss of deciduous cheek teeth may upset this harmonious development (*see* Chapters V and VI).

The upper first premolar is usually the first tooth of this series to erupt, followed closely by the lower canine. Apart from the third molars, the upper canine and the lower second premolar are usually the last of the series. The developmental position of the upper canine is under the floor of the orbit and its long path of eruption is one of the factors contributing to its frequent aberration. With the eruption of the cheek teeth all the spacing in the incisor region tends to close. At this stage the overbite is approximately one-third to one-half the length of the crowns of the lower incisors.

Late Changes in the Dentition.—During the eruption of the second molars the dentition does not call for any special comment. At the time of eruption of the third molars certain late changes in the dentition may become evident. Both Björk and Lande, by examining lateral radiographs of individuals at the age of 12 and 21 years, have shown that there is a tendency for the mandible to become more prognathic than the maxilla towards the end of the growth period. Björk's sample dealt with a particular ethnic group, but Lande had a mixed sample. This growth trend may produce a decrease in the incisor overbite but this is not found in all cases. Another change which occurs in relation to this relative prognathism of the mandible is that the angle between upper and lower incisors tends to increase (*see Fig.* 14).

In approximately 90 per cent of the British population the lower incisors show a tendency to become imbricated in the late teens. This is an expression of crowding and is not directly related to the eruption of the third molars because it can occur where these teeth are absent. Such crowding is usually forecast by slipped contact points at an earlier stage in the dentition. It may well be that the continued growth of the dental bases carries the apices of the incisors downwards and forwards but their crowns are prevented from moving into a wider arc by limitations imposed by the tissues of the facial mask which shows increasing tension with age.

A dentition with all 32 teeth in normal occlusion is relatively rare in the British Isles. The overbite is a little less than the one-third found in the 14-year-old. There is a slight curve in the occlusal plane so that the incisal edges are not in the same line as the occlusal surfaces of the lower cheek teeth. There is an outward tilting of the upper buccal segments and a slight lingual tilting of the lower buccal segments.

Although the dentition is designed to carry out the incision of food and powerful movements of mastication, these can be achieved in a variety of ways by variations in the dentition which are perfectly normal for the individual, and the concept of an ideal occlusion is really a myth and not consistent with biological variation.

The Growth of the Soft Tissues surrounding the Dental Arches.—The soft tissues of the tongue, lips, and cheeks act like a rubber mould into which the dento-alveolar structures develop.

The shape and size of these soft-tissue features and their attachment to the bony base are all part of the general pattern of development. Their shape changes considerably from infancy to adult life. In the newborn infant the tongue is large relative to the size of the mouth cavity and rests in contact with the lower lip. The lower lip forms most of the anterior boundary of the mouth, the upper lip being short, flaccid, and everted. As the jaws grow downwards and forwards, the teeth and alveolar process form within these boundaries (*Fig.* 15). Brodie has

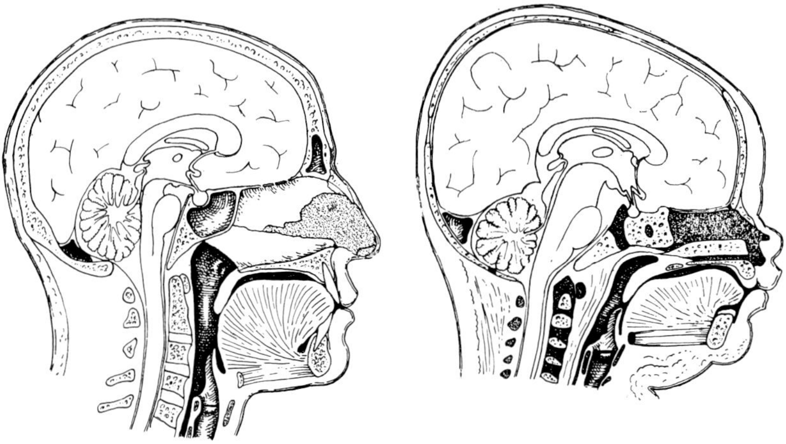

Fig. 15.—Section through head of adult and infant, showing soft tissues.

stressed the importance of the muscular band composed of the buccinator which becomes contiguous with the superior constrictor and anteriorly with the muscles of the lip. This leash of muscles is attached to the cranial base and must grow coincidentally with the downward and forward growth of the jaws as part of the general growth pattern. The tongue is a particularly important organ in moulding the dental arches centrifugally. Its size may vary considerably but is usually related to mandibular size. It reaches its maximum size at about the age of 12 years and it is possible that its influence on the arches diminishes after this time. As previously stated, the facial soft tissues become more tense and active with age and probably have a more important influence than the tongue on the eventual arch perimeter in the later stages of growth (*Figs.* 14 and 15). Normal activities of lips and tongue will be discussed in Chapter III.

Cephalometric Studies.—Following the pioneer work of Broadbent in the Bolton Study, many cephalometric appraisals have been made of the growing facial skeleton. Attempts to produce a rigid plan of normal development have failed. However, from cephalometric research by Brodie and Broadbent it is possible to make the following generalizations (*Fig.* 16):—

1. The cranial base angle BSN between basion, sella, and nasion as shown in *Fig.* 16 varies only very slightly during growth.

2. The pterygomaxillary fissure is a fairly constant landmark in the facial area. It does not appear to vary anteroposteriorly.

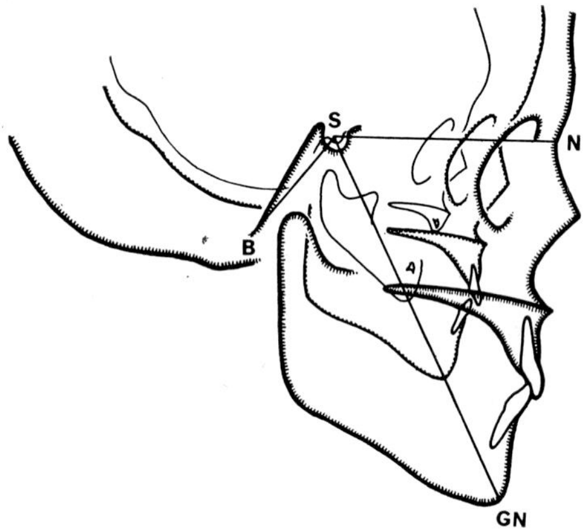

Fig. 16.—Diagram to show growth trends and constancy of pattern. Note many landmarks all grow along relatively straight lines and the angle NSGn varies very little. (*After Broadbent.*)

3. The chin point moves downwards and forwards along a fairly constant axis. This growth axis or 'Y' axis is expressed as a line drawn from the centre of the sella turcica to the chin point. Therefore the angle NSGn is fairly constant for the individual, although there are certain slight deviations.

4. The descent of the palatal plane remains fairly constant and parallel.

5. The Frankfort plane (a plane passing through the lower borders of the orbits and the upper margins of the external auditory meatus) cannot be regarded as a reliable constant, owing to the difficulty in locating the porion accurately.

Details of the essential points in cephalometric research are omitted from this chapter and will be found in the APPENDIX.

In the following quotation Brodie makes it quite clear that there cannot be a rigid concept of facial growth: 'The individual cannot be judged against a statistical yardstick that has been derived from a group.

Viewed in this light it is absurd to think that one can arrive at a diagnosis on the basis of a single angle or even a combination of angles. We have not arrived at the stage as yet where such means of appraisal are possible. We are only beginning to understand dimly the nature of the phenomena that yield the infinite variety we see in the human countenance.'

BIBLIOGRAPHY

BALLARD, C. F. (1957), 'The Aetiology of Malocclusion. An Assessment', *Dent. Practit.*, **8**, 42.

BAUME, L. J. (1950), 'Physiological Tooth Migration and its Significance for the Development of Occlusion', *J. dent. Res.*, **29**, 123.

BJÖRK, A. (1951), 'Discussion on the Significance of Growth Changes in Facial Pattern and their Relationship to Changes in Occlusion', *Dent. Rec.*, **71**, 197.

— — (1955), 'Facial Growth in Man studied with the Aid of Metallic Implants', *Acta odont. scand.*, **13**, 9.

BONNAR, M. E. (1956), 'Aspects of the Transition from Deciduous to Permanent Dentition', *Dent. Practit.*, **7**, 42.

BRASH, J. C. (1928), 'Growth of the Alveolar Bone and its Relation to Movements of the Teeth including Eruption', *Int. J. Orthod.*, **14**, 196.

BROADBENT, B. H. (1931), 'A New X-ray Technique and its Application to Orthodontics', *Angle Orthodont.*, **1**, 45.

— — (1941), 'Ontogenetic Development of Occlusion', *Ibid.*, **11**, 223.

BRODIE, A. G. (1940), 'Some Recent Observations on the Growth of the Face and their Implications to the Orthodontist', *Amer. J. Orthodont.*, **26**, 471.

— — (1941), 'Growth Patterns of the Human Head from the Third Month to the Eighth Year of Life', *Amer. J. Anat.*, **68**, 209.

— — (1953), 'Late Growth Changes in the Human Face', *Angle Orthodont.*, **23**, 146.

CHAPMAN, H. (1935), 'The Normal Dental Arch and its Changes from Birth to Adult', *Brit. dent. J.*, **58**, 201.

CHARLES, S. W. (1925), 'The Temporomandibular Joint and its Influence on the Growth of the Mandible', *Ibid.*, **46**, 845.

CLINCH, L. M. (1954), 'Analysis of Serial Models between Three and Eight Years of Age', *Trans. Brit. Soc. Orthodont.*, 13.

DIXON, A. D. (1958), 'The Development of the Jaws', *Ibid.*, 10.

FRIEL, S. (1954), 'The Development of Ideal Occlusion of the Gum Pads and the Teeth', *Amer. J. Orthodont.*, **40**, 196.

HUNTER, J. (1771), *The Natural History of the Human Teeth.* London: J. Johnson.

LANDE, M. J. (1952), 'Growth Behaviour of the Human Bony Facial Profile as revealed by Serial Cephalometric Roentgenology', *Angle Orthodont.*, **22**, 78.

LEIGHTON, B. C. (1959), 'Early Development of the Deciduous Dentition', *Trans. Brit. Soc. Orthodont.*, 100.

MOORREES, C. F. A. (1959), *The Dentition of the Growing Child.* Cambridge, Mass.: Harvard University Press.

MOSS, M. L., and SALENTIJN, L. (1969), 'The Primary Role of Functional Matrices in Facial Growth', *Amer. J. Orthodont.*, **55**, 566.

POWELL, T. V., and BRODIE, A. G. (1963), 'Closure of the Spheno-occipital Synchondrosis', *Anat. Rec.*, **147**, 15.

RIX, R. E. (1953), 'Some Observations on the Environment of the Incisors', *Dent. Rec.*, **53**, 427.

RUSHTON, M. A. (1958), 'Some Aspects of Anteroposterior Growth of the Mandible', *Ibid.*, **68**, 80.

SCOTT, J. (1948), 'The Development and Growth of the Upper Jaw', *Trans. Brit. Soc. Orthodont.*, 71.

— — (1953), 'Cartilage of the Nasal Septum', *Brit. dent. J.*, **95**, 27.

— — (1958), 'The Analysis of Facial Growth', *Amer. J. Orthodont.*, **44**, 507.

SICHER, H. (1947), 'Growth of the Mandible', *Ibid.*, **33**, 30.

SILLMAN, J. H. (1951), 'Serial Study of Good Occlusion from Birth to Twelve Years', *Amer. J. Orthodont.*, **37**, 481.
SYMONS, N. B. B. (1951), 'Studies on the Growth and Formation of the Mandible', *Dent. Rec.*, **71**, 41.
THOMPSON, J. A. (1946), 'The Rest Position of the Mandible and its Significance to Dental Science', *J. Amer. dent. Ass.*, **30**, 151.
TULLEY, W. J. (1957), 'Observations on the Path of Eruption of the Incisors', *Trans. europ. orthod. Soc.*, 279.
WEINMAN, J. P., and SICHER, H. (1947), *Bone and Bones.* St. Louis: C. V. Mosby.

CHAPTER III

THE DEVELOPMENT OF THE ORAL CAVITY AS A FUNCTIONAL UNIT

In textbooks describing the detailed physiology and anatomy of the oral cavity there is little reference to the development of the various oral functions as the child grows and matures. The orthodontist needs to know something of these milestones in development if he is to appreciate where oral function deviates from the normal to the point of being a problem related to treatment. These functions must be discussed in conjunction with the changing anatomical relationships in the mouth and pharynx.

The oral cavity is essentially the cephalic end of the alimentary canal, designed to take in food. This is a primitive vegetative function which is all that is required of the newborn infant. As the child develops, the more complicated patterns of mastication and speech are superimposed on this simple vegetative function. The movements of the articulator elements in mature speech are among the most complicated voluntary movements to be found anywhere in the body.

The development of oral function has been studied by Gesell, Whillis, Gwynne-Evans, Rix, Ballard, Bosma, and Tulley.

It is proposed to deal with oral and pharyngeal function under the following headings:—

1. Airway maintenance.
2. The mouth used for exploration.
3. Feeding.
    a. Suckling.
    b. Spoon-feeding.
    c. Chewing.
    d. Swallowing.
4. Speech.
5. Facial expression.

Airway Maintenance.—Breathing is spontaneously evoked at birth. If the infant is to survive, a posture of the mandible and the hyoid bone must be established to ensure that the airway is maintained. This comes well before the reflexes which enable the child to orientate its head in space. (Some children born with so-called micrognathia may not have a very small mandible, but lack the integrity of the reflex mechanism required to establish this postural position. The tongue may fall back and obstruct the airway, if they are not carefully nursed and safeguarded.)

The newborn infant is essentially a nasal breather. The lips may be just together or slightly parted. The upper lip and facial musculature is rather flaccid and immobile compared with the more active lower lip. The laryngeal skeleton is high in the neck and there is a relationship between the dorsum of the tongue, the soft palate, and the epiglottis

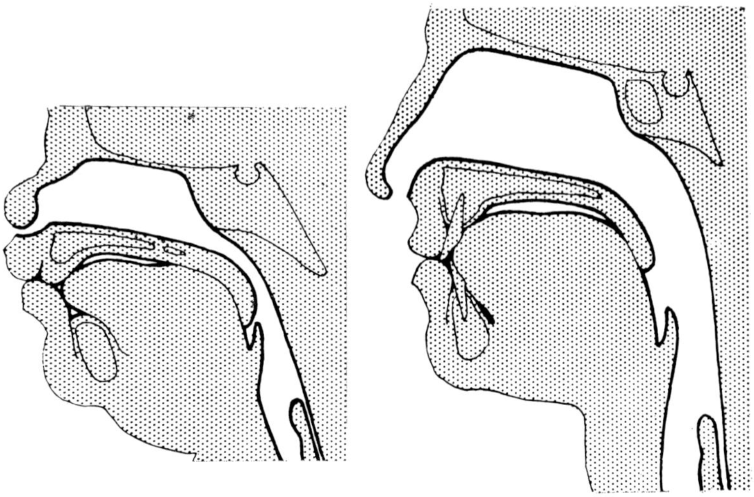

A B

Fig. 17.—A, Lateral view of the head at birth showing tongue to lower lip resting position with the gum pads widely separated at rest. B, Lateral view of the adult head at rest showing: (i) teeth and alveolar process dividing the mouth into oral cavity and vestibule; (ii) tongue no longer in contact with lower lip; (iii) descent of laryngeal skeleton.

which makes oral breathing extremely difficult (*Fig.* 17 A). Any temporary stoppage of the nasal passages in infancy embarrasses respiration and the newborn infant has to learn to mouth breathe.

At this time the infant's tongue fills most of the oral cavity and is in contact laterally with the cheeks and anteriorly with the lower lip. The tongue is blunt and has no tip, but this develops later coincident with the need for increasing mobility. The tongue has a strong sensory affinity for the lower lip—if the lower lip is drawn forward the tongue is seen to follow.

The mandible comes to take up a definite postural position in the first six months of life, as the child gains control over the muscles supporting its head and back and sits up. The gum pads at this stage are widely separated at rest. With the eruption of the deciduous teeth and the development of the alveolar process, the space between the jaws is taken up until the teeth come to lie 2–3 mm. apart at rest. Ballard refers to this mandibular posture as the innate or built-in postural position to distinguish it from habitual postural positions which may

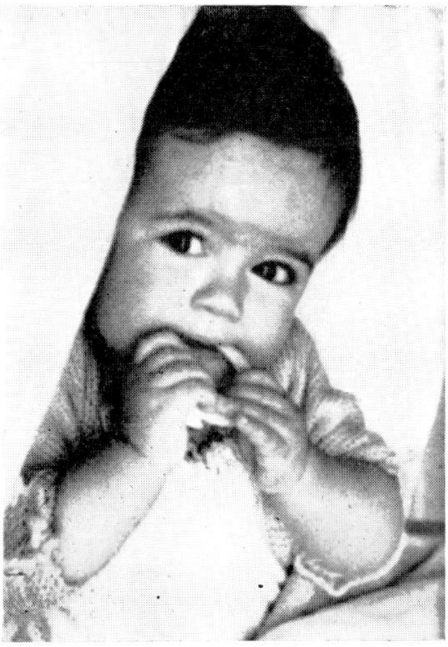

A

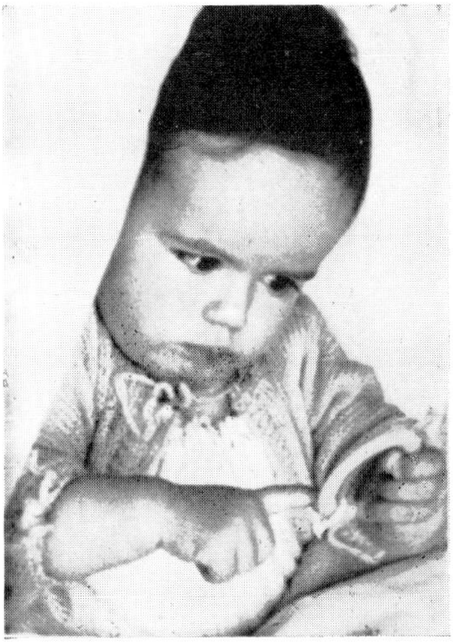

B

Fig. 18.—A, Hand-to-mouth behaviour, mouth used to explore objects. B, Signs of co-ordination between hands and eyes. (*By kind permission of Mr. E. Gwynne-Evans.*)

develop to compensate for variations in skeletal and dental form. (*See* Chapter V.)

As the child grows, the laryngeal skeleton descends in the neck. Although the tongue remains in contact with the soft palate the glottic opening is no longer in close proximity to the uvula (*Fig.* 17 B).

Exploration of Objects.—Before the hands and eyes are fully co-ordinated, the mouth is used for a primitive type of exploration. All objects are placed in the mouth and this is known as 'hand-to-mouth' behaviour. It is used to gain a sense of size and shape and thus any harmful objects must be kept out of the child's grasp. *Fig.* 18 A, B shows how the child learns to appreciate shapes and how co-ordination of eyes and hands is taking over.

Feeding.—

Suckling.—Infant feeding takes place by a rhythmic pumping and squirting action. The mechanism has been studied by analysis of cine films in slow motion by Gwynne-Evans, and by the use of cine fluoroscopic films by Ardran and Kemp.

Suckling with ingestion of amniotic fluid occurs before birth. In the first few days after birth the lips are not readily poised on presentation to the breast. When a child is naturally fed, the nipple and areola are grasped between the upper gum pad and the dorsum of the tongue

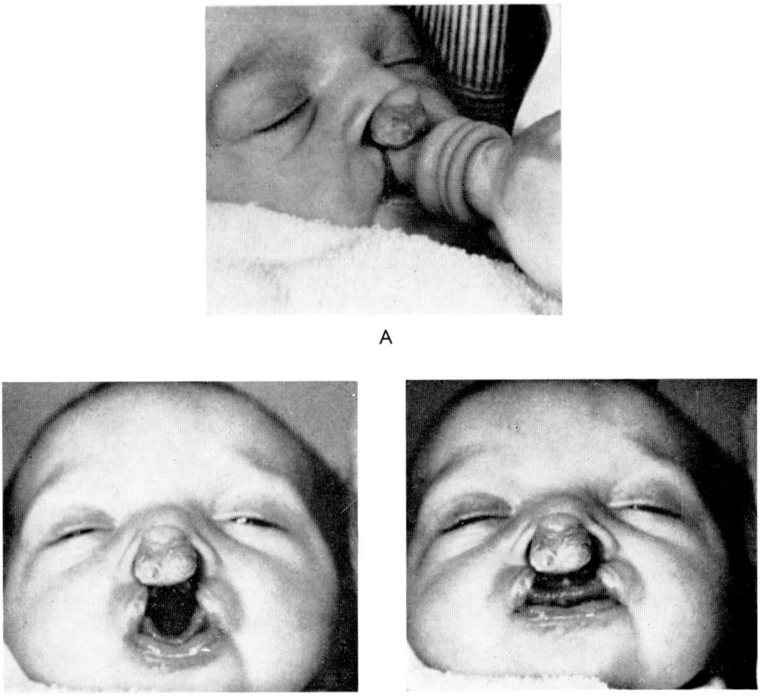

A

B C

Fig. 19.—A, Infant being bottle-fed. B, Cleft lip revealing grooving of tongue and lowering of mandible to receive teat. C, Elevation of the front of the tongue and mandible.

which comes forward over the lower gum pad. The lips form a seal around the breast, and the mouth cavity is enlarged as the jaw is lowered. The central portion of the tongue is deeply grooved anteroposteriorly and its edges everted. As the tongue is raised anteriorly this groove is obliterated from before backwards and this is followed by firm elevation of the jaws. The nipple is considerably extended and taken well back into the mouth and the squeezing action is completed by contraction of the floor of the mouth. *Fig.* 19 shows stages in this action of the tongue and mandible and *Fig.* 20 shows drawings based on the analysis of movements from cineradiography. Milk is squirted back into the oropharynx by a rhythmic peristaltic type of activity in the tongue and floor of the mouth assisted by the mandibular elevators. This action is

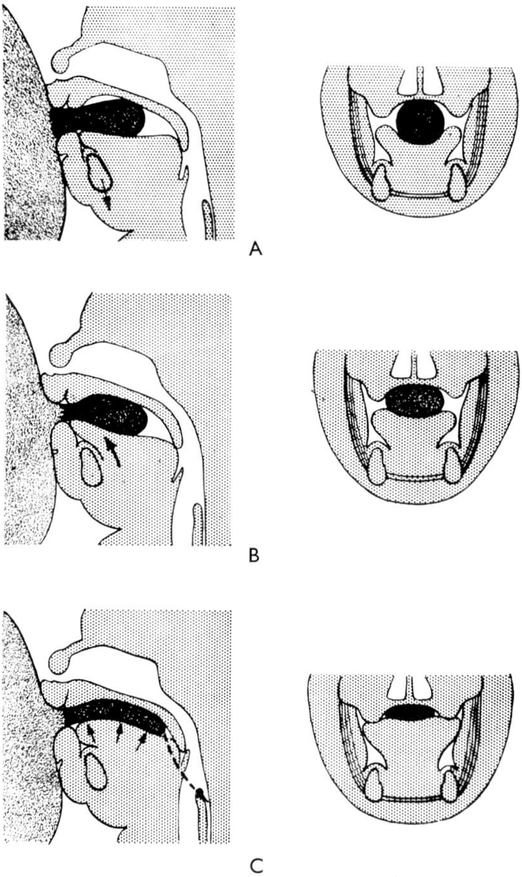

Fig. 20.—The suckling cycle. A, Mandible lowered and tongue forward to receive nipple and areola of breast. Note growing of tongue in transverse view. B, Elevation of tongue tip followed by mandible, groove in tongue becoming obliterated. C, Completion of squeezing with expression of milk. The cycle repeats as mandible is lowered; there is some intra-oral negative pressure created in movement.

called suckling to differentiate it from sucking which is the creation of an intra-oral negative pressure. In suckling, there is an intra-oral negative pressure created by the depression of the mandible at one stage of the cycle but there is also this pumping and squeezing action which is typical of 'milking'.

Spoon-feeding, Weaning.—Mixed feeding commences between 4 and 6 months. At this time the lips are becoming more active. Gesell states that this lip activity manifests itself in a spluttering kind of lip play which delights the parents.

The lips are not poised when first presented with the spoon. Semi-solid foods and liquid foods are taken into the mouth and the tongue movements are still primitive, the infant tries to suckle the spoon (*Fig.* 21). The lips are not completely competent to keep food within the mouth and it leaks out and runs down the chin. Between 4 and 6 months, co-ordination of lip movements brings about a change in the feeding pattern. The child soon begins to pout and smack the lips and the upper lip is drawn over the spoon so that the infant learns to suck in semi-solid food and sip from a cup. The lower lip also becomes more active and is indrawn to prevent escape of food. This makes the mother's task in feeding the child considerably easier (*Fig.* 22).

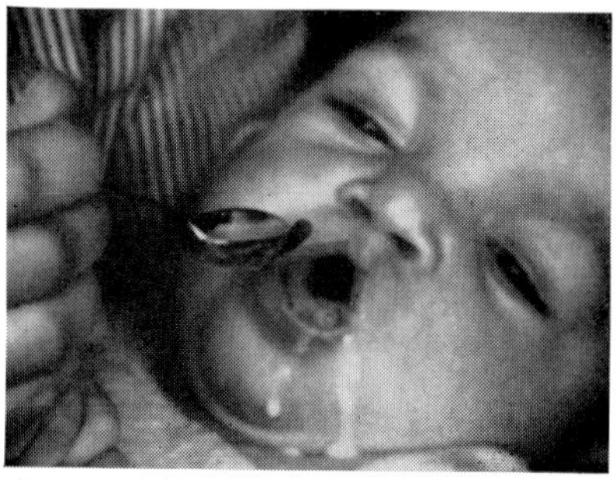

Fig. 21.—Persistence of suckling action of tongue when spoon-feeding commences. The upper lip deficiency gives clear view of the tongue.

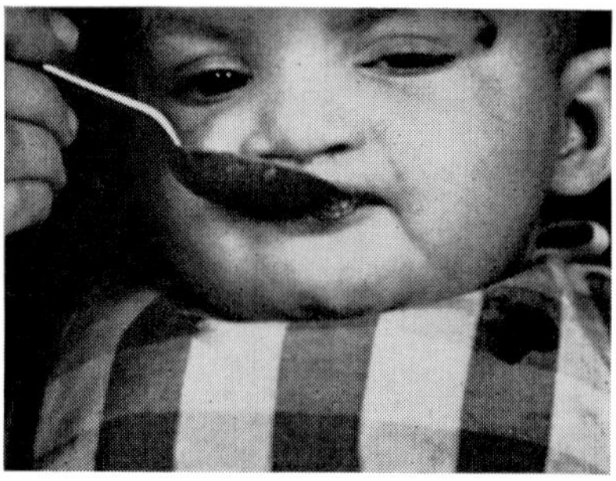

Fig. 22.—Increasing lip activity enables food to be cleanly sucked from the spoon.

The lips and cheeks contract rhythmically to move food about the mouth and are active during swallowing which takes place with the gum pads widely separated.

Chewing.—Mastication is the complex pattern of jaw movements which are used to move food about the mouth to prepare it for swallowing and to perfect insalivation. Premasticatory movements of the jaw can be seen before the eruption of the teeth. These movements are at first mainly in the vertical plane but protrusive movements occur with the eruption of deciduous canines and lateral movements follow, becoming more purposeful with the eruption of the deciduous molars. Gesell states that the infant pattern of chewing becomes well defined by the end of the first year. By 18 months the child is able to enjoy meat and other tough foods and the lateral excursions of the jaw are more marked. From cine-film analysis Gesell states, 'to the 18-month-old child, chewing is a complicated process which requires effortful attention on his part. The 2-year-old child chews more automatically, and by 3 years the pattern is comparatively mature.'

There is considerable variation in this pattern of chewing just as there is considerable variation in the walking gait from one individual to another. It is modified to the particular occlusion of the teeth and the relationship of the jaws and the form of the articular surfaces of the temporomandibular joint. It requires practice, but the pattern is probably built up on an underlying innate co-ordinating pattern and once it is established it does not require concentration but is easily disturbed by the presence of a painful tooth or the sudden encountering of hard objects and food. The details of the movements of the jaws in mastication are to be found in other texts and will not be described here.

Swallowing.—

Swallowing in the Infant: When the child is being breast- or bottle-fed some authorities maintain that the peristaltic type of action already described produces a stream of milk which passes down lateral food channels on either side of the laryngeal skeleton and is prevented from entering the aditus to the larynx by a flap valve mechanism operating between the soft palate and the dorsum of the tongue. The high position of the epiglottis behind the soft palate is thought to enable suckling to occur without cessation of breathing (Gwynne-Evans). Ardran and Kemp, and others, however, describe a cycle where after every two or three intra-oral suckling movements there is a discrete swallow with nasopharyngeal closure. Certainly the anatomical arrangement in the oropharynx of the newborn infant could make suckling possible without interruption of the airway (*Figs.* 19, 23).

Swallowing in the weaned infant does not follow the same pattern as that seen in the older child or in the adult. The teeth are not yet present or are just erupting and the gum pads are widely separated. The food is scooped directly on to the dorsum of the tongue. The tip has developed and this facilitates the movements of food about the mouth. Swallowing behaviour is the same for semi-solids as for fluids at this age. As food is passed back into the oropharynx, the gum pads are not placed together and the lips and cheeks contract to meet the tongue spread.

As the deciduous teeth erupt and the alveolar processes develop, the mouth is divided into the vestibule and the mouth cavity proper. Alveolar bone and teeth now form the anterior and lateral rigid boundaries to the mouth when the teeth are occluded. Occlusion of the teeth during swallowing becomes more frequent and the lips usually play less and less a part in the swallowing of masticated food and saliva.

Mature Swallowing Behaviour: Rix and Whillis have suggested that the significant difference between the infantile swallowing action and

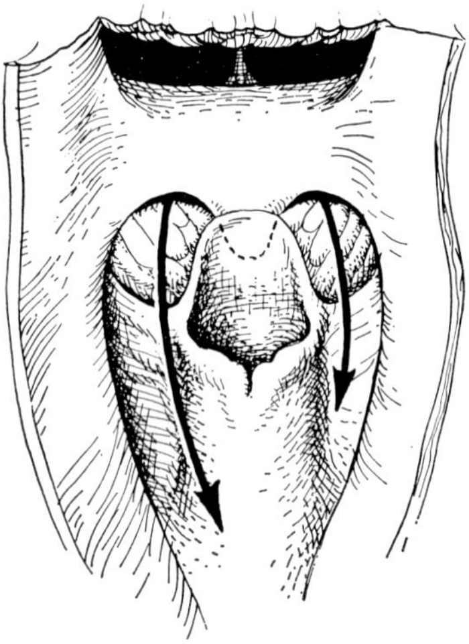

Fig. 23.—Posterior view of pharynx in the infant showing high position of epiglottis in relation to uvula. Lateral food channels prevent easy inhalation of milk. Soft palate and dorsum of tongue act as a flap valve.

that of the adult is the firm occlusion of the teeth at the moment of transfer of food into the oropharynx.

Swallowing action can be divided into three phases: first, the intra-oral mechanism by which the food is transferred from the anterior to the posterior part of the mouth; secondly, the passage of food through the isthmus of the fauces into the oropharynx; and thirdly, the continuation of food down the oesophagus. The intra-oral phase of swallowing will differ in detail according to the type of food and the state in which it is swallowed.

Rix coined the term 'basic swallow' when referring to the swallowing of saliva. This activity continues at intervals through the day and night. Lear and Kincade have studied this under a variety of circumstances. Several factors control the frequency of this act and it will differ from one person to another. During speech it is probably as frequent as at any other time.

Whillis made a detailed study of the intra-oral movements in swallowing of both fluids and solids. He divides the intra-oral phase of swallowing into two stages. First, the action which moves the substance to be swallowed posteriorly and the second or 'mylohyoid phase', when the transfer of food is made into the oropharynx. In swallowing fluids this first stage is again divided into two parts. The fluid is taken into the mouth and swept on to the dorsum of the tongue and held in a groove formed by the eversion of the lateral margins and central depression. This trough is obliterated from before backwards by progressive contraction of the transverse muscle-fibres—the fluid is thus moved into the swallow-preparatory position on the posterior aspect of the dorsum of the tongue. At the 'mylohyoid phase' or second stage of swallowing the teeth are firmly occluded to fix the mandible, allowing a firm base for the contraction of the mylohyoid muscles elevating the floor of the mouth. The tongue is compressed against the palate and against the lateral and anterior rigid walls of the cavity bounded by the teeth and alveolar process. Where this occlusion of the teeth is seen, the lips and cheeks play little actual part (*Fig.* 24).

Semi-solid food or food reduced by mastication is usually insalivated to a paste, very rarely is there a true bolus. This is collected on the dorsum of the tongue and massaged against the palate posteriorly. There is no definite grooving and squirting effect such as that seen in the swallowing of fluids, but the mylohyoid phase may be described in the same manner with firm occlusion of the teeth.

Although this swallowing behaviour is usually accompanied by firm occlusion of the teeth, there are exceptions. For example, when sipping and swallowing from a cup, the teeth are not occluded and the tongue acts as a simple conveyor belt in the floor of the mouth; fluid is sucked on to the tongue by the use of the lips and the creation of an intra-oral negative pressure.

The teeth are not firmly occluded when swallowing soft and succulent foods. The pattern of swallowing here is similar to that used by the infant—the lips and cheeks contract to resist the spread of the tongue and the swallow is more in the nature of a gulp.

As will be shown in Chapter V, Rix considered that the tongue, acting in a rigid-walled cavity, was an important factor in the centrifugal moulding of the dental arches and of the palatal vault. He showed that some children with high arched palates and various forms of malocclusion did not occlude their teeth at any time during the swallowing action and there was excessive circumoral contraction. Atypical swallowing action will be considered later.

The Involuntary Phase: As food and liquid enter the pharynx the muscular activity is no longer under voluntary control. Two protective mechanisms come into play. First, nasopharyngeal closure is effected by the elevation of the soft palate and the contraction of the musculature surrounding the upper part of the pharynx which has been described as the sphincter of Whillis. Secondly, the laryngeal aperture is protected by the epiglottis, elevation of the laryngeal skeleton, and contraction of

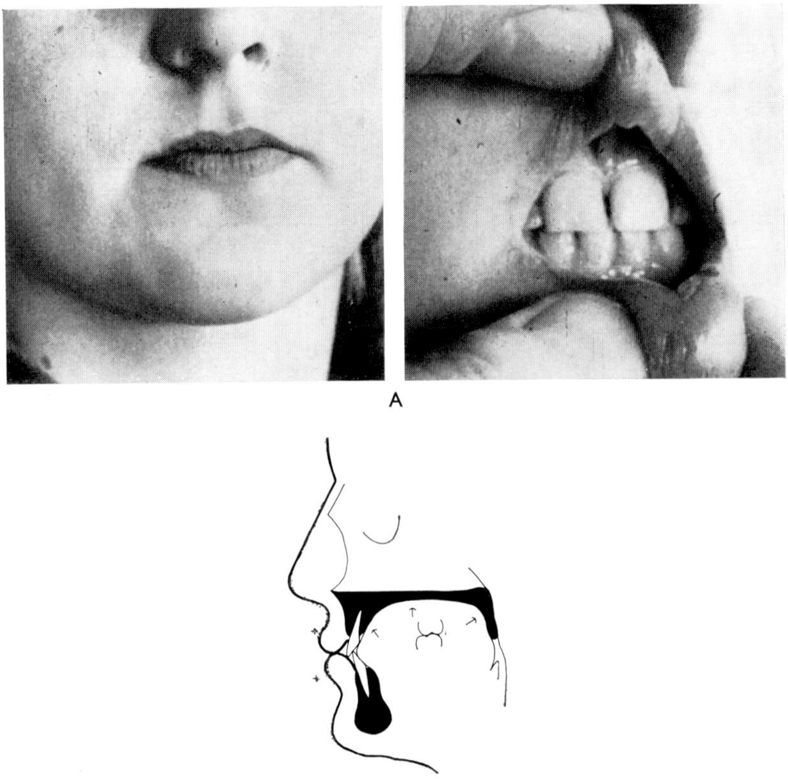

Fig. 24.—Swallowing with teeth together. A, Extracted cine frames showing no excessive activity of lips, teeth together at the mylohyoid phase of swallowing. B, Diagram illustrating the tongue moulding the palate and dental arches during swallowing. The teeth form a rigid anterior and lateral wall at this stage.

the muscles surrounding the laryngeal inlet with momentary apposition of the vocal folds.

Speech.—The first sounds are made at birth, being those of 'baby cry'. At 1 month throaty noises are heard as a variation of cry and by 2–3 months vowel sounds appear. Between 6 and 7 months syllables with plosive consonants preceding the vowels are heard, coincident with increased lip play in feeding. These are soon collected together to give the typical 'dada', 'baba', etc. Although these sounds bring delight to fond parents, they have no meaning. By repetition and copying parents, brothers, and sisters, sounds begin to take on a meaning. By 1 year the infant may say several simple words and understand many more. Comprehension certainly precedes the articulation of speech sounds. Between 15 months and 2 years the child has his own jargon, but by 2 years he can put several words together. He talks incessantly and is quick to imitate. Speech may be an acquired skill, but it is none the less built up on unchanging co-ordinating patterns of motor activity. It is a complicated process involving the production of basic notes in the larynx, known as phonation, and modification of these notes by changing the shape of the cavities in the mouth, nose, and throat which is known as articulation. Although there are classic descriptions of position of the tongue and other articulating elements in various speech sounds, there is considerable individual variation, particularly when one takes into consideration the variations in the shape and size of the oral cavity. The different ways in which sounds are put together in connected speech will determine the articulatory movements.

Acquisition of normal speech relies on a normal receptor mechanism —good hearing—normal central connexions, and a normal effector mechanism. Quite gross defects in the dentition will not impair speech as the normal child is usually extremely versatile. Severe oral disabilities, e.g., cleft palate, count as defects in the effector mechanism. A normal sensory feed back from the mouth and pharynx is essential for normal speech.

The aspects of abnormal speech in relation to malocclusion will be discussed in Chapter V.

Facial Expression.—It has already been pointed out that in the newborn infant the facial musculature, particularly that of the middle-third of the face, is rather flaccid. Only the lower lip is active The lips may be either just together or slightly parted at this time and this may not be related to their future posture. In the normal child the lips should be of adequate length to effect an anterior oral seal without any obvious contraction of the orbicular sphincter.

The initial grimaces of the child's face express only gross discomfort or displeasure, but soon expressive movements become meaningful. Facial expression will depend to some extent on the shape and configuration of the soft tissues which are part of the overall pattern for the individual. Huber has made an extensive study of the anatomy of facial expression. A somewhat flaccid facial expression remains in some children until after puberty—others show animated reactions in childhood and revert to somewhat passive facial expression in the age range

9–12 years. In most adults the facial mask reflects the strain of modern living and the musculature becomes more tense. When the lips are normally sealed at rest without effort, there should be approximately one-third coverage of the upper incisors by the lower lip.

This quotation from Kingsley's *Oral Deformities*, written in the last century, is still very relevant:

'These various movements around the angle of the mouth require careful observation for their full comprehension; and it must have already become apparent that this knowledge is of vital importance to him who would succeed in the art of dentistry.'

BIBLIOGRAPHY

ARDRAN, G. M., and KEMP, F. H. (1951), 'The Mechanism of Swallowing', *Proc. R. Soc. Med.*, **44**, 1038.

— — and LIND, J. (1958), 'A Cine-radiographic Study of Breast-feeding', *Brit. J. Radiol.*, **31**, 156.

BALLARD, C. F. (1955), 'Consideration of the Physiological Background of Mandibular Posture and Movement', *Dent. Practit.*, **6**, 80.

GESELL, A. (1942), 'Morphologies of Mouth and Mouth Behaviour', *Amer. J. Orthodont.*, **28**, 367.

GWYNNE-EVANS, E. (1951), 'Organisation of the Oro-facial Muscles in Relation to Breathing and Feeding', *Brit. dent. J.*, **91**, 125.

HUBER, E. (1931), *Evolution of Facial Musculature and Facial Expression.* Baltimore: Johns Hopkins Press.

KINGSLEY, N. W. (1879), *Oral Deformities.* New York: Appleton.

LEAR, C. S. C., FLANAGAN, J. B. jun., and MOORREES, C. F. A. (1963), 'The Frequency of Deglutition in Man', *Arch. Oral Biol.*, **10**, 1.

RIX, R. E. (1946), 'Deglutition and the Teeth', *Dent. Rec.*, **66**, 105.

— — (1948), 'Deglutition'. 25th Ann. Congr. of the Europ. Orthod. Soc., July, 1948. *Trans. europ. orthod. Soc.*, 191.

SILLMAN, J. H. (1951), 'Serial Study of Good Occlusion from Birth to 12 Years of Age', *Amer. J. Orthodont.*, **37**, 481.

TULLEY, W. J. (1962), 'An Electromyographic Study of the Oro-facial Muscles in Relation to the Form of the Jaws and Occlusion of the Teeth', Ph.D. Thesis, University of London.

— — (1963), 'The Development of the Oro-facial Musculature', Clinics in Developmental Medicine, No. 13.

WHILLIS, J. W. (1946), 'Movements of the Tongue in Deglutition', *Trans. Brit. Soc. Orthodont.*, 121

CHAPTER IV

CLASSIFICATION OF DENTAL IRREGULARITIES

A SHORT introduction to a broad classification of dental irregularities is required before discussing their aetiology. There have been many classifications described in the literature. Those which are based on aetiology are too complex and vague. Bennett's classification, which was widely used for some time, was based on the false assumption that dental irregularities are due to developmental defects in bone growth and not part of the infinite variation of facial form. However, the list of factors operating locally on the dental arches which was compiled by Bennett has been modified and is still used in current teaching. (*See* Chapter V.)

Morphological classifications are used as a means of providing a shorthand description of both the occlusal relationship and the jaw relationship.

Classification of Occlusal Relationship of the Teeth.—The classification used in this book is derived from Angle's original, but is less rigid in its application. It refers to the crowns of the teeth only, and is based on the anteroposterior relationship of the upper and lower cheek teeth in occlusion. This assessment is not confined to the relationship of the first permanent molars owing to the local changes in position which may have occurred following extractions.

Class I.—Cases with normal anteroposterior relationship of the cheek teeth with other abnormalities of occlusion are described as Class I malocclusions (*Fig.* 25 and Chapter X).

Class II.—Cases with an anteroposterior error in arch relationship where the cheek teeth in the lower arch are 'postnormal' relative to the upper are described as Class II malocclusions.

There are two broad divisions which may be differentiated by the incisor positions and relationships:—

Class II, division 1: in which there is an overjet of all the upper incisors (*Fig.* 26 and Chapter XI).

Class II, division 2: in which the central incisors are closely applied to the lower incisors whilst the upper lateral incisors overlap the centrals (*Fig.* 27 and Chapter XII).

In both division 1 and division 2 there is usually a deep overbite, though in division 1 this is not invariably the case.

Class III.—Cases where there is an abnormal anteroposterior relationship of the cheek teeth with a lower arch which is prenormal relative to the upper are described as Class III (*Fig*. 28 and Chapter

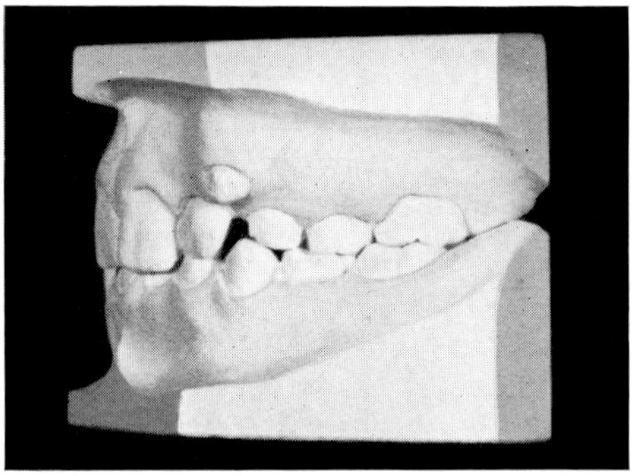

Fig. 25.—A Class I malocclusion. A normal anteroposterior relationship of the cheek teeth with crowded arches.

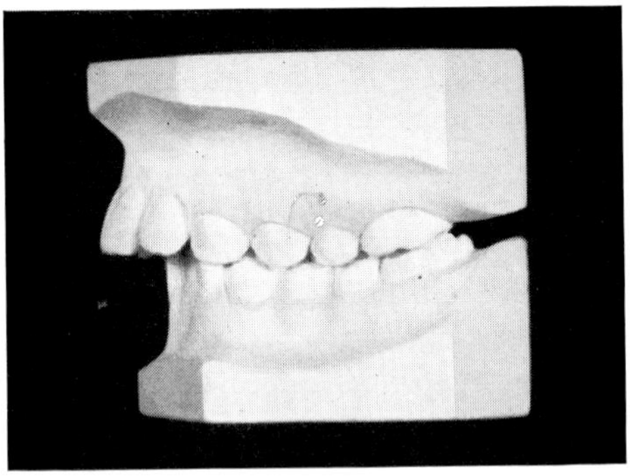

Fig. 26.—A Class II, division 1 malocclusion.

XIII). Frequently the lower incisors occlude in front of the upper incisors.

In each class abnormalities of occlusion may be found associated with crowding, spacing, or of arch relationship in a radial or vertical direction.

The term 'radial relationship' refers to the buccolingual and labiolingual relations of one arch to the other. A cross-bite is when the normal relationship is reversed, e.g., upper buccal segments occluding lingually to the lowers. A similar situation may present in the incisor region.

Abnormalities in the vertical relationship of the incisors are described in terms of overbite. This may be increased to the point of it being exceedingly deep with contact of the lower incisors with the cingulum of the upper incisors or, in fact, making contact with the palatal mucosa. The overbite may be reduced or show an edge-to-edge

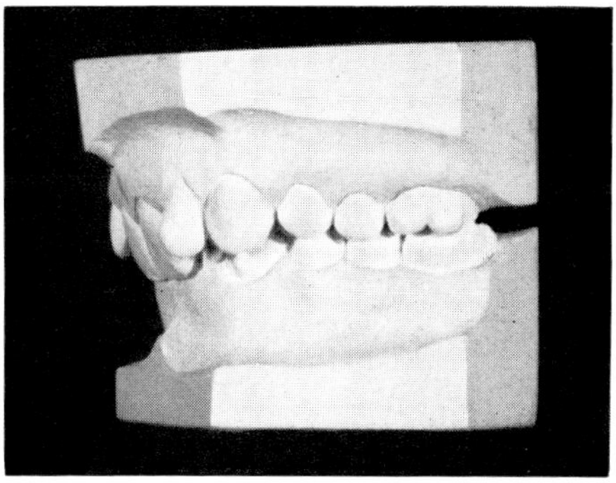

Fig. 27.—A Class II, division 2 malocclusion.

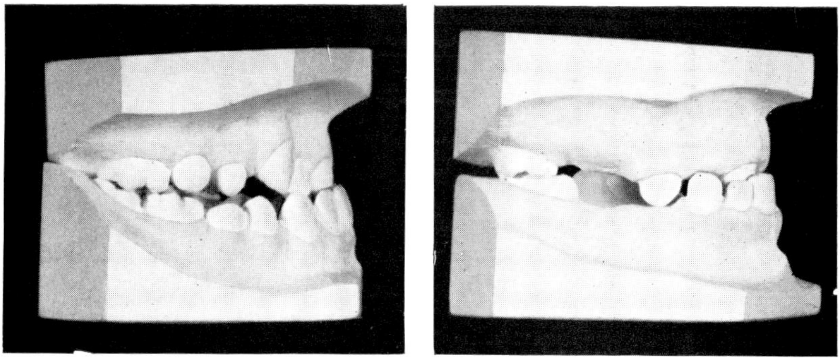

A B

Fig. 28.—Class III malocclusions. A, A true Class III malocclusion; B, A pseudo-Class III malocclusion with mandibular overclosure.

position. Where the incisors overlap but fail to make contact, this is referred to as an 'incomplete overbite'. The term 'anterior open bite' is used when upper and lower incisors fail to meet in the vertical plane without any overlap.

Classification of Anteroposterior Dental Base Relationship (Skeletal Pattern).—The term 'skeletal pattern' was first coined by Ballard and has come to be used in a similar way to Angle's classification of occlusal relationship. This term will be used throughout the book. There are many ways in which the anteroposterior relationship of the tooth-bearing areas of the jaws can be assessed. Any major discrepancy is obvious clinically when the patient is viewed in profile (*Fig.* 29).

Skeletal 1: where there is normal anteroposterior relationship of the dental bases (*Fig.* 30 A).

Skeletal 2: where the mandibular dental base is postnormal relative to the maxillary dental base (*Figs.* 29 A, 30 B). (There could be a maxillary protrusion, a mandibular retrusion, or both.)

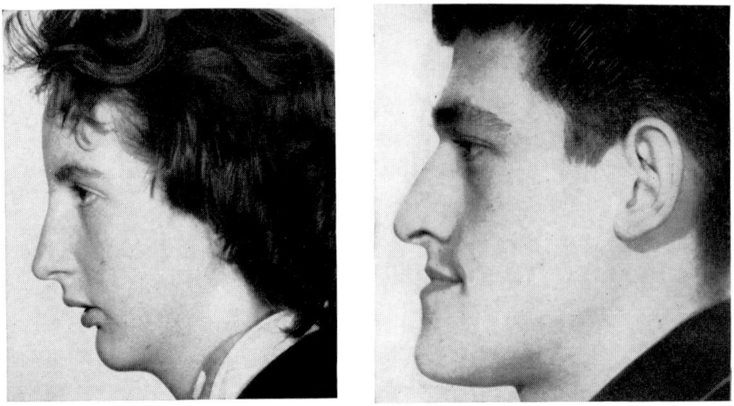

A B

Fig. 29.—A, Obvious Skeletal 2 facial pattern. B, Obvious Skeletal 3 facial pattern.

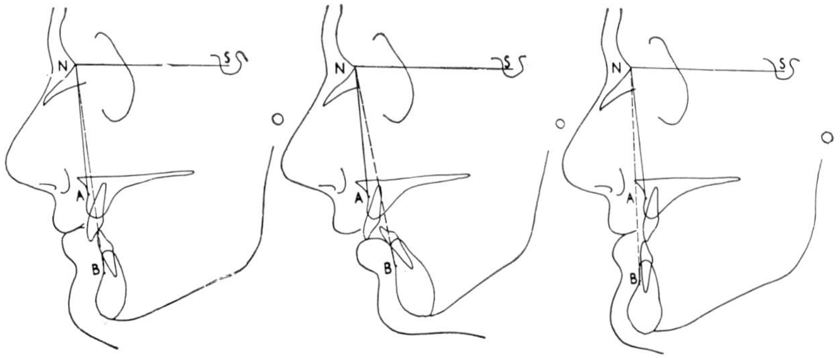

A B C

Fig. 30.—A, *A Skeletal 1 Relationship.* The angle SNA is 80° and the angle SNB is 78°. These are the average values found where the dental bases are normally related to each other and to the cranial base. B, *A Type of Skeletal 2 Relationship.* In this case the angle SNA is 80° and the angle SNB is 73°. There is a mandibular retrusion with a maxilla normally related to the cranial base. C, *A Type of Skeletal 3 Relationship.* The angle SNA is 80° and the angle SNB is 83°. There is a mandibular protrusion in this case with a maxilla normally related to the cranial base.

Skeletal 3: where the mandibular dental base is prenormal relative to the maxillary dental base (*Figs.* 29 B, 30 C). (There could be a mandibular protrusion, a maxillary retrusion, or both.)

A number of methods of analysing tracings of lateral skull head-plates have now been published. Some of these are extremely complex and are not included in this text, but a short section of cephalometrics is included in the APPENDIX. *Fig.* 30 illustrates a simple part of Down's analysis where points A and B which are the deepest points on the concavity of the alveolar bone taken from tracings of lateral radiographs are related to the cranial base to illustrate the difference in angular measurement between points SNA and SNB, N being the nasion and S the centre of the sella turcica. This method has some disadvantages as these points are difficult to identify accurately and they are not truly representative of the apical position of the upper incisors.

In a Skeletal 1 relationship there is only about 2° difference in these angles (*Fig.* 30 A). In a Skeletal 2 relationship there is a significant difference of more than 3° (*Fig.* 30 B), and in a Skeletal 3 relationship there may be no difference in the angles or there may be a negative difference (*Fig.* 30 C).

By this means it is possible to assess whether there is a maxillary or mandibular discrepancy or both, by comparing these angles with 'average' values.

An approximate adaptation of this method can be used clinically by palpating these bony points with the fingers, viewing the patient in profile, and making a subjective assessment. This is described in Chapter VI.

Another method which has been described by Ballard also involves the use of tracings of lateral skull radiographs. See Chapter VI and APPENDIX.

In the following chapters the many variations of occlusal and dental base relationships will be discussed.

BIBLIOGRAPHY

ANGLE, E. H. (1899), 'Classification of Malocclusion', *Dent. Cosmos*, **41**, 248.

BALLARD, C. F. (1948), 'Some Bases for Aetiology and Diagnosis in Orthodontics', *Trans. Brit. Soc. Orthodont.*, 27.

— — (1951), 'Recent Work in North America as it affects Orthodontic Diagnosis and Treatment', *Dent. Rec.*, **71**, 85.

BENNETT, N. (1914), *Science and Practice of Dental Surgery*, Vol. 1. London: Oxford University Press.

DOWNS, N. B. (1948), 'Variations in Facial Relationship. Their Significance in Treatment and Prognosis', *Amer. J. Orthodont.*, **34**, 812.

CHAPTER V

THE AETIOLOGY OF DENTAL IRREGULARITIES

THE study of dental deformities has interested dentists, biologists, and anatomists for many years but the question of their aetiology was given little consideration until the eighteenth century.

The various concepts that have led up to current views on the aetiology of dental irregularities will be dealt with under three main headings:—

1. Factors affecting the size and shape of the jaws.
2. Factors influencing jaw relationship.
3. Factors affecting the form of the dental arches with particular reference to the moulding effect of the soft tissues surrounding them.

The Form of the Jaws.—John Hunter's classic work, *The Natural History of the Human Teeth*, published in 1771, contains many valuable observations on the normal and abnormal growth of the jaws. This remarkable man was well ahead of his time.

In the middle of the nineteenth century many writers, including Tomes, attributed abnormalities of jaw form and dental malalinement to lack of function. Bottle feeding and mastication of soft foods were cited as causes of underdevelopment of the jaws. There were, however, a few clinicians who did not fully agree with these dogmatic views, but nevertheless they were perpetuated at the turn of the century by Angle in the several editions of his book. Also there were many writers in Europe who contributed to the belief that postnatal environment was mainly responsible for jaw malformations, interpreting Wolfe's Law as being simply that form is dependent upon function. Sim Wallace was one of the greatest protagonists of this theory and laid particular stress on the importance of mastication.

While most of the textbooks written between 1900 and 1920 did not completely ignore the inheritance of facial form they again stressed the influence of environment. For example Bennett stated: 'Whatever may be the extent of the influence of heredity, there can be no doubt that the effect of environment in its widest sense during the growth of the individual is of vast importance.'

Typical of the writings of this time is Bennett's statement: 'the local effect of lack of function is more important than results of general malnutrition—function stimulates growth. This is particularly true of muscle and also of bone in so far as it is the means of muscular attachment. The length of a long bone will not be increased by excessive use, although it should be remarked that after such a disease as infantile paralysis normal length is not usually attained wholly.'

It was common practice at this time to quote extreme pathological cases as examples of the effect of lack of function. These examples were hardly relevant to the jaws, but Bennett continued thus: 'The size, density, and form of such bone as the maxilla and mandible vary according to the extent to which they are used during the period of growth. The dependence of the structural formation of the inner as well as the superficial parts of the mandible upon muscular tension has been demonstrated by Walkjoff.'

In his other writings Norman Bennett gives the impression that he is somewhat unsure about this dogma. At this time, Baker published the results of experiments limiting function which were performed on animals by mutilating the dentition on one side or by unilateral removal of the muscles of mastication. These experiments introduced a pathological element and could not be considered as valid evidence.

There were many other writers in the first quarter of this century who stressed the cause and effect relationship between mouth-breathing and the small maxilla, but Bennett expressed considerable doubt over this. He states: 'It is rather curious that most of the gross forms of abnormal occlusion—superior and inferior protrusion and retrusion—may be associated with nasal obstruction and mouth breathing, although it should be recognized on the one hand that these forms of malocclusion may occur independently of mouth breathing and, on the other hand, that mouth breathing is not always followed by any obvious deformity of the maxilla or mandible or dental arches.'

The less known works on the heredity of facial form by William J. Brady and Martin Dewey were not put in perspective until Brash published his classic Dental Board Lectures on 'The Aetiology of Irregularity and Malocclusion of the Teeth'. In this work he carefully analysed the study of facial form and dental development in twins. He also emphasized the genetic facial pattern of some of the royal families in Europe where there had been intermarriage. Brash pointed out that the study of the jaw form and occlusion in monozygotic and dizygotic twins gave the best evidence to support the part played by inheritance and the minor role of local environment.

He further goes on to state in relation to function and form: 'No doubt, size of jaws and size of muscles that move them, like skeleton and musculature in general, are correlated, but the extent of the correlation, like all other biological correlations, is to be measured not in the individual but in the mean, and it by no means follows that in the individual the size of the jaws is caused by the amount of activity of the muscles. Certainly the convincing evidence that it is so has yet to be produced and the contrast between the great strength of an achondroplasic dwarf and the great muscular weakness of an acromegalic giant may well give us pause before adopting such a simple conclusion.' This was the beginning of the understanding of how small a part environment plays in the growth of the jaws.

Brash comes to grips with the environmentalists and states: 'It appears that at the back of all this discussion about the lack of use of the jaws is the erroneous assumption that growth and size of bones must be in some direct ratio to the magnitude of the forces applied to them and the frequency of that application; whereas it is more than probable that there is a very wide range of activity within which growth will proceed in a perfectly normal manner, and that it requires an altogether exceptional degree of lack of use, amounting almost to cessation of use altogether, to affect in any degree the growth of the bones concerned. No amount of exercise, on the other hand, can possibly induce any part of the skeleton to grow beyond the limits to which it is congenitally predetermined. It may be that in time Man may find it possible, by taking thought in the form of pituitary extract, to add one cubit unto his congenital stature, but it is highly improbable that he will ever be able, by taking exercise in the form of hard crusts, to add a fraction of that anatomical unit to congenitally narrow jaws.'

Murray's observations on transplants of chick embryo femurs show that the architecture of the bones is an inherent property; only the refinements of surface markings are absent where there is no muscle attachment or pull. In his general summary and conclusions, Brash states: 'It is no novel suggestion that inheritance may be the main factor in determining the form of the jaws and the position of the teeth. Over and over again the importance of inheritance in this problem has been stressed, and insisted upon, and now that evidence is beginning to accumulate it seems to be more and more obvious that that is the chief line of investigation to be pursued. Environmental agencies are, of course, the complement of inheritance. Necessarily and incidentally they must be investigated at the same time, but it may make a great deal of difference if they are considered in relation to the genetic constitution of the individual upon whom they act.'

In a paper published in 1925 Axel Lundström was probably the first to use the term 'apical' (dental) bases and he pointed out that the size and shape of the tooth-bearing areas of the jaws and the teeth were genetically determined. When the size of the dental bases and the size of the teeth were not correlated, problems of spacing or crowding could arise. This could not be considered as simply a local lack of development as Bennett had tended to suggest. (*See* p. 62.)

In 1931, Broadbent, working in the Bolton Study, Western Reserve University, Cleveland, developed the X-ray technique with standardized head-positioning which made a serial study of facial growth possible.

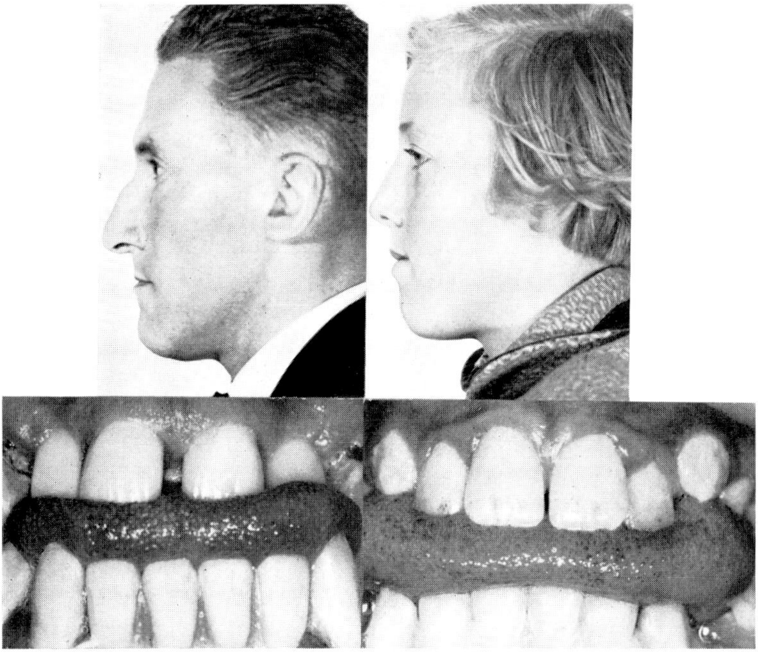

Fig. 31.—Father and daughter with Class III malocclusions. Note the similar facies and the tongue position at rest. Both have an open bite and lisp.

Thus, for the first time, a really scientific appraisal of facial growth could be made by superimposing tracings of the lateral skull radiographs taken at yearly intervals. From this work and that of Brodie and his co-workers, the concept of an inherited growth pattern arose. The evidence for the influence of heredity on the facial pattern is overwhelming and may be summarized as follows:—

Facts indicating the Major Influence of Heredity.—

1. Facial characteristics are dominant in certain families through generations. *Fig.* 31 shows father and daughter with similar facial characteristics. The classic example is the Hapsburg jaw and protruding lower lip.

2. There are dominant jaw characteristics in pure races, despite change in environment.

3. There may be marked differences in the form and size of the teeth and jaws of fraternal twins with similar intra-uterine and postnatal environment, as compared with the identical development of uniovular twins.

4. The evidence derived from cephalometric research shows a relatively fixed pattern of facial development for each individual.

5. Experimental cross-breeding in animals demonstrates that various jaw structures can be transmitted, producing, for example, the upper jaw of one animal type and the lower jaw of another.

6. Tissue-culture experiments show that the intrinsic characteristics of a bone may develop without functional stimulus.

Minimal Influence of Environment.—Environmental agencies can be discounted as having any effect on the growth pattern in the ordinary everyday problems of orthodontics. This leaves rare pathological and unusual environmental stimuli which deserve brief mention.

Prenatal Influences.—It may be possible that certain factors influencing development are transmitted by the placenta. Some congenital abnormalities of the jaws are due to intra-uterine disturbances but their numbers are relatively few. (*See* APPENDIX.)

Moulding of the head in the birth canal does occur, but it is transitory. Only in extremely rare cases is gross injury responsible for disturbances of growth patterns.

Postnatal Influences.—Abnormal pressures from burn scars or orthopaedic appliances may deform the mandible if these pressures are intense and persistent.

It is unlikely that habits such as leaning on the hand at school and sleeping in an abnormal position, which are reputed to produce compression of the jaws, have the intensity or constancy to do so.

Pathological conditions may affect growth sites. One example is the interference with the growth of the mandible due to trauma or infection of the temporomandibular joint following otitis media. Endocrine dysfunctions and gross nutritional defects are extremely rare, but when they occur they do have an effect on jaw growth, e.g., acromegaly and cretinism.

The Relationship of the Jaws.—Following the development of this concept of a fixed pattern of facial growth, detailed studies have been made of the position of the mandible in relation to the skull base. It had been assumed for many years that the position of the mandible was not static and could be changed by external factors and by orthodontic treatment.

The significance of the rest position of the mandible, slung from the skull by the attached musculature, was mentioned by Norman Bennett, but Thompson and Brodie appraised this in a new light. They found, using cephalometric recordings, that the resting posture of the mandible is relatively constant for the individual. This has been further emphasized by Ballard to the extent that he suggests that the rest position should be called the 'endogenous postural position' to distinguish it from 'habit postural positions' which may be acquired by the patient.

Sicher and Last, from the anatomists' point of view, have maintained that the rest position varies with different head positions. Prosthetists have shown evidence that it can be changed, but in the older age ranges of patients with loss of teeth, other factors come into play.

Further research work by Thompson and Perry and others have established that from the clinical point of view the individual rest position is relatively fixed after the first few months of life.

The path of closure of the mandible from the true resting posture into the position of maximum cuspal interdigitation is normally a simple hinge movement. There is no evidence to show that orthodontic treatment can produce any permanent change in jaw relationship 'by bringing the mandible forward'.

There are certain dental irregularities associated with deviation from the normal hinge movement from rest to occlusion.

1. *Forward Displacement.*—Rix described a type of pseudo-Class III malocclusion due to adverse guiding of deciduous canine teeth following loss of deciduous cheek teeth at a critical stage of dental development where there is a mild Class III tendency. There is no doubt that this can also occur without premature loss of deciduous teeth. (*See* p. 69.) Hopper and Nevakari have shown that any initial forward movement of the mandible soon disappears. Because of lack of normal incisor contact, the mandibular elevators may not reciprocally relax and the permanent cheek teeth are temporarily prevented from reaching their full occlusal height (*Fig.* 32). The clinical implications of this are dealt with in Chapter XIII.

2. *Lateral Displacement.*—A lateral displacement in the path of closure producing a unilateral cross-bite may result when the upper arch is slightly too narrow to receive the lower arch in a centric position. (*Fig.* 33.) The clinical implications of this are dealt with in Chapter X.

3. *Posterior Displacement.*—Clinicians have described a distal displacement of the mandible with a degree of overclosure which might be responsible for the condyle impinging on the posterior aspect of the joint, producing painful symptoms. Current views are that these cases are extremely rare. Ballard, Hovell, and others have described a forward

position which is adopted in many Class II cases to overcome inability to seal the lips and also to mask the retrusive appearance. Brodie refers to this as the 'Sunday face'. This is in fact a forward position of rest established by habit and when the patient closes his teeth there would

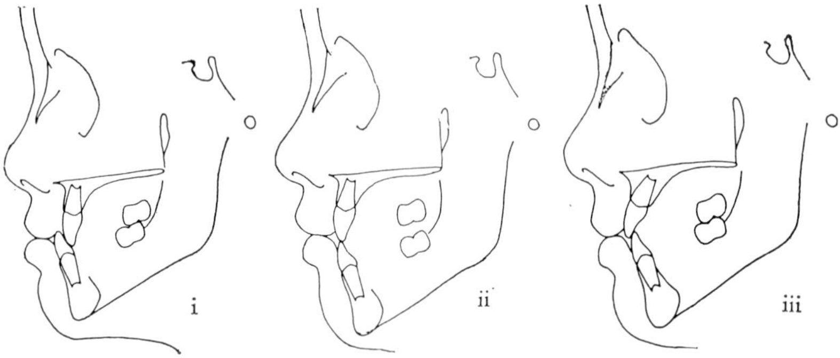

Fig. 32.—(i) Tracings of lateral radiographs showing initial overclosure; (ii) Possibility of biting edge-to-edge on incisors; (iii) Upper incisors moved over the bite.

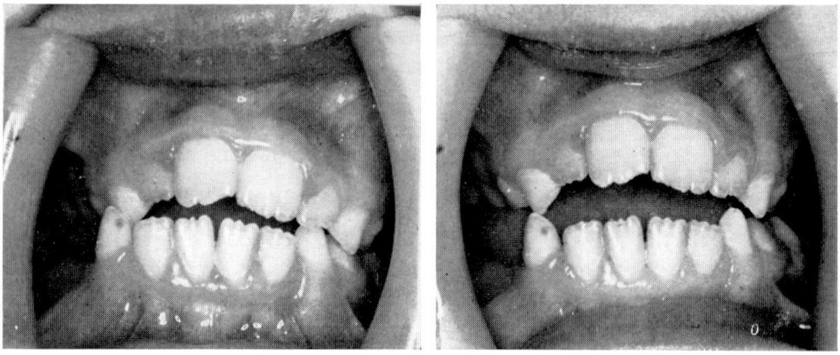

A B

Fig. 33.—A, Patient with unilateral cross-bite. Upper arch is slightly too narrow and there is a mandibular displacement to the right. B, Note premature contact of right deciduous canines when closing in centric position.

appear to be an upward and backward displacement of the condylar head which is much more common than the true distal displacement previously mentioned. The implications of this mandibular displacement will be mentioned in Chapter XII.

With the concept of a relatively fixed position of rest for the mandible and the concept of a fixed pattern of facial growth, it is logical next to consider the role of the soft tissues surrounding the developing dento-alveolar structures in determining their position on the dental bases.

The Form of the Dental Arches and their Soft-tissue Environment.—Much has been written concerning the effect of the tongue, lips, and cheeks which act as a mould into which the teeth and alveolar process develop. It is interesting to review the literature briefly.

One of the earliest references to the influence of the tongue is that of Lefoulen in 1839 who describes 'sounds of speech in which the tongue strikes against the upper anterior teeth pushing them forward'.

Désirabode, writing in 1843, is the first traceable reference to the fact that the lips on the outside and the tongue on the inside of the mouth constitute a balance of forces that determine the position of the teeth. Shortly after this Bridgeman introduced the 'lateral pressure theory' and described the significance of external muscle forces from the lips and cheeks and internal muscle forces from the tongue.

In 1864 Ballard attributed excessive cheek contractions of 'fruitless sucking' as being a factor producing dental irregularities. Apart from the obvious local and temporary effects of the insertion of digits between the teeth, the effect of sucking habits producing lateral contraction of the arches had a wide following in the early literature.

In 1865 Alfred Coleman stated: 'When we remember that resistance to our efforts is not only afforded by the bone itself but probably to some extent also with other bones composing the face and cranium, nor must we forget also the influence of muscular resistance, not only tending to counteract our effort but also to restore the former conditions upon withdrawal of the expansive force.'

A little after this time Tomes, describing the V-shaped upper arch, considered it to be due to excessive cheek pressure without counter pressure from the tongue, due to its low resting position in mouth-breathing, and at this time considerable thought was given to this factor by Donders and others. Tomes stated: 'It will generally be found that this malformation is associated with greatly enlarged tonsils which necessitate breathing being carried out with the mouth open.' Kingsley did not agree with Tomes's theory. He states: 'My own observation has not shown this association of enlarged tonsils with this kind of deformity so generally as to enable me to accept Mr. Tomes's theory, even if I could believe that the muscular contraction of the cheeks could produce such results under such circumstances, neither is it quite conceivable that the pressure of the orbicularis oris at the centre, with the mouth open, would not exert a counteracting influence upon the incisors and thus restore the equilibrium.

'The pinched or V-shaped dental arch I believe to be nearly always of congenital origin—that is—an inherited tendency, favoured in all probability by like circumstances with those which initiated it in the ancestry.'

At the turn of the century, Angle recognized the problems of the muscular environment of the dental arches, but would not accept the fact that in certain cases they might form an insurmountable difficulty in preventing permanent alinement of the teeth. In the appendix of the 7th edition of *Malocclusion and the Teeth*, he states: 'We are just beginning to realise how common and varied are the vicious habits of the lips and tongue, how powerful and persistent they are to overcome. The period of retention of the teeth after they have been moved into normal occlusion is one of the most important in treatment and so complicated and persistent are the delicate forces that tend to derangement of the established occlusion as to necessitate the most thoughtful consideration of the problems involved and a degree of skill in overcoming them which much experience alone can develop even among those with talent for the work.'

Bennett showed an understanding of the problem: 'The teeth are constantly subject to the play of forces acting upon them in all directions. The muscles of mastication produce conditions of vertical and lateral stress, the use of the tongue in mastication and speech reacts upon the teeth internally and the lips and cheeks in their every movement, even of transient emotion, bring pressure to bear externally. Many of these forces are too slight and of insufficient duration to produce any definite movement of the teeth but others are constantly acting; with the mouth shut and the teeth closed the buccal cavity is obliterated, and the teeth are compressed between the tongue and the lips and cheeks. Very little experience in the movement of teeth by mechanical means is enough to show that even quite a small force acting continuously will produce a considerable movement, and it becomes clear that the teeth in their arches are but passive objects kept in a state of equilibrium under the influence of the muscles that react upon them directly and indirectly.'

At this time, Bennett appreciated the fact that the teeth were guided by these muscle functions during eruption but maintained that once in occlusion, the effect of these forces was counterbalanced by occlusal lock. He discussed Sim Wallace's theory that tongue size is dependent on tongue function and that this is a dominant factor in determining the size of the dental arches, but he rather dismissed the tongue as an important factor in arch development.

Brash, in his Dental Board Lectures, did not place emphasis on the effect of the soft tissues of the tongue and lips but he went so far as to state: 'There is a correlation between the growth of the soft parts and the growth of bones but neither is mechanically determined by the other. The growth of the tongue and the mandible are no doubt correlated but it is improbable that the tongue exercises any important mechanical influence on the general form and size of the mandible or in moulding the form of the growing palate.'

Alfred Rogers was a great believer in the relationship between function and form and developed a series of exercises designed to improve muscle function with the belief that this could improve the form and relationship of the jaws. He paid some attention to lip and tongue function and had a following in his muscle-retraining technique.

Van Thal in 1935 studied speech in relation to malocclusion and found that abnormal movements of the tongue and lips in speech could not be directly related to malocclusion. Froeschels found that lisping and open bite originated from a general abnormality of tongue activity. Trusdell and Trusdell focused attention on abnormal habits in deglutition but did not follow up their original work.

There was naturally a break in investigations during World War II and renewed interest in the soft-tissue environment of the dentition was stimulated by Rix in a paper 'Deglutition and the Teeth' and this was followed by a series of papers by Rix, Ballard, Gwynne-Evans, and others.

Two basic concepts were put forward which rather highlighted the particular function of deglutition. The first—that swallowing patterns, showing excessive lip activity during the swallowing of saliva and masticated food, without firm occlusion of the teeth, might be a residual infantile characteristic reminiscent of the infantile swallow described in Chapter III. The other theory was that these patterns of behaviour were innate characteristics of the individual and they were descriptively labelled 'visceral' swallowing movements.

These various abnormal contraction patterns of the lips and the lack of tongue pressure moulding the teeth centrifugally were suggested as being primary aetiological factors in certain forms of malocclusion.

Many of the older clinicians were frankly sceptical of these theories, finding that their empirical treatment plans were in no way affected by this concept of soft-tissue behaviour. At this time it was not appreciated that the writers were really describing a relatively small number of difficult cases of the type that had always showed a tendency to relapse. Rix and others were explaining these relapses by referring to the fact that certain orthodontic procedures moved the teeth out of balance with their soft-tissue environment.

In order to investigate oral and facial behaviour, a Clinic was started at the Queen Victoria Hospital, Tite Street, London, in 1946.

This Clinic incorporated the fields of otolaryngology, orthodontics, and speech therapy. Myofunctional appliances and exercises were given a trial. A similar unit was started at Guy's Hospital in the Anatomy Department to make a detailed serial investigation of a number of cases by cine-film analysis.

It is convenient to describe the present-day view of the relationship between orofacial function and the occlusion of the teeth by considering the functions of the mouth and the pharynx under the same headings used to describe the development of normal behaviour in Chapter III, namely Breathing, Feeding, Speech, and Facial Expression.

Abnormalities in Breathing.—As described in Chapter III, the facial and lingual musculature take no active part in the normal breathing process although the posture of the mandible and the hyoid bone are important in airway maintenance. The lips should be together at rest without conscious contraction of the orbicular sphincter and the tongue and soft palate are in contact. Many children have lips which are either too short or flaccid to achieve lip seal without conscious effort, but they are not necessarily breathing through the mouth. Contact of the tongue and palate forms a secondary sphincter mechanism closing off the airway.

Despite the frequency of upper respiratory infections associated with a narrow upper dental arch there is no clear-cut cause-and-effect relationship (*Fig.* 34). Emslie in a symposium on mouth-breathing summarizes what Bennett had suspected many years before: 'Recent observations suggest that too much importance has been attached to mouth-breathing *per se* as an aetiological factor in the maldevelopment of the face and jaws and not enough to the predisposing genetic factors. Where the genetic pattern produced a narrow maxilla with concomitant narrow nasal passages the effects of oedematous mucosa and adenoid tissue in the postnasal space will be much more likely to produce partial obstruction.'

The false assumption that mouth-breathing is directly related to the contracted dental arch with a Class II incisor relationship was emphasized by Ballard, Gwynne-Evans, and Leech as a result of their findings from the Upper Respiratory Clinic. Gwynne-Evans states: 'In my view the theory of adenoidal facies has resulted from a purely subjective approach and a lack of knowledge of the extent of inherited variations. I should also like to be so bold as to suggest that if our observations are sound and can be applied to the remainder of the body then much time is probably being wasted and feelings of frustration induced in parent and child by treatment or training and perhaps unnecessary surgical procedures performed because the extent of genetically determined variations in our population is not appreciated.' *Fig.* 35 shows a patient with the 'adenoid facies' where there is no history

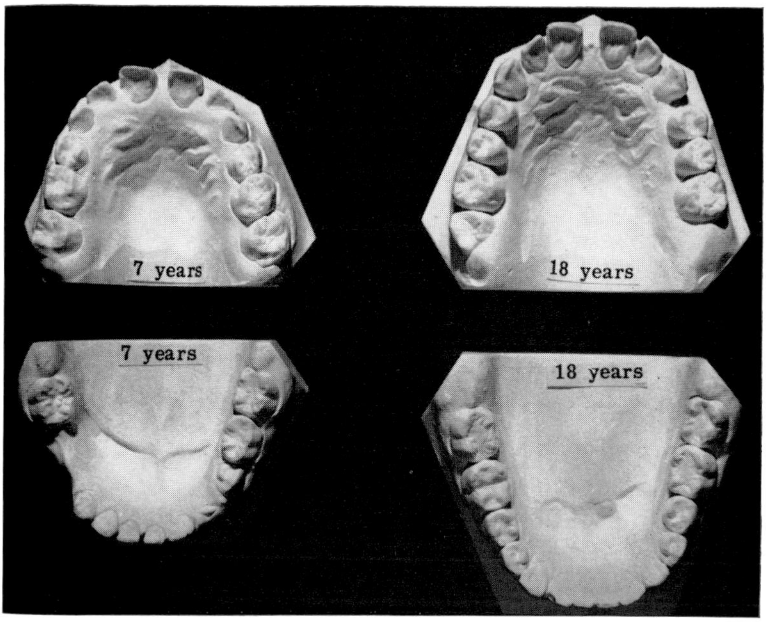

Fig. 34.—Models of patient at 7 years and at 18 years showing well-developed jaws and dental arches despite history of very marked upper respiratory symptoms and obstruction in childhood.

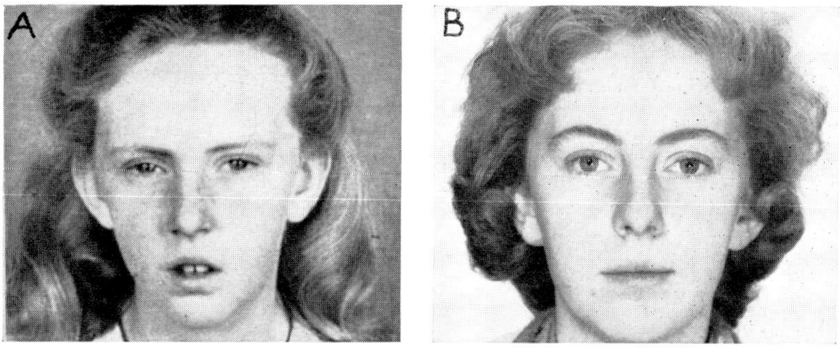

Fig. 35.—A, Patient showing so-called 'adenoid facies' aged 10 years. There is no history of upper respiratory obstruction. B, The same patient, aged 16 years, showing more mature face. Lips are being held together by conscious effort but they fail to seal when relaxed. There was no orthodontic treatment.

of nasal or postnasal obstruction. As the patient developed her expression changed dramatically.

As previously stated, failure of the lips to seal at rest does not necessarily indicate mouth-breathing. There may be a posterior barrier formed by contact between the tongue and soft palate. The term 'lip incompetence' was first used by Ballard to describe lips which are anatomically too short or which have an abnormal posture and do not effect an anterior oral seal when the mandible is in the true rest position. The use of the term 'incompetence' when applied to the orbicular sphincter is not strictly comparable to the physiological terminology used when referring to other sphincters in the alimentary

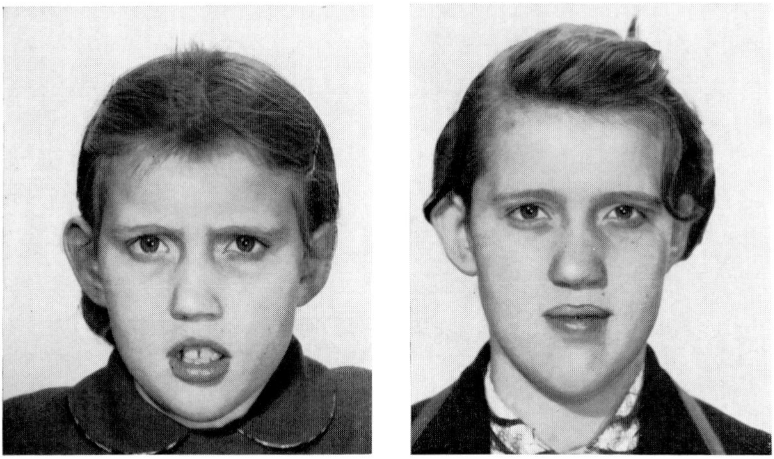

A B

Fig. 36.—A, Patient, aged 8 years, showing lack of lip seal. The upper lip is short and the lower lip flabby. B, The same patient at 15 years, showing conscious contraction of lips to effect a seal.

tract which are under the control of the autonomic nervous system. It is, however, a useful descriptive term. Examples are shown in *Fig.* 36 A and B and *Fig.* 37 A. Where a patient is a true mouth breather, the lips may or may not be 'incompetent' but merely be habitually held apart with the mandible adopting a low resting position. When the cause of nasal obstruction is removed a lip seal may or may not be established immediately.

Where the lips are separated by the incisor teeth, but will come together at rest when the dental interference is removed, they may be described as 'potentially competent' (*Fig.* 37 B).

The authors have shown that from an epidemiological survey, approximately 50 per cent of English school children at the age of 11 years have some degree of lip incompetence. Walther, however, gives a figure as high as 80 per cent in a similar survey.

It is quite possible to have a perfectly normal occlusion with incompetent lips if the skeletal pattern is excellent (*see* p. 54).

Feeding.—*Bottle Feeding*: There is no positive evidence to show that the jaws and dental arches of the bottle-fed child will be smaller or less well related than those of the breast-fed child. The facts can best be expressed by the following quotation from a report published by the Ministry of Health in 1943: 'The dental irregularity technically known as postnormal occlusion is equally common amongst breast- and bottle-fed children. The adverse mechanical effects of artificial feeding have

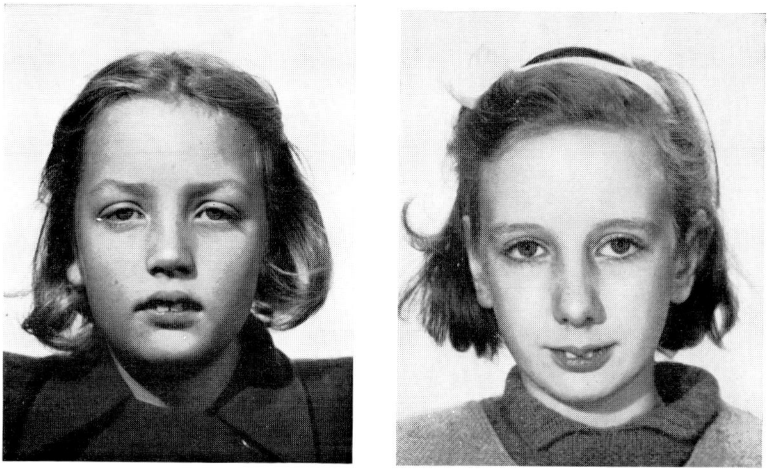

A B

Fig. 37.—A, Patient with short upper lip is not able to effect an anterior seal without conscious effort after the incisors are retracted. Incompetent lips (Ballard). B, Patient with lips of adequate length which are obviously able to make an anterior seal at rest when the incisors are retracted. Potentially competent lips (Ballard).

been greatly exaggerated. There is no evidence that breast feeding will ensure good arches in good relationship.'

Straub, in California, still maintains that bottle feeding does not provide the correct stimulus for normal oral function and therefore, indirectly, has an adverse effect on the development of the dental arches. Rogers, however, points out that a very small proportion of American children on the West Coast are breast fed. Certainly convincing proof has yet to be produced that bottle feeding has an adverse effect in any way.

Swallowing: The one aspect of feeding behaviour which has certainly received the greatest emphasis is that of deglutition. Rix described children with a swallowing action in which the teeth were not occluded at *any* time and the lips showed differing patterns of activity. He visualized this as an infantile type of swallow reminiscent of the transitional stage of swallowing found in the weaned infant. Rix described swallowing activity where the 'dispersing' action of the tongue

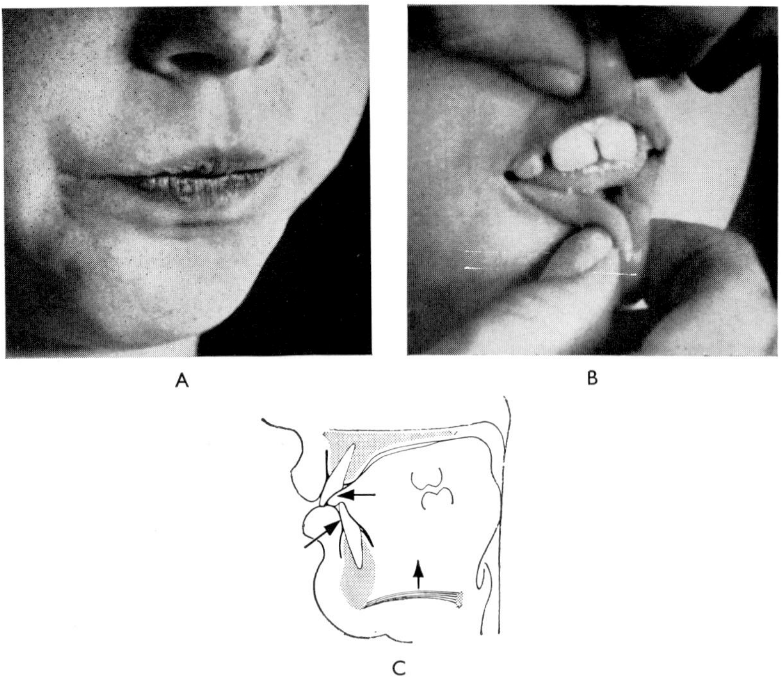

Fig. 38.—Example of excessive circumoral contraction, the strong activity of the lower lip scooping under the upper incisors to meet the tongue-thrust. This type of adverse behaviour of the lips and tongue may be an additional factor increasing the overjet of the upper incisors. A, Extracted cine frame to show excessive lower lip contraction. B, Tongue-thrust. C, Diagram to show action of lips and tongue in effecting an anterior oral seal.

and lower lip caused the upper incisors to be splayed forward and/or the lower incisors retroclined. This imbalance of forces was also related to a disturbance in the cheek–tooth relationship fostering forward movement of the buccal segments and a tendency to cross-bite (*Fig.* 38).

Rix described another group where upper and lower arch perimeters were not disturbed but where the tongue, acting in a larger space with the teeth separated, failed to give general centrifugal moulding of the dental arches and palate. In some of the cases in this group there might be a passive compression of the incisor segments fostering retroclination of the incisors and anteroposterior crowding of the arches.

In such cases the tongue appeared not to exert a commensurate forward thrust but maintains the normal buccolingual relationships with the cheek teeth.

In the light of recent knowledge it would seem that many of these lip and tongue activities described as atypical swallowing actions are adaptations to morphological features. When there is a marked degree of mandibular retrusion and there is lip incompetence, the anterior oral seal has to be obtained by the mandible coming forward and the lower lip contracting to meet the tongue (*Fig.* 39). This places the incisors in an unfavourable environment as they erupt and these adverse muscle

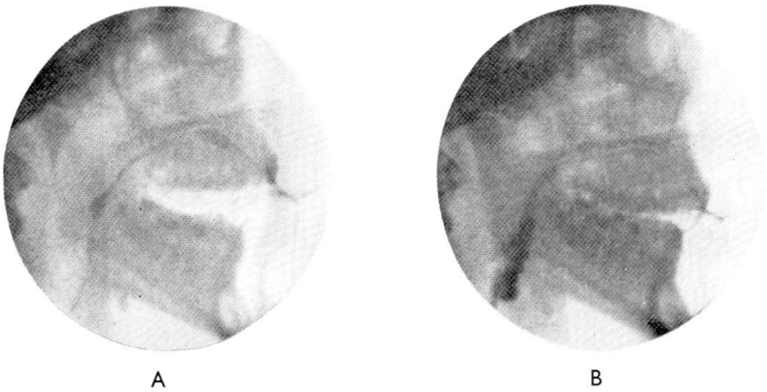

Fig. 39.—'Abnormal' swallowing sequence (patient with Class II, division 1 malocclusion). A, Prior to swallowing with barium on dorsum of tongue. B, Mylohyoid phase of swallowing as barium is transferred into the mesopharynx. Note that the teeth are not together and the tongue protrudes between the upper and lower incisors in contact with the contracting lower lip. (Extracted cine frames.)

forces may have the effect of increasing or maintaining an overjet. This is the type of activity which Rix describes as the 'infantile swallow'. It must be emphasized that marked circumoral contraction with the tongue participating in the anterior oral seal will not have an adverse effect on the incisor relationship if the skeletal pattern is I or tending to III as the lower lip may contract against the labial surfaces of the upper incisors.

This pattern of behaviour does not necessarily mean that the upper labial segment cannot be retracted (*see Fig.* 41).

Mastication: Although our modern diet requires little effort in mastication there is no evidence to show that in the individual who inherits jaws of adequate size to accommodate all the teeth, lack of masticatory effort in any way diminishes the size of the jaws. There is also no evidence that a child who inherits small jaws will influence the dental arch development in any way by chewing exercises or a specially arranged diet. Mastication is described in Chapter III as a complicated process and is related to the specific form and relationship of the jaws.

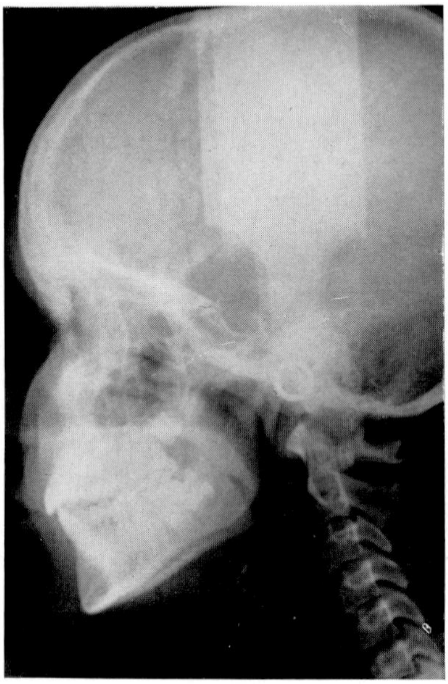

A

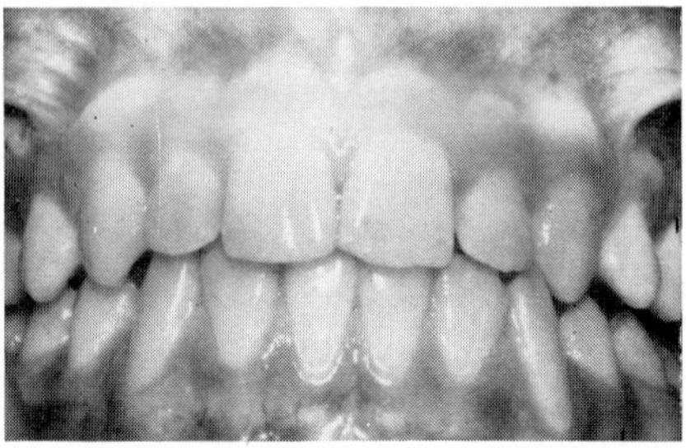

B

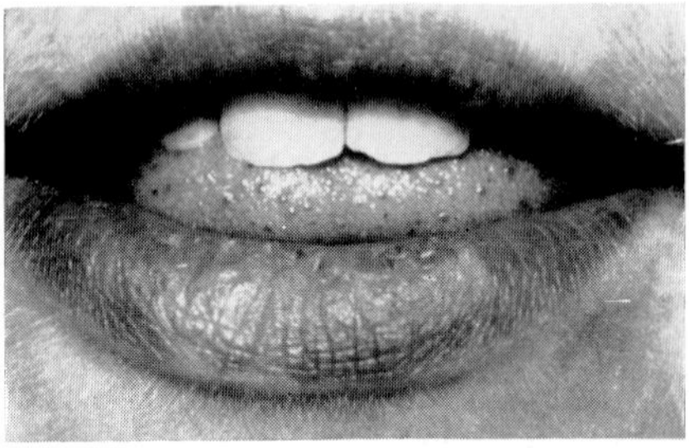

C

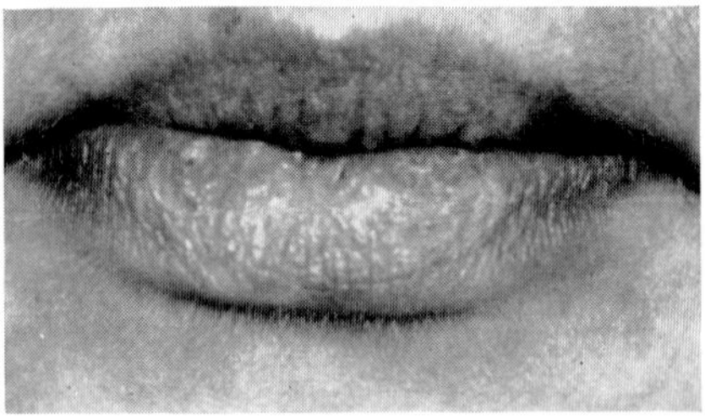

D

Fig. 40.—Example of a schoolchild with A, excellent skeletal form, B, excellent occlusion, but with strong tongue-thrust in speech and circumoral contraction in swallowing (C and D).

Speech.—Speech, being an acquired behaviour and requiring extremely complicated movements, is more likely to show marked variations and these may be due to faults in the receptor, connector, and effector mechanisms. The findings of van Thal and others that malocclusion is not a cause of speech defect and that speech defects are rarely a cause of malocclusion have been reinforced by Hopkin and McEwen, and Ballard. Tulley has shown that marked defects of speech with anterior tongue-thrust can be found where there is a perfectly normal occlusion (*Fig.* 40). In a study of 1500 schoolchildren aged 11 years, only 40 (2·7 per cent) were shown to have lisping speech with anterior tongue-thrust and only half of this group of 40 children had any form of malocclusion (*Fig.* 41).

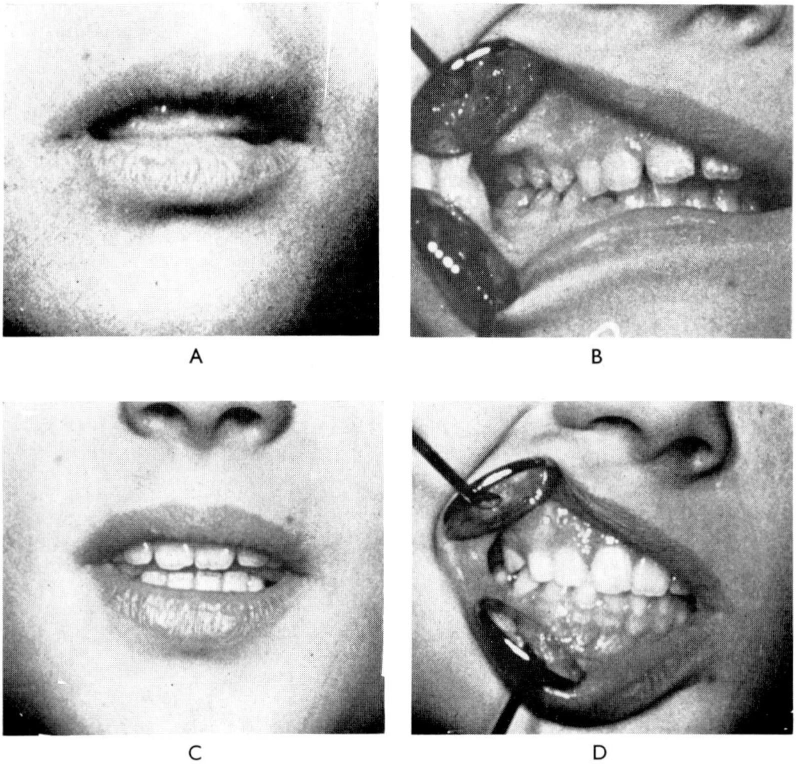

Fig. 41.—Patient showing how anterior tongue-thrust in speech, associated with an increased incisor overjet, disappeared following orthodontic treatment. A, Extracted cine frame of tongue position in 'S' sound before treatment. B, Increased overjet before treatment, age 10 years. C, Extracted cine frame to show absence of tongue-thrust in 'S' sound after treatment. D, Position of incisors after treatment, age 11 years.

A number of these anterior tongue-thrusts have been described by Ballard as being a compensating mechanism where there is an abnormal skeletal and soft-tissue morphology. For example, as in *Fig.* 42, where there is a high angle between the lower border of the mandible (the mandibular plane) and the maxillary plane, the posterior face height is short. Ballard has shown that the tongue may adopt a forward resting posture and, where there is lack of lip seal, the tongue may thrust forward in swallowing and in speech.

Tulley, studying a group of patients with a marked interdental lisp associated with a malocclusion, found that they all had the type of facies shown in *Fig.* 43. There was a coarse middle-third or lower half of the face, the lips were incompetent, there was an anterior open bite or incomplete overbite, and a tongue-thrust both in swallowing and speech which was very resistant to change. It would be quite wrong to state that the tongue-thrust was the primary cause of the malocclusion or that the malocclusion was the cause of the tongue-thrust. In the

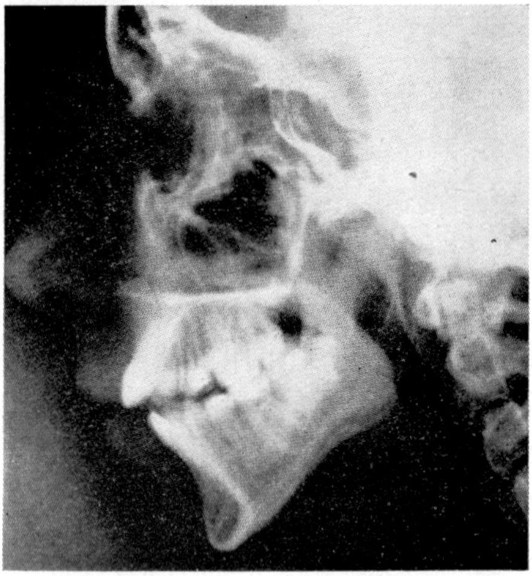

Fig. 42.—X-ray of patient with high maxillary-mandibular-plane angle showing forward resting position of tongue.

sample of 1500 children only 0·6 per cent had this type of facies and this puts the problem in its true perspective.

Ballard has described some form of anterior tongue-thrust as being 'built-in' or 'endogenous'. Some authorities have denied the possibility of inheriting patterns of behaviour but there is considerable evidence to support this theory as a neuro-anatomical variation. It could be said that imitation could be a possible way of transmitting such a speech defect, but the authors have seen many families where there is clear evidence of a familial pattern of behaviour in some of the children but not in others (*see Fig.* 44). Further investigations are required before we understand the nature of some of these variations and it must be made quite clear that we are not dealing with a pathological entity in these cases.

It is of course possible to find a very persistent tongue-thrust in children who have a neurological impairment with sensory or motor deficit or both, but these are extremely rare.

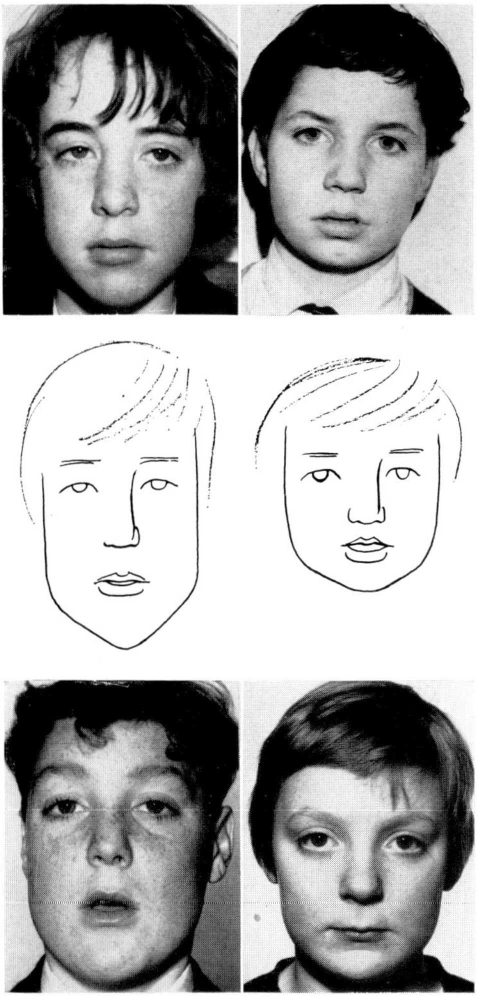

Fig. 43.—Artist's impression of the facies of the problem case with a selection of actual cases from the hospital and school groups. The two lower pictures are brother and sister.

Some children appear to have a tongue which is less agile in performing the delicate movements required for certain speech sounds, of which the 'S' sound is one of the most precise. In children where this so-called endogenous tongue-thrust is found, there need be no associated malocclusion where the skeletal and soft-tissue form is good.

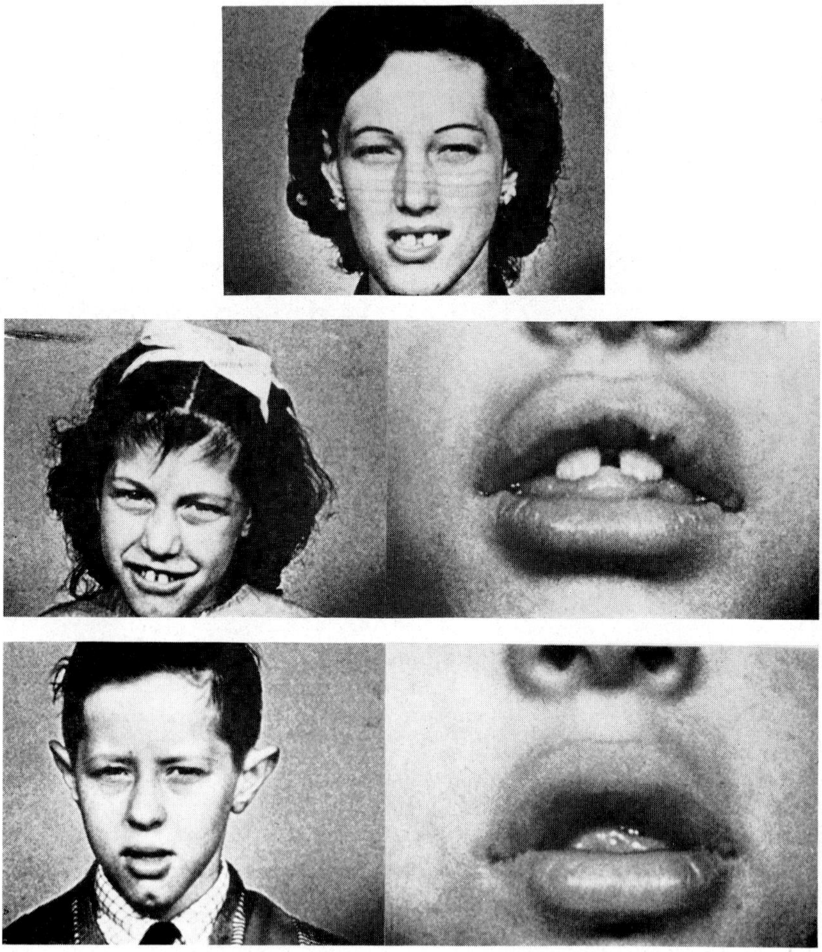

Fig. 44.—Mother, daughter, and son all with lisping speech. Father and younger son have a normal occlusion. Note the daughter has a Class II, division 1 malocclusion with persistent lisp. The son has a Skeletal 3 dental base relationship with anterior open bite. Note similarity in lip morphology. (Extracted cine frames.)

Facial Expression.—Certain movements of the lips in facial expression would tend to foster abnormal incisor relationship but many of these expressive movements stem from the anatomical configuration of the soft tissues and the relationship of their attachment to the bony bases. For example, where there is a retrusive mandible there may also be a taut lower lip musculature and in expressive behaviour this is drawn up in the form of a sling perpetuating proclination of the upper incisors and is secondary to the jaw relationship (*Fig.* 45). It is not found

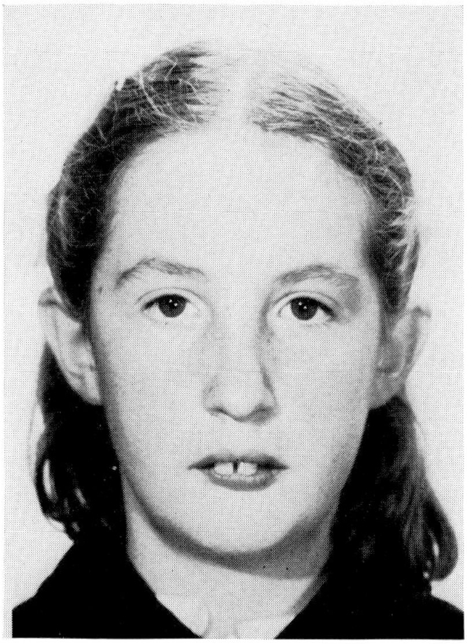

Fig. 45.—Patient showing very tight 'sling-like' lower lip.

very frequently, but when it does occur it may be a major factor preventing improvement in the incisor overjet.

Habit activities abound in expressive behaviour as is only to be expected. Lips which are anatomically too short to meet at rest may show increased activity in facial expression. Some cases with Class II malocclusions make a deliberate attempt to seal with the upper lip in the normal manner by posturing the mandible forward whereas others may fail to make this adaptive modification. *Fig.* 46 shows identical twins where one has adopted the forward mandibular posture at rest to seal the lips with conscious effort so that her incisors are less prominent than her sister's.

Summary of Major Aetiological Factors.—Before turning to a description of the factors operating to produce local dental irregularities a brief summary should be made of the major factors. There is no doubt that heredity largely dictates the form and relationship of the jaws. This will, in turn, have a primary influence on the size, shape, and relationship of the dental arches developing on this basic scaffold.

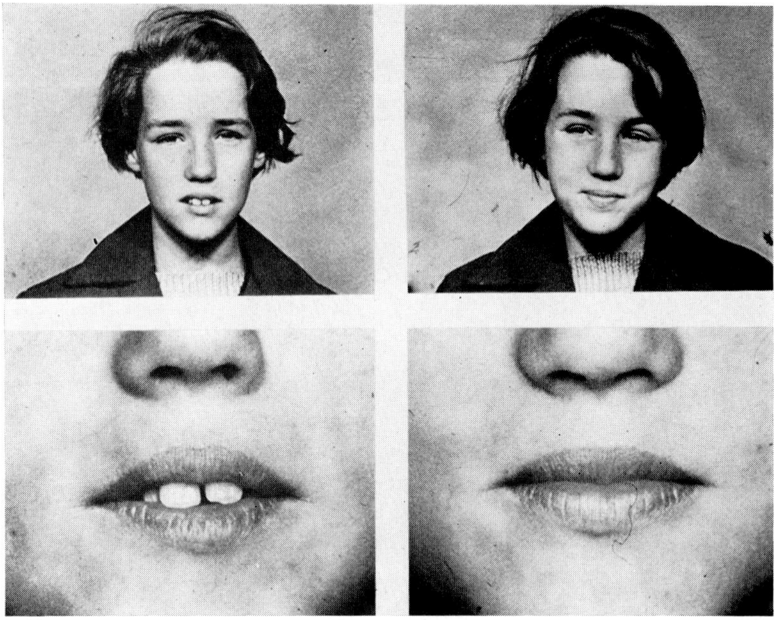

A B

Fig. 46.—Extracted cine frames of identical twins. Twin A shows lip incompetence and there is an increased overjet so that the lower lip scoops under the upper incisors to meet the tongue when an anterior oral seal is effected. Twin B has adopted a downward and forward habitual posture to conceal the upper incisors and her overjet is less marked. Note active conscious contraction of lips.

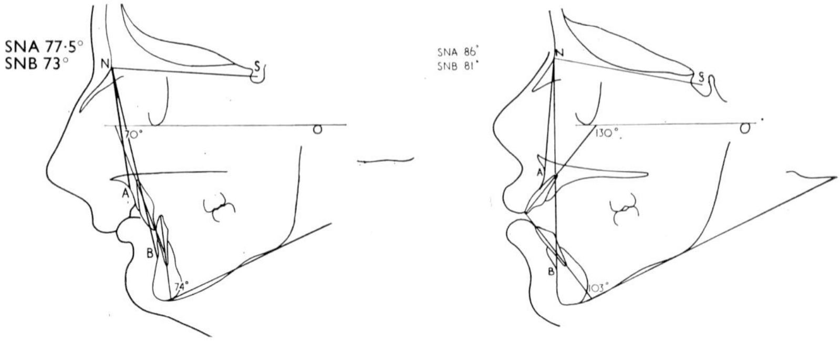

A B

Fig. 47.—Soft-tissue outlines related to axial inclination of incisors. A, Exaggerated Class II, division 2 malocclusion with tight short lips. The tongue is small in this case. B, Bimaxillary proclination with anterior open bite. The lips are flabby and the tongue is large.

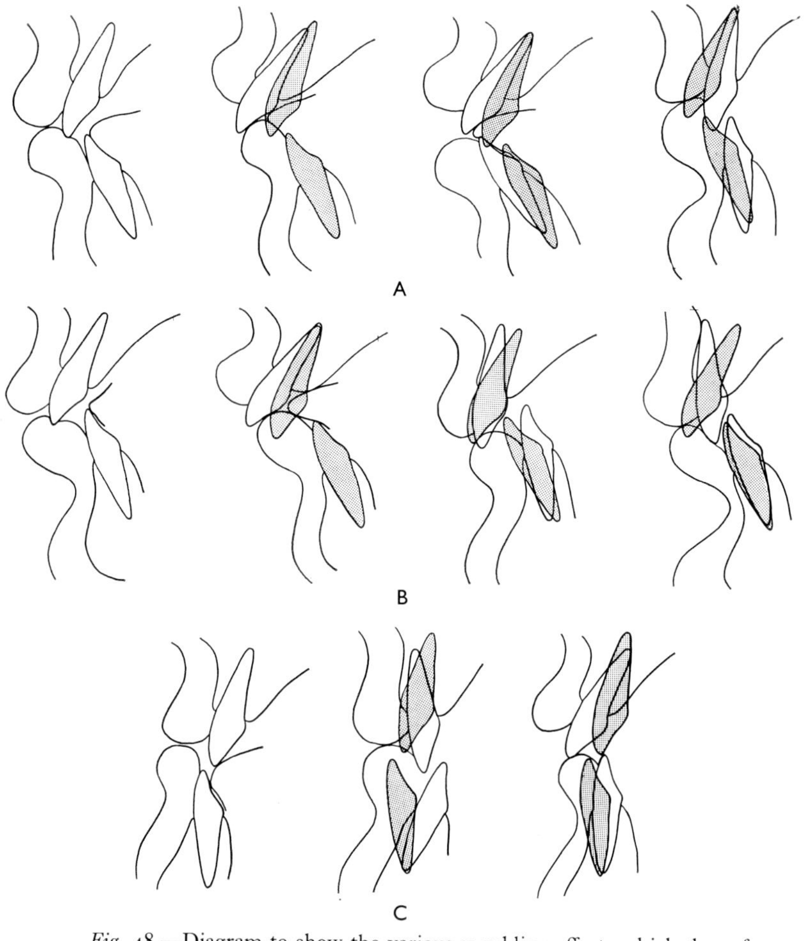

Fig. 48.—Diagram to show the various moulding effects which the soft tissues could have on the axial inclination of upper and lower incisors where there is a Skeletal 1, Skeletal 2, or Skeletal 3 dental base relationship. (*Note*: All these diagrams are in the position of rest. The stippled teeth show the normal inclinations which would have prevailed but for the soft-tissue moulding.) A, i, Incisor relationship showing normal axial inclination of incisors. Skeletal 1 dental base. ii, Due to habit, lower lip trapped under upper incisors maintaining an increased overjet. iii, Bimaxillary proclination of incisors with associated soft-tissue morphology. iv, Retroclination of upper and lower incisors showing associated lip morphology. B, i, Skeletal 2. Incisors with normal inclination showing increased overjet. ii, Increased proclination of upper incisors through lip action. Tongue posture preventing lower incisors from erupting. iii, Unusual type of Class II, division 1 with strong lower lip action causing retroclination of lower incisors. Upper incisors upright. iv, Class II, division 2 type of lip morphology causing retroclination of both upper and lower incisors. C, i, Skeletal 3 showing position of upper and lower incisors with normal inclination. ii, Retroclination of upper and lower incisors by moulding of soft tissues on Skeletal 3 base. iii, Class II incisor relationship established with increased overjet despite Skeletal 3 base.

The tongue, lips, and cheeks serve as a mould into which the dento-alveolar structures develop. The shape and size of these soft-tissue structures is also part of the inherent pattern. A large tongue is often associated with large and well-developed jaws and dental arches. Where there is a small oral fissure and small tongue, the jaws are often small and there is insufficient room for all the teeth. *Fig.* 47 illustrates two diametrically opposed types of facial pattern and dental arrangement. Despite the prolific literature concerning abnormal function of the soft tissues, this aspect should not be over-emphasized. Tulley has shown that of a sample of 1500 schoolchildren of whom 400 required some form of orthodontic treatment, in only 71 of these cases could the tongue and lips be regarded as a factor to be reckoned with in orthodontic treatment. *Fig.* 48 demonstrates how the axial inclinations of the incisors may vary under the influence of the soft-tissue moulding.

Long-term studies of developing faces put the changing shape of the facial skeleton and the soft tissues in their proper perspective in relation to the developing dentition. Brodie has shown how the tongue stops growing at puberty and any early adverse influence it may have had reduces. In the teens there is an increasing desire to obtain a lip seal, and even the most flaccid lips become more active in adult life (*Fig.* 49).

Examination of patients in the age range 6 to 10 years gives an altogether biased view of the importance of both the shape and function of the soft tissues. Patients with a major defect in lip length in relation to anterior face height do not show natural improvement with growth but they do make compensating efforts to achieve lip seal.

Factors Operating Locally on the Dental Arches.—There are a number of well-defined factors originally included in Bennett's classification which operate locally on the dental arches. Some of these factors are definitely inherited, others may be more realistically described as environmental.

Their immediate effect will vary according to whether there is a basic abnormality in skeletal form or whether they are operating in a situation which would otherwise produce a normal dentition.

INHERITED FACTORS OPERATING LOCALLY ON THE DENTAL ARCHES.—(1) Abnormalities in the size and number of teeth. (2) Large persistent labial fraenum. (3) Abnormal developmental position of crypts.

1. *Abnormalities in the Size and Number of Teeth.*—

a. Small Teeth and Missing Teeth: Teeth which are much smaller than normal and teeth which are missing show a familial incidence.

Missing or small teeth, in large or normal sized arches, may cause spacing (*Fig.* 50). The upper lateral incisors, the lower second premolars, and the lower third molars are the most commonly missing. A number of

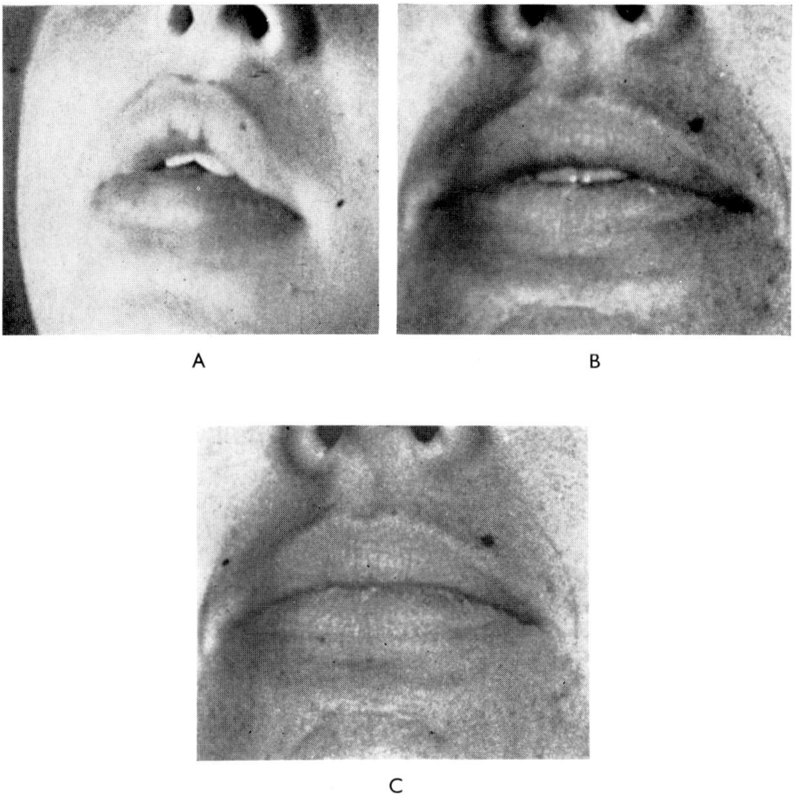

Fig. 49.—Shows examples of extracted cine frames from the authors' clinical research. There is a change in lip posture over a 12-year period. A, 10 years, lips at rest; B, Lips at rest, 22 years; C, Lips held together, note muscle effort.

surveys have been made in various parts of the world and the incidence of missing teeth, including missing molars, varies from 1·5 to 6·1 per cent. The samples vary both in content and number as to whether they represent a true cross-section of the child population or a sample chosen from orthodontic patients as in *Fig.* 51. Rose showed that 258 (4·3 per cent) of these 6000 patients had one or more missing teeth. The practical problems created in such cases will be discussed in Chapter VIII.

b. Large Teeth and Extra Teeth: Large teeth and supernumerary teeth also have a familial incidence. Such teeth in normal or small arches will inevitably produce crowding (*Fig.* 52). Supernumerary

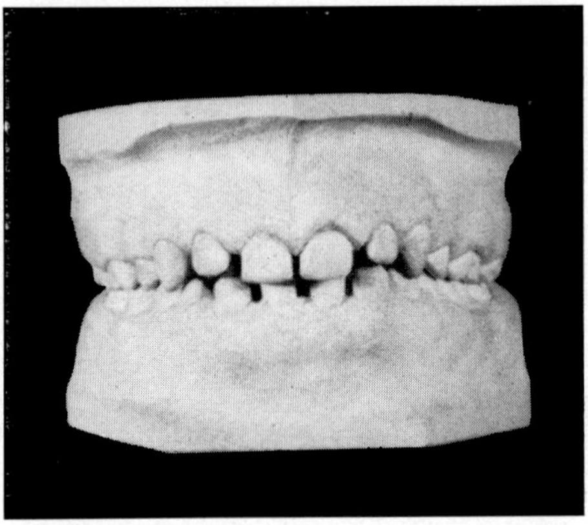

Fig. 50.—Model showing small *permanent* teeth and missing lower incisors in normal size arch.

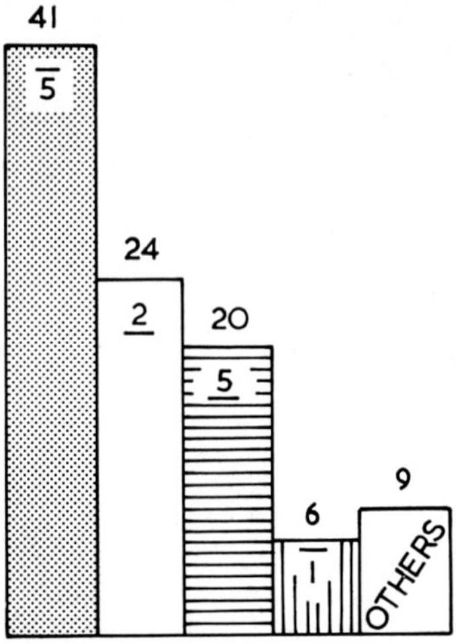

Fig. 51.—Order of missing teeth (excluding third molars) in 6000 London orthodontic patients. Expressed as a percentage of the 258 with missing teeth. (*After Rose.*)

teeth may or may not resemble those of the normal series and can occur anywhere in the jaws. They are generally found in the upper incisor region and can prevent incisor eruption or deflect them from the normal path of eruption. (*See* Chapter VIII.)

2. *The Labial Fraenum.*—A large superior labial fraenum which is attached to the alveolar crest and also between the incisors by a thick fibrous band to the palatal mucosa has been considered as a local cause of a central diastema. The present-day view is that the fraenum is rarely the primary cause of a median diastema. The implications of a large fraenum in relation to treatment are described on p. 91. *Fig.* 53 shows a large fraenum in both mother and daughter. No space is present between the mother's incisors, and the daughter's incisors are still erupting.

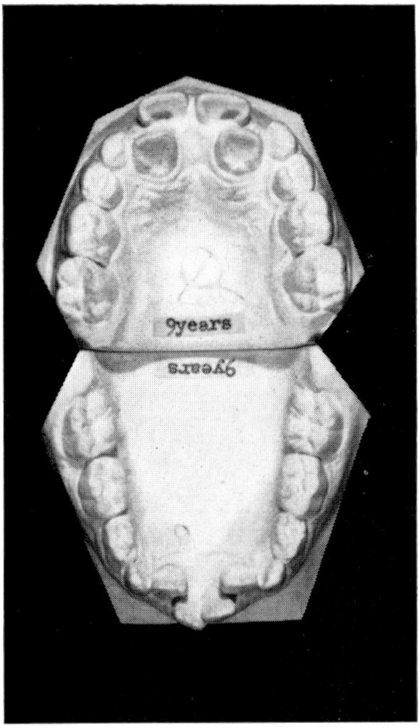

Fig. 52.—Large teeth in normal size arch.

3. *Abnormal Position of Crypts.*—Teeth may develop in a grossly abnormal position and thus erupt into an unusual part of the arch, for example, an upper canine erupting in the molar region.

ENVIRONMENTAL FACTORS OPERATING LOCALLY ON THE DENTAL ARCHES.—(1) Premature loss of deciduous teeth. (2) Early loss of permanent teeth. (3) Retention of deciduous teeth. (4) Sucking habits. (5) Trauma (direct displacement of permanent teeth or teeth damaged prior to eruption). (6) Pathological factors displacing teeth, e.g., cysts.

1. *Premature Loss of Deciduous Teeth.*—The premature loss of deciduous incisors has little effect on the permanent dentition. This

section is concerned with the premature loss of deciduous cheek teeth, including the deciduous canines.

There is a diversity of opinion concerning the importance of the deciduous dentition in dental arch development. If the dental arches are developing on jaws with a good inherent growth and the arches are developing in a satisfactory muscular environment, the effects of early loss of deciduous teeth will be very slight.

However, in most mouths these ideal conditions do not exist. In cases with potential crowding, one of the effects of early loss of

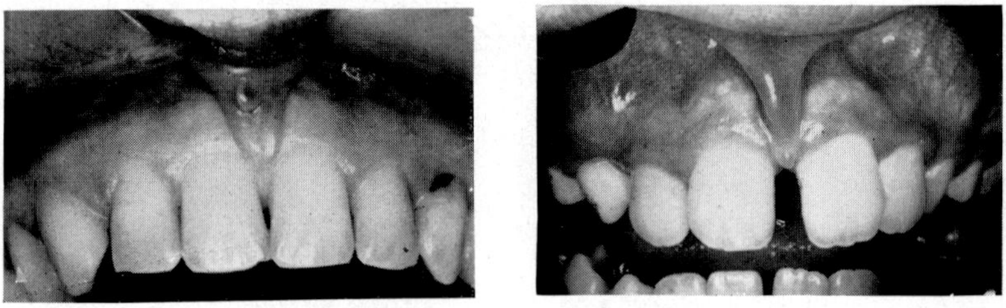

A B

Fig. 53.—(A) Mother and (B) daughter with large labial fraenum. Note that the fraenum has not prevented the diastema from closing in the adult. The child still has permanent canines to erupt and the incisors are being proclined by the thumb which can account for the diastema which is not caused primarily by the fraenum.

deciduous teeth is to reveal and localize the crowding. The smaller the arch, and the more restricting the circumoral musculature, the more rapidly will space be lost. This loss of space is also related to the age at which the extractions occur; the earlier the extraction, the greater the space lost. It can sometimes be regained in part, but this may be at the expense of crowding elsewhere in the arch.

The various effects of early loss may be divided into: (*a*) The effects on the individual arch. (*b*) The effects on the incisor relationship owing to the interdependence of the arches.

a. Local Effects on the Arch.—

i. There is forward drift of posterior teeth. Space for successional teeth is lost and they are deflected from the arch (*Fig.* 54).

ii. Anterior teeth tend to spread around the arch into the space made available. If the extractions are unilateral there will be a shift of the centre line towards that side (*Fig.* 54 C).

Theoretically a break in the continuity of the arch could have a local narrowing and shortening effect as shown in *Fig.* 55. This does not have the same clinical significance as has been thought hitherto.

Details of the Local Effects.—

Early Loss of Second Deciduous Molar: If the second deciduous molar is extracted before eruption of the first permanent molar this tooth will erupt in a more anterior position. This will result in the

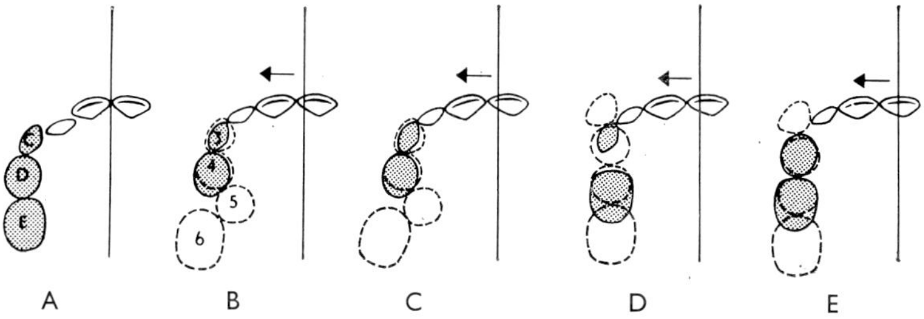

Fig. 54.—Showing movement of teeth in one arch following the premature loss of deciduous cheek teeth. A, Arch before extraction. B, Effect on neighbouring teeth of loss of second deciduous molar before eruption of the first permanent molars. C, Effects on the neighbouring teeth of loss of second deciduous molars after eruption of the first permanent molars. D, The effects on neighbouring teeth of the loss of the first deciduous molars. E, The effects on the neighbouring teeth following the loss of the deciduous canine.

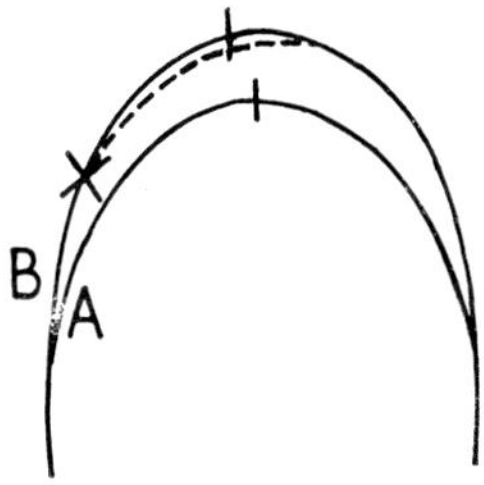

Fig. 55.—Diagram showing the effects of unilateral extraction of deciduous cheek teeth on the front of the dental arch when there is an adverse soft-tissue environment. A represents the occlusal form of the arch before extraction; B the form of the arch as it would move forwards with growth of the jaws.

The dotted line indicates a possible effect on arch form that can occur under certain circumstances. It certainly does not operate in every case although centre-line shift, as indicated by the anterior mark, almost invariably occurs.

second premolar being excluded from the arch when it erupts (*Fig.* 54 B). In the upper arch the second premolar commonly erupts into the palate. In the lower arch it is usually displaced lingually, but it may impact vertically between the first molar and the first premolar.

Where the second deciduous molar is extracted after the first molar has fully erupted, the upper first molar will rotate forward as shown in *Fig.* 54 C. In the lower arch there will be a mesial and sometimes a lingual tilt of the first molar. There will be a drift of the anterior teeth around the arch towards the site of extraction.

Early Loss of First Deciduous Molar: Where the first deciduous molar is lost prematurely the first molar and the second deciduous molar will drift forward without rotation or tilting and the anterior teeth spread around the arch. In the upper arch this usually means that the first premolar will erupt in the arch but the canine will be outlocked (*Fig.* 54 D). In the lower arch either the first premolar or the canine may be outlocked, depending on the sequence of eruption.

Early Loss of First and Second Deciduous Molars: If the first and second deciduous molars are lost prematurely, there is increased opportunity for forward drift of the first molar and distal drift of the incisors.

Early Loss of Deciduous Canine: When the deciduous canine is shed early it is usually due to the fact that overcrowding causes the lateral incisor to resorb its root. There is a distal movement of the lateral incisor to encroach on the space occupied by the deciduous canines, and the permanent canine is excluded from the arch (*Fig.* 54 E). (The deliberate extraction of deciduous canines as a temporary relief of crowding in the incisor region will be mentioned in Chapter VIII.)

b. Effects of Premature Extractions on Incisor Relationship.—

α. Where there is a normal dental base relationship, well-developed jaws, and normal muscle forces labial and lingual to the incisor segments, the extraction of deciduous cheek teeth will have a minimal effect on incisor relationship.

β. In Class I or Class II, division 1 malocclusions on a Skeletal 1 base, the lower lip resting under the upper incisors, early loss in the lower dental arch has been said to increase the overjet by removing the buttress to the lower labial segment and thus allowing the overbite to deepen. However, in most instances the lower incisors are held in lingual facial balance and Mills has shown that there is no so-called 'collapse' of the lower labial segment. In cases where there is a sufficiently deep overbite, as in Class II, division 2, some authorities will maintain that premature loss of deciduous cheek teeth may cause the overbite to deepen and in the present state of knowledge it is better to heed the clinical impression that an intact lower dental arch in Class II, division 2 is important. Early loss in the *upper* arch has little effect on the incisor relationship and only adds to the problems of treatment by allowing forward drift of upper molars. This also applies where there is a Class II, division 1 malocclusion with a Skeletal 2 dental base relationship.

Where there is a marked Skeletal 2 dental base relationship and the mandible is short anteroposteriorly the tongue may prevent further lingual movement of the lower incisors following early loss in the *lower* arch, particularly if there is a passive lower lip.

γ. In cases with a Skeletal 3 dental base relationship with a reduced overbite or an edge-to-edge bite, early loss in the *upper* arch *may* allow the upper incisors to fall inside the lowers, owing to the antero-posterior shortening of the upper arch relative to the lower. Early loss in the lower arch in true Class III cases may have little effect on the incisor segment if there is a large tongue resting low in the arch. However, in some cases with slight crowding it may allow slight relative lingual movement of the lower incisors and thus maintain an overbite if the upper arch is kept intact.

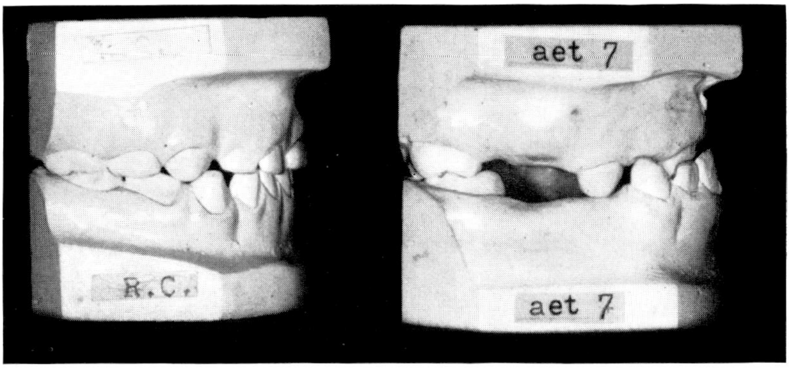

Fig. 56.—Models at 5 years and 7 years illustrating how loss of deciduous molars prior to eruption of permanent incisors and first permanent molars may initiate overclosure with consequent reverse overbite and production of pseudo-Class III malocclusion on a Skeletal 1 base or exaggeration of the malocclusion on a Skeletal 3 base.

In Class III cases where several deciduous teeth are lost in both upper and lower arches, mandibular overclosure may be encouraged at the time when the deciduous incisors are being shed and the first permanent molars are not yet in occlusion. It can also occur in a Class I case tending towards Class III. *See Fig.* 56 and Chapter XIII.

Too many dogmatic statements have been made about the actual effects of premature loss of deciduous cheek teeth on the labial segment of the dental arches. It must be appreciated that every case must be judged on its merits. There is strong statistical evidence in support of the fact that there is little change in labial segment relationship and no real local collapse of the lower incisors. *One of the most important aspects of unilateral loss of deciduous teeth will be the shift of centre line.*

2. *Early Loss of Permanent Teeth.*—The untimely loss of permanent teeth due to caries has the same general effect on arch form and incisor relationship as the premature extraction of deciduous teeth. The main difference is that, whereas early loss of deciduous teeth may have little effect when the dentition is developing favourably, the extraction of permanent teeth under the same circumstances may allow considerable drifting, rotation, and tilting of neighbouring teeth. If the arches are large the space created may not close.

The whole problem of compensating for untimely extractions by balancing extractions in other segments is dealt with in Chapter VIII.

3. *Retained Deciduous Teeth.*—Prolonged retention of deciduous incisors may deflect a permanent upper incisor palatally owing to its developmental position, so that it becomes trapped by the opposing lower teeth. In a crowded arch the other incisors may drift to encroach on the space which the inlocked tooth should occupy. Occasionally a central incisor is deflected labially and again may fail to fall back completely into the arch when the deciduous tooth is removed owing to the mesial movement of the neighbouring teeth. Only rarely does prolonged retention of deciduous molar teeth permanently deflect their successors.

4. *Sucking Habits.*—There is some difference of opinion concerning the role of these sucking habits in the aetiology of malocclusion but there is no doubt that they do cause local abnormalities, if only of a temporary nature. It is possible that the part they play has been rather minimized in recent years. Examples are shown in *Fig.* 57.

If a persistent thumb-sucking habit is capable of proclining the incisors on one side of the dental arch and the cheek teeth move forward to follow the incisors where there is some crowding, this could occur bilaterally and thus produce the Class II, division 1 malocclusion where there are normally related dental bases.

It is quite certain, however, that habits have neither the force nor the constancy to hold back the mandible to produce a Skeletal 2 relationship (true mandibular retrusion).

Where the sucking habits are superimposed on a dentition which is developing well on large and well-related jaws, they will have no ultimate ill effect on the occlusion.

It is where these habits are superimposed on dental arches which are not developing well, and where there are abnormalities in the size and relationship of the jaws and abnormalities in form and function of the soft tissues, that the contribution made by the habit towards the malocclusion is difficult to assess. Lower lip sucking is a habit which is almost always secondary to a retrusive mandible because the lip naturally falls under the upper incisor teeth.

One particular question which still remains unanswered is whether the excessive contraction of the cheeks which accompanies persistent

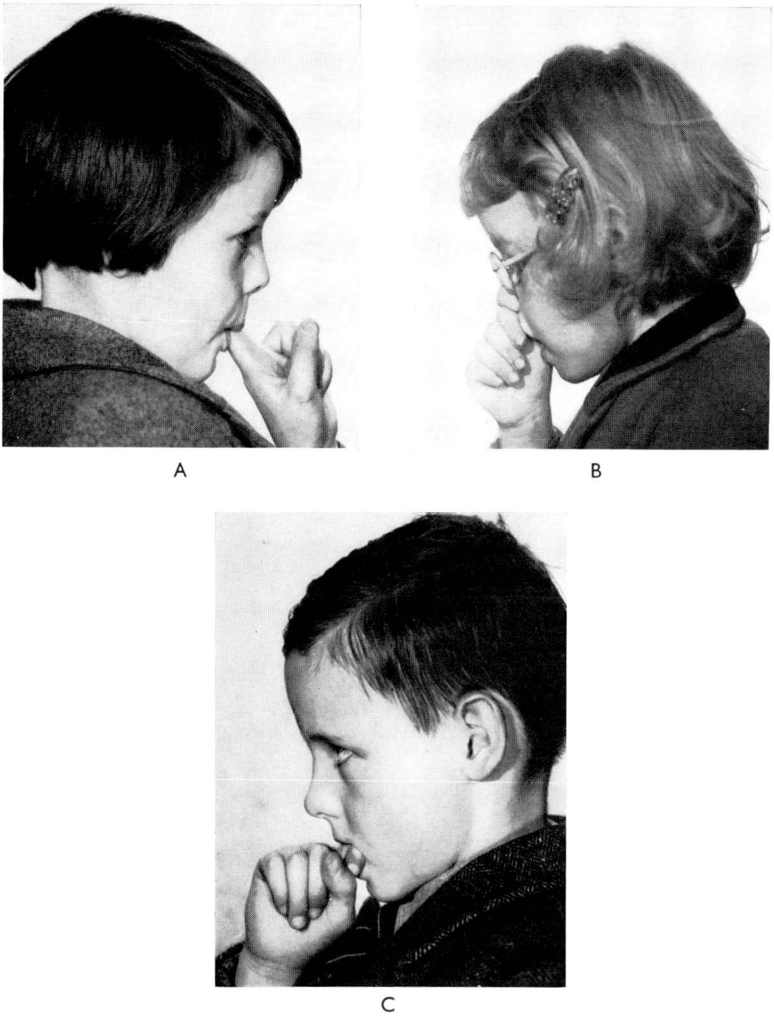

Fig. 57.—Some of the variations of the sucking habit.

digit sucking has, *per se*, any constricting effect on the dental arches. This question is bound up with the fact that a high proportion of these digit suckers exhibit an atypical swallowing behaviour with excessive circumoral contraction, so that it is virtually impossible to assess to what extent the sucking habit alone is responsible for contraction of the arches.

The literature is full of conflicting views on all these points. Clinical experience indicates that apart from a few very persistent cases, adult

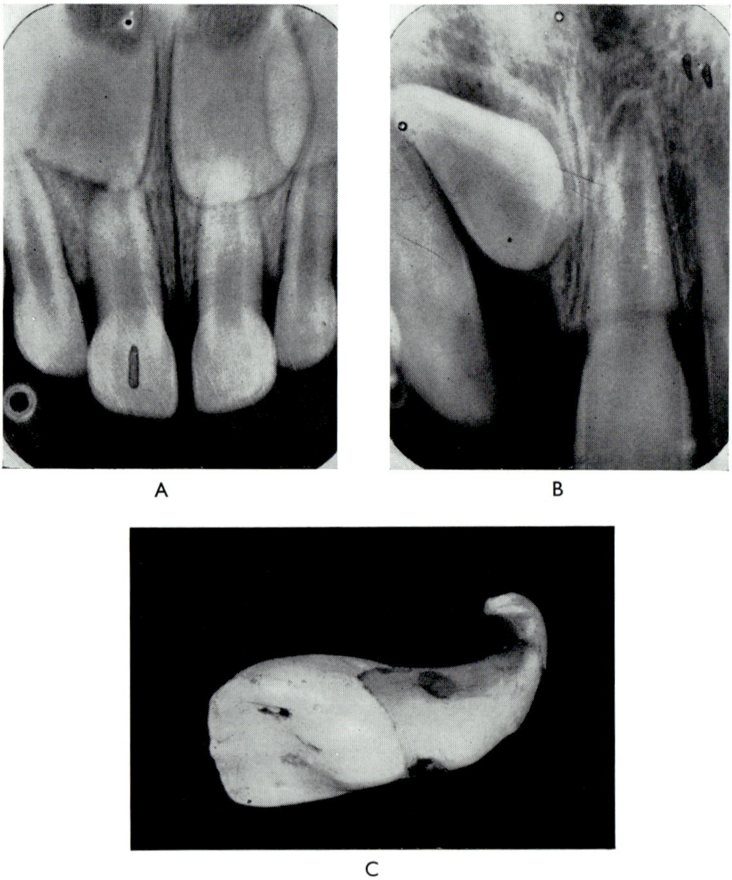

Fig. 58.—A, X-ray of a deciduous incisor at the time of injury to A| aged 3½ years. B, X-ray of same patient showing dilaceration of central incisor aged 8 years. C, A dilacerated incisor removed surgically.

dentitions show little or no effects following digit sucking. Where defects appear to remain there are usually other adverse soft-tissue forces still at work and well-defined skeletal discrepancies.

5. *Trauma.*—Blows on the mouth with displacement of or injury to the incisors are common during infancy. Injury to the deciduous

incisors may cause damage to the forming permanent incisors, which varies in degree. It may produce a marked disturbance in the development of the crown or root, as shown in *Fig.* 58, which is known as a 'dilaceration'. Whether the incisor tooth is able to erupt and become a useful tooth in the normal series depends on the severity of the damage.

Permanent incisors are frequently injured directly. They may be displaced without loss of vitality, they may have to be extracted, or they may be completely knocked out.

6. *Local Pathological Lesions.*—Lesions likely to affect the position of one or more teeth in the developing dental arches such as a cyst or a fibro-osseous dysplasia must be included in the local environmental factors, but their incidence is rare.

SUMMARY.—The malocclusions which are the everyday concern of the orthodontist are mainly due to inherited jaw and facial characteristics. They are variations of normal development and are not due to any pathologically abnormal growth.

There are infinite variations of jaw size, shape, and relationship. The tongue and lips may foster an acceptable dentition on abnormally related dental bases when the discrepancy is not very marked. For example, a mild Skeletal 3 dental base relationship is frequently seen where there is an excellent occlusion of the teeth, the significant effect being a slight reduction in overbite.

Where there is a major discrepancy in jaw relationship in the antero-posterior plane, normal function of the soft tissues cannot succeed in maintaining a normal occlusal relationship. For example, in cases with a marked Skeletal 2 relationship the lower lip is under the upper incisor teeth even though it may play a passive role.

When there are adverse muscle forces acting around the dental arches it has been seen that they can produce an abnormal occlusal relationship on normally related dental bases. When a combination of abnormal muscle forces and a discrepancy in dental base relationship occurs, the prognosis for treatment of the resulting malocclusion is at its poorest.

The effects of local factors enumerated in this chapter vary according to the individual case and must be related to the particular individual situation.

BIBLIOGRAPHY

ANGLE, E. H. (1900), *Malocclusion of the Teeth*, 6th ed. Philadelphia: S.S. White Dental Manufacturing Co.

BALLARD, C. F. (1962), 'The Clinical Significance of Innate and Adaptive Postures and Motor Behaviour', *Dent. Practit.*, **12**, 219.

— — and WALTHER, D. P. (1953), 'Some Cases to illustrate the Relationship between Aetiology, Prognosis and Treatment Planning in Orthodontics', *Dent. Rec.*, **73**, 669.

BRADY, W. J. (1905), 'The Influence of Heredity on Malocclusion', *Trans. Amer. Soc. Orthodont.*, 117.

CHAPMAN, H. (1950), 'Tooth Extraction as an Orthodontic Measure', *Int. Dent. J., Lond.*, **1**, 101.

COOKSON, A. M. (1968), 'Tongue Resting Position', *Trans. Brit. Soc. Orthodont.*, 119.

FOX, J. (1803), *The Natural History of the Human Teeth.* London: Thomas Cox.

HOPKIN, G. B., and MCEWEN, J. D. (1955), 'Speech and the Orthodontist', *Dent. Practit.*, **6**, 123.

HUNTER, J. (1771), *The Natural History of the Human Teeth, explaining their Structure, Use, Formation, Growth and Diseases.* London: J. Johnson.

KJELLGREN, B. (1948), 'Serial Extraction as a Corrective Procedure in Dental Orthopaedic Therapy', *Trans. Europ. Orthod. Soc.*, 134.

LAST, R. J. (1954), 'The Muscles of the Mandible', *Proc. R. Soc. Med.*, **47**, 571.

LUFFINGHAM, J. K. (1969), 'Lip and Cheek Pressure exerted upon Teeth in Three Adult Groups with Different Occlusion', *Archs oral Biol.*, **14**, 337.

LUNDSTRÖM, A. F. (1925), 'Malocclusion of the Teeth regarded as a Problem in Connection with the Apical Base', *Int. J. Orthod.*, **11**, 591.

MILLS, J. R. E. (1968), 'The Stability of the Lower Labial Segment. A Cephalometric Survey', *Dent. Practit.*, **18**, 293.

PERRY, H. T. (1954), 'Role of the Neuromuscular System in Functional Activity of the Mandible', *J. Amer. dent. Ass.*, **48**, 665.

PRINGLE, K. E. (1938), 'The Relationship between Incisor Overlap and the Extraction of Upper Temporary Teeth', *Dent. Rec.*, **59**, 190.

RIX, R. E. (1953), 'Some Observations on the Environment of the Incisors', *Ibid.*, **73**, 427.

ROGERS, A. P. (1939), 'Evolution, Development and Application of Myofunctional Therapy in Orthodontics', *Amer. J. Orthodont.*, **25**, 1.

ROGERS, J. H. (1961), 'Swallowing Patterns of a Normal Population Sample compared to those of Patients from an Orthodontic Practice', *Amer. J. Orthodont.*, **47**, 674.

ROSE, J. S. (1966), 'A Survey of Congenitally Missing Teeth, excluding Third Molars, in 6000 Orthodontic Patients', *Trans. Brit. Soc. Orthodont.*, 75.

SICHER, H. (1954), 'Position and Movements of the Mandible', *J. Amer. dent. Ass.*, **48**, 120.

SMITH, D. I. (1957), 'The Eruption of the Third Molars following Extraction of Second Molars', *Trans. Brit. Soc. Orthodont.*, 55.

STRAUB, W. J. (1960), 'Malfunction of the Tongue', *Amer. J. Orthodont.*, **46**, 404.

VAN THAL, J. (1935), 'Tongue Thrusting in Relation to Sigmatism', *J. Coll. Speech Therapist*, **18**, 1.

THOMPSON, J. R., and BRODIE, A. G. (1946), 'The Rest Position of the Mandible and its Significance to Dental Science', *J. Amer. dent. Ass.*, **33**, 151.

TOMES, C. S. (1872), 'On the Developmental Origin of the V-shaped Contracted Maxilla', *Month. Review. D. Surg.*, **1**, 2.

TULLEY, W. J. (1962), 'An Electromyographic Study of the Oro-facial Muscles in Relation to the Form of the Jaws and the Occlusion of the Teeth', Ph.D. Thesis, University of London.

— — (1964), 'The Tongue: That Unruly Member?', *Dent. Practit.*, **15**, 1.

TWEED, C. H. (1944), 'Indications for the Extraction of Teeth in Orthodontic Procedure', *Amer. J. Orthodont.*, **30**, 405.

WILKINSON, A. A. (1942), 'The Early Extraction of the First Permanent Molar as the Best Method of preserving the Dentition as a Whole', *Trans. Brit. Soc. Orthodont.*, 13.

CHAPTER VI

EXAMINATION AND CASE ASSESSMENT

BEFORE deciding on the form of treatment it is obviously essential to make an assessment of the case. A method is outlined in the following paragraphs.

History.—This should include:—

Relevant Medical History.—

a. Note of serious illnesses with sequelae.

b. Factors which might affect the extraction of teeth under local or general anaesthetic, e.g., cardiac or respiratory abnormalities, or diseases, or haemorrhagic diseases.

c. Note allergies and possible contra-indications to therapy.

d. Upper respiratory infections and whether colds are frequent.

The general health of the child may not affect the treatment planning but attendance may be poor.

Relevant Dental History.—

a. Inherited features, particularly where there are Class II or Class III malocclusions.

b. The date of extractions and note any difficulties.

c. The date and nature of any traumatic incidents, either to the deciduous or permanent teeth, or to the jaws. It is helpful to know whether the patient indulges in sporting activities and is particularly accident prone.

d. The nature of sucking habits and their duration.

Examination.—A routine and detailed general examination of the mouth should be made. From the orthodontist's viewpoint, the examination should also include:—

1. The form of the dental arches and their relationship.
2. An assessment of the skeletal form and relationship.
3. The form and function of the soft tissues of the lips and tongue surrounding the dental arches.

The Dental Arches and their Relationship.—Impressions should be taken and models constructed as a record. They are also useful in explaining treatment to the patient and parents and for planning appliance design. The following aspects should be noted:—

1. *Presence, Position, and Quality of each Individual Tooth.*—It is important to estimate the prognosis for teeth that have been heavily

restored or require restoration. This will perhaps point to the most desirable teeth to be extracted, where extractions are required as part of the plan of treatment.

2. *Shape of the Dental Arches.*—Note must be taken as to whether the arches are broad or V-shaped and whether the vault of the palate is high.

3. *Disproportion between Arch Size and Size and Number of Teeth.*—It is important to decide whether there is potential crowding or spacing. Few patients are able to accommodate all 32 teeth in good alinement.

4. *Anteroposterior Relationship of the Dental Arches* as judged by the relationship of the cheek teeth. This is recorded under the modified Angle's classification described in Chapter IV taking into account possible mesial drift of one buccal segment in relation to another.

5. *Anteroposterior Relationship of the Incisors.*—It is necessary to assess whether the overjet is within the average limits of 2–3 mm. or whether it is increased or reduced to an edge-to-edge position or whether in fact there is a reversed overjet which might be described as an anterior cross-bite.

6. *Lateral Relationship of the Dental Arches* together with an assessment of the relationship of the upper and lower centre lines to each other and to the median plane.

The buccolingual relationship of the cheek teeth may be disturbed so that in the old terminology there may be a 'cross-bite' where the upper dental arch is narrow in relation to the lower dental arch. This may affect the whole buccal segment or one single tooth. Another form of abnormality in the lateral relationship may be that the upper cheek teeth may be in total buccal occlusion to their lower counterparts.

7. *Vertical Relationship of the Incisors.*—Note should be taken whether the incisor overbite is within the range of normality, namely that the upper incisors overlap the lowers by one-third of their clinical crowns. An increase in this overbite should be noted and particularly whether there is any contact of lower incisors with the palatal gingivae. The overbite may be reduced, edge to edge, or there may be a frank open bite where there is no overlap of the incisors and no contact. Where the overbite exists but where the lower incisors are not in contact with their upper counterparts or with the palate, this is referred to as an 'incomplete overbite'.

Radiographs.—Routine radiographs should be taken of all areas where teeth are unerupted, together with an occlusal view of the anterior part of the upper arch. The main objects of radiographs prior to the formulation of a treatment plan are to ascertain:—

1. Whether the full complement of permanent teeth is developing.

2. Whether there are any unerupted supernumerary teeth.

3. The position, angulation, and formation of unerupted teeth, e.g., upper canines, and lateral incisors having deep cingulum pits.

4. Periapical conditions and the presence of pathological lesions.

Methods have been advocated using both intra- and extra-oral films. Intra-oral films provide the information required and show

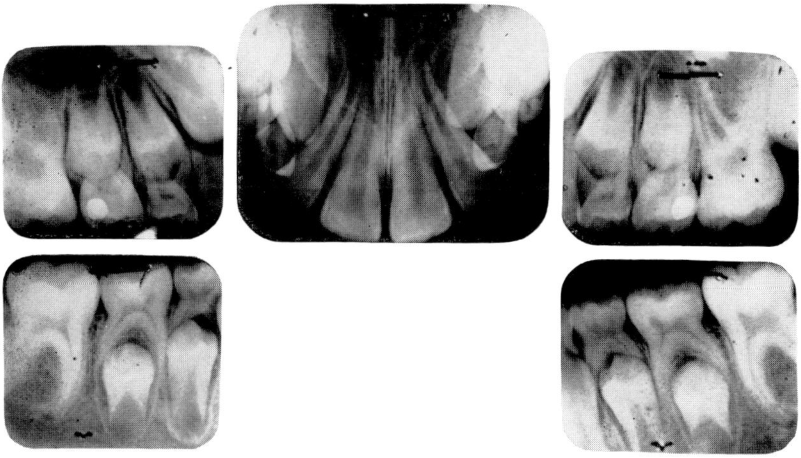

Fig. 59.—Intra-oral films taken as a routine measure in orthodontic cases seen in the mixed dentition.

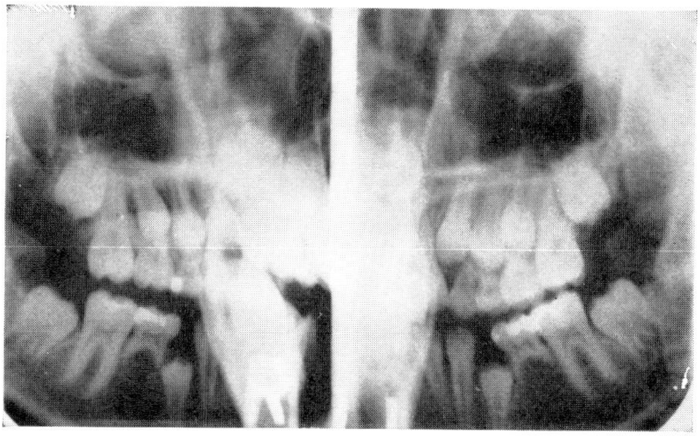

Fig. 60.—Extra-oral film, oblique lateral, of left side showing the detail of tooth position which can be obtained from the canine to second or third molar.

great detail regarding individual teeth (*Fig.* 59). However, extra-oral films in cassettes obviate the discomfort which young patients often associate with the intra-oral films. They also provide a better picture of the relative positions of all the cheek teeth from the first premolar to the third molar (*Fig.* 60).

Where accurate localization of an unerupted tooth is required prior to surgical exposure or removal, special views may be necessary. The use and interpretation of occlusal, stereoscopic, and lateral views are discussed in the Appendix.

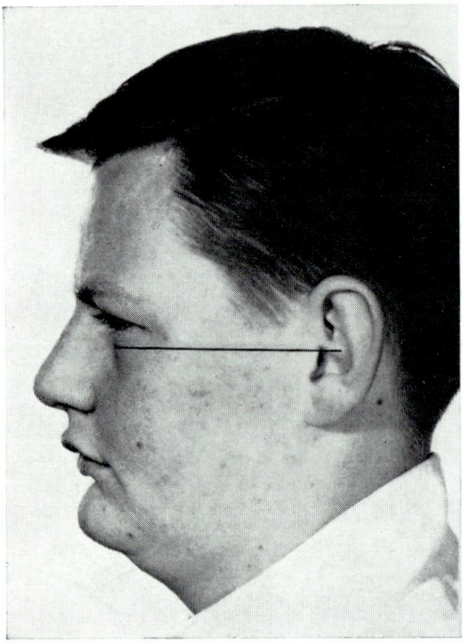

A

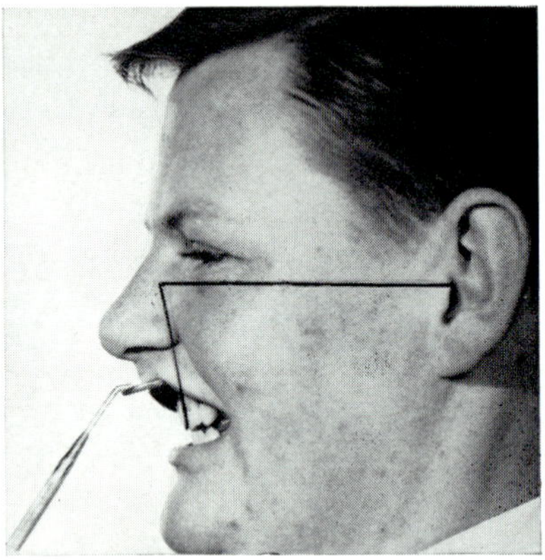

B

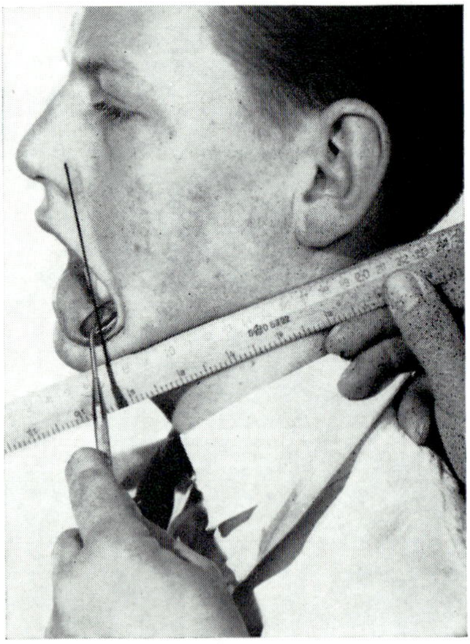

C

Fig. 61.—A, Patient with head orientated so that the Frankfort plane is horizontal. B, Clinical estimation of axial inclination of upper incisors to Frankfort plane. C, Clinical estimation of angle of lower incisors to mandibular plane. (*Continued on* p. 79.)

Skeletal Relationship.—Examination of the skeletal pattern should include an assessment of whether there is any major facial asymmetry when the patient is viewed in full face. Note should also be taken of whether there is any obvious narrowness of one jaw in relation to the other. This can usually be achieved by clinical assessment and the authors do not consider a postero-anterior skull radiograph to be necessary in all clinical cases.

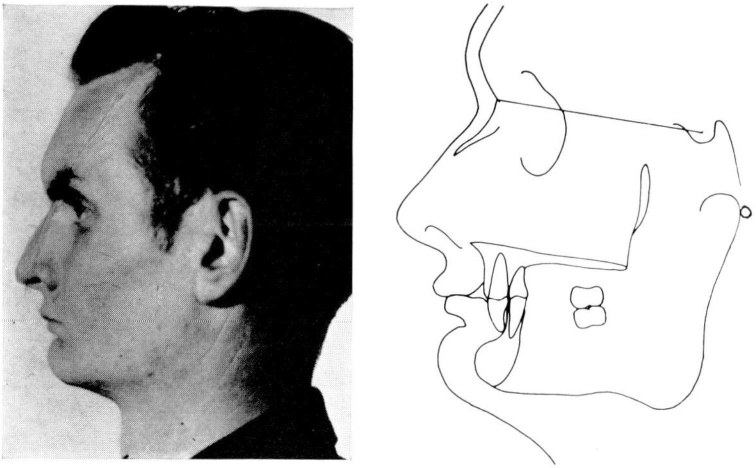

D

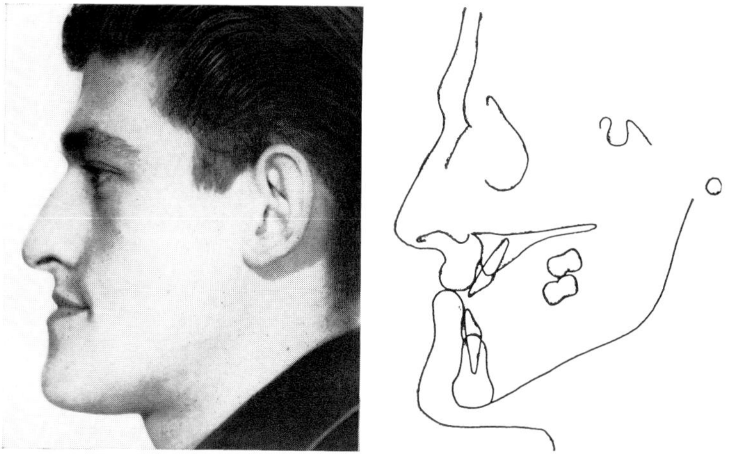

E

Fig. 61 (*continued*).—D, Profile and tracing of patient with low Frankfort-mandibular-plane angle and very deep overbite. E, Profile and tracing of patient with high Frankfort-mandibular-plane angle and open bite. (*Continued on* p. 80.)

The most important aspect of the skeletal pattern is the antero-posterior relationship of the dental bases. Many methods have been described of assessing this but any major discrepancy in bony profile can be readily identified clinically by observation when the patient is sitting upright with the Frankfort plane horizontal (*Fig.* 61 A).

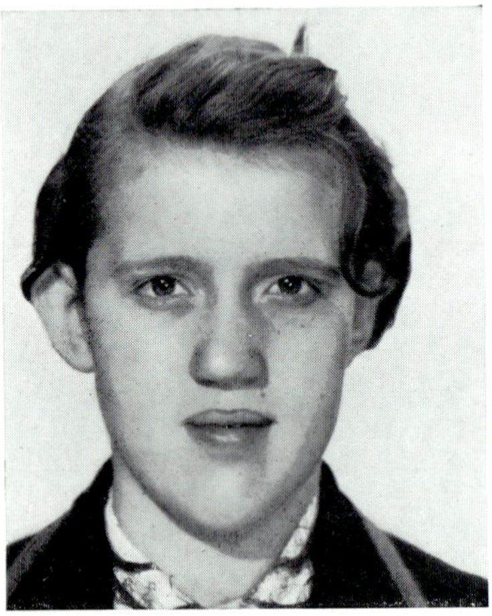

F

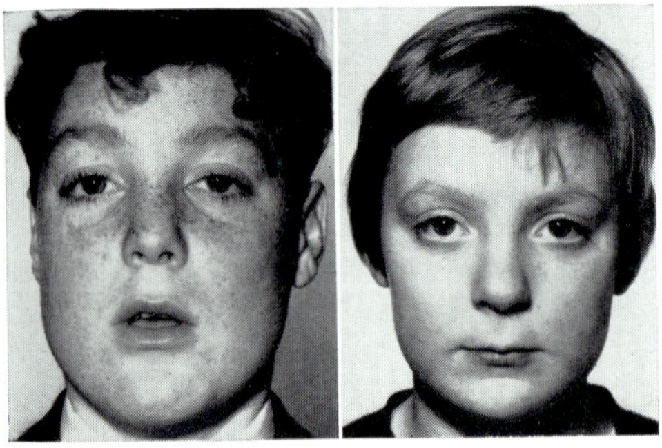

G

Fig. 61 (*continued*).—F, Patient consciously pursing up the lower lip to effect a lip seal. G, Examples of different morphology and posture.

The soft-tissue profile may be deceptive, particularly when there is a very thick upper lip and a prominent mental eminence has also to be discounted.

If the lips are separated when the patient is viewed from the lateral aspect and the area of bone in the region of the apices of upper and lower incisors is palpated, it is possible to make an estimate of the degree of skeletal abnormality.

It is necessary to judge whether the tooth-bearing areas of the mandible are approximately normally related (Skeletal 1) to that of the mandible or whether there is a relatively large disproportion. Where there is a relative mandibular retrusion they are labelled as Skeletal 2, and where there is a relative mandibular protrusion they are labelled as Skeletal 3.

Another important aspect of skeletal form is to establish the shape of the mandible, which may vary from a high to a very low angle. Those with high Frankfort-mandibular-plane angles tend to have open bite in the occlusal pattern whereas those with low angles may have very deep overbites (*see Fig.* 61 D). With practice it is possible to estimate the axial inclination of the incisor teeth, the uppers being related to the Frankfort plane and the lowers to the mandibular plane (*see Fig.* 61 A, B, and C).

The average angle which the upper incisors subtend to the Frankfort plane is $105° \pm 2$ and the lower incisors subtend an angle of $90° \pm 2$ when the Frankfort-mandibular-plane-angle is within average limits (25°–28°). It is necessary to appreciate whether the incisor over-jet is caused merely by errors in incisor inclination or whether there is a fundamental abnormality in jaw relationship. (*See* APPENDIX.)

The lateral cephalometric radiograph is becoming widely used as a diagnostic tool and cephalometric tracings are made to study various linear and angular measurements. This is dealt with in detail in the APPENDIX.

The Surrounding Soft Tissues.—

1. *The Lips at Rest.*—The size and shape of the lips and their position in relation to the incisor teeth are important, noting particularly the presence or absence of lip seal. If the lips are sealed, note whether this is being achieved without effort, or by consciously pursing the lips (*Fig.* 61 F). Lips which are unable to affect an anterior oral seal without conscious effort and are not impeded from doing so solely by the incisor teeth are referred to as incompetent. (*See* Chapter V.)

The size of the oral fissure and the texture of the lips should be noted. They may vary from the extremely 'tight' lips which are sealed at rest to the rather flabby everted lips compared in *Fig.* 61 G.

2. *The Tongue at Rest.*—The shape and size of the tongue are difficult to assess as it is such a mobile organ. If really large, it may be able to touch the nose when extruded. Its resting position in relation to the incisors and lower lip is important. Forward resting posture of the tongue can usually be seen when the patient is observed without disturbing the lips.

3. *The Lips and Tongue in Activity.*—The size, shape, and posture of the lips and tongue may well dictate the way they function. Lips which are incompetent will show an increased activity when forming an anterior oral seal. In the moment of swallowing, the tongue may come forward to participate in this seal, particularly if there is a forward movement of the mandible to compensate for some degree of mandibular retrusion.

It is important to note the pattern of lip contraction in relation to the upper incisors and whether the tongue is participating in this anterior oral seal. Many of the more rapid movements of the tongue, for example in speech, may not be of any major importance provided there is no forward tongue posture at rest.

In certain instances, morphological features of the lower lip cause it to be drawn upwards in expressive behaviour. The contour of the lower lip and its rest position in relation to the upper incisors and the occlusal level may well determine whether treatment of an increased overjet can be permanently maintained by the lower lip. *See* Chapters V and X.

The Path of Closure from the Rest Position to Occlusion.—The normal path of closure of the lower incisors from the rest position to centric occlusion is the result of a simple hinge movement at the condyle. Deviations in the path of closure should be noted. They may be divided as follows:—

1. *Lateral Displacement* (deviation of the mandible to one side or the other).

2. *Forward Displacement*: There may or may not be a forward displacement where there is an overclosure associated with a pseudo-Class III malocclusion.

3. *Posterior Displacement*: True distal displacements are rare. It is desirable to try to assess whether there is any habitual mandibular posture which differs from the 'endogenous postural position'. Where the patient adopts a habit posture in a Skeletal 2 case the mandible is held forward at rest to try to mask the overjet of the incisors. The path of closure from this forward position to occlusion gives a false picture of distal displacement of the mandible.

Having followed this method of examination and case assessment, the application is explained in the ensuing chapters.

CHAPTER VII

LOCAL FACTORS: THEIR IMPLICATIONS IN TREATMENT PLANNING

FROM Chapter V it is obvious that the form and relationship of the dental arches is largely controlled by the size and relationship of the jaws. Other factors act locally to produce minor variations in arch form and modifications in incisor relationship. The effects of these will depend very much on the basic morphological features of the case.

There are a number of interceptive procedures of a simple nature which may ameliorate or prevent further deterioration, and knowledge of these factors will assist the general dental practitioner who sees a large number of children through the stages of their dental development.

It is important that these factors be viewed in the light of the whole dentition, and it will be seen that the treatment measures which will be briefly mentioned here will have to be part of a more comprehensive treatment plan.

Premature Loss of Deciduous Teeth.—The effects of early loss of deciduous cheek teeth have been described in some detail in Chapter V. These manifestations occur in mouths where the development of the jaws and the influence of the soft tissues surrounding the dentition do not allow a favourable development of the arches. Where there is good development of the jaws and good radial development of the dental arches, fostered by normal tongue size and activity, many of the effects of the early extraction are minimized.

In the British Isles many children have dental arches which are inadequate to accommodate all the teeth, and the effects of early loss of deciduous teeth present a common problem. *It is therefore the usual practice to conserve the deciduous dentition where possible until these teeth are shed naturally.*

When deciduous teeth have been removed prematurely the decision has to be made as to whether the space should be maintained. In some cases the extraction can be looked upon as a helpful measure in the early treatment of the case, allowing some easement of incisor crowding. In other cases consideration has to be given to compensating extractions in contra-lateral or opposing quadrants, bearing in mind the possible effects on the overbite and centre-line. (*See* Chapter VIII.)

Space Maintenance.—The whole question of whether space maintainers should be fitted following premature loss of deciduous cheek teeth is open to considerable debate. There are domestic difficulties in inflicting an appliance on a child at a very early age and in

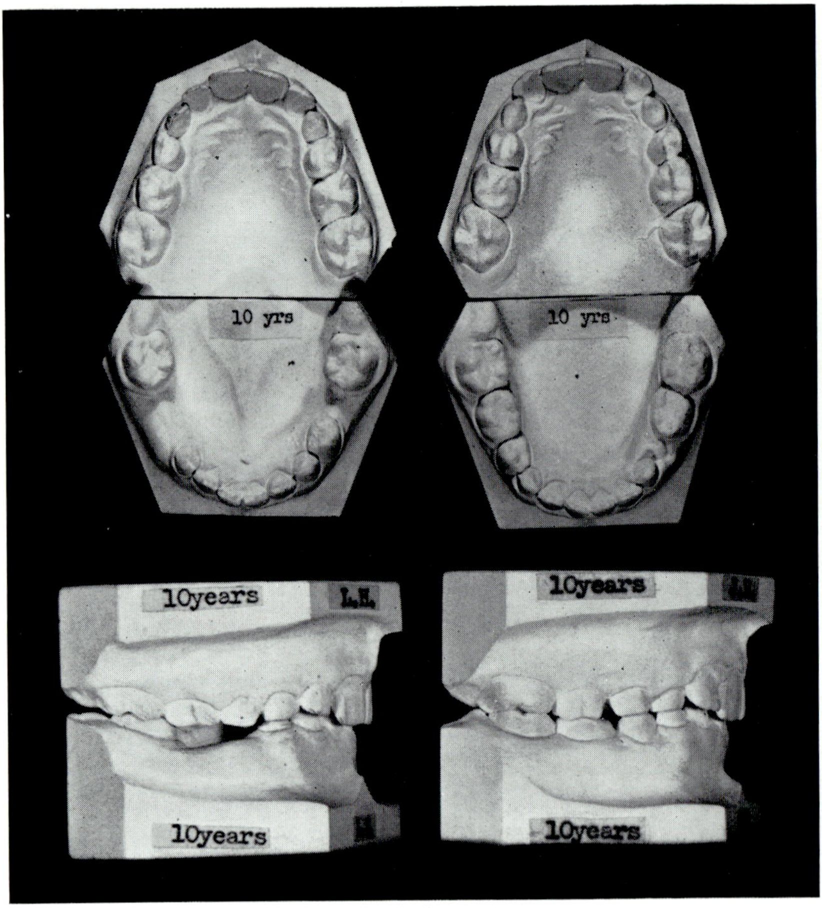

A

persuading the patient to wear this appliance continuously for a number of years when there is no guarantee that it will actually prevent the need for orthodontic treatment later. Prolonged use may also increase the caries incidence.

Small space retainers which are fixed in the mouth require regular inspection as their distortion or disappearance may cause anxiety.

The situations in which space may be maintained with some advantage are as follows:—

1. *In a patient with a dentition which is not perfect, but acceptable, where early loss occurs in one or both quadrants of the lower arch.* In such a case it may tip the balance between an acceptable incisor alinement and a degree of malocclusion which requires treatment. This

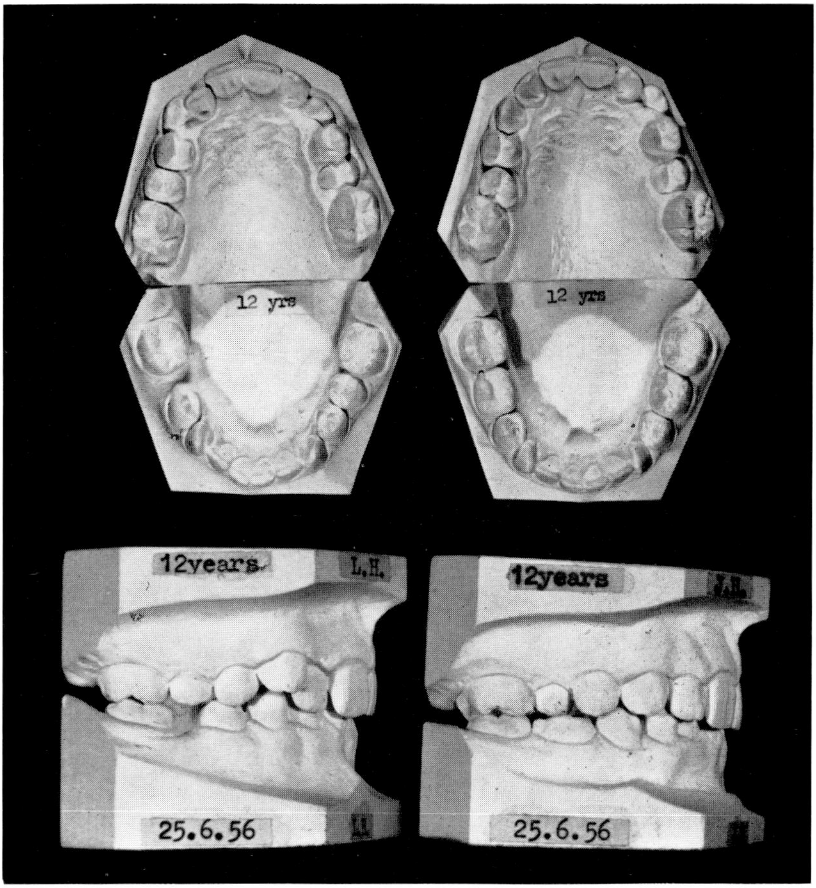

B

Fig. 62.—Models of identical twins where one (L.H.) had $\overline{ED|E}$ extracted at 7 years of age. The other twin (J.H.) was used as a control and had an acceptable but not perfect alinement. Use of a lower space maintainer here might have prevented the need for extractions. Models at (A) 10 and (B) 12 years.

Note: (1) Flattening of the lower dental arch on the side that $\overline{ED|}$ were extracted; (2) Loss of space for $\overline{5}|$; (3) Secondary effect on the upper arch so that there is an irregularity of $\underline{32}|$.

situation is illustrated by reference to models of identical twins (*Fig.* 62) one of whom has lost lower first and second deciduous molars on the right side. The one without extractions shows acceptable but slightly crowded arches which act as a control. The other shows the result of the lower arch on the right side with secondary effect of the upper incisors on that side.

2. *In an Angle's division 2 malocclusion with early loss in the lower dental arch.* A space maintainer may be used to prevent deterioration in incisor relationship with possible deepening of the overbite in the face of lower lip pressure. Such a procedure is only acceptable if there is a reasonable expectation that it will obviate the need for lower premolar extractions at a later date.

This whole concept is now open to question as Mills has shown that extractions do not necessarily remove support for the lower labial segment and the use of lower space maintainers should be restricted to those cases where the overbite might be deepened to the point of becoming traumatic to the soft tissues by a very slight change in axial inclination of the lower incisors.

3. *In Angle's Class III malocclusions with early loss in the upper dental arch.* The anteroposterior length of the *upper* arch should be maintained as far as possible. An upper appliance designed to move the upper incisors forward will act as a space maintainer and prevent forward drift of the upper first molars following early loss. Hence the appliance should not be removed immediately the incisors are over the bite.

At one time bite blocks were used to maintain the occlusal level if deciduous molars were removed before the eruption of the first permanent molars. This was said to prevent overclosure and a pseudo-Class III occlusion developing when the dental base relationship was tending towards Skeletal 3 (*Fig.* 63); because these bite blocks are not well tolerated over a long period of time, and as they cannot prevent the forward drift of the unerupted permanent molars, they were not a very practical form of preventive treatment. The established pseudo-Class III incisor position is simple to treat when the first molars have erupted.

Delayed Shedding of Deciduous Teeth.—Where there is a delay in the normal shedding of a deciduous tooth the permanent tooth may be deflected from its normal path of eruption. In most cases this deflexion is not permanent. The lower incisor erupting lingual to the deciduous incisor is commonplace (*Fig.* 64). It will generally move forward into alinement in due course if there is sufficient space. If, however, shedding of an upper deciduous incisor is delayed, the permanent incisor may be deflected palatally (*Fig.* 65.) It may be trapped inside the bite and space lost for its alinement if the arch is crowded. The timely extraction of the retained deciduous teeth will prevent this.

Where a tooth has become deflected in this way and there is sufficient room for it to be moved over the bite, this is often achieved with a wooden tongue spatula or the handle of a spoon used as a lever, the lower incisors being the fulcrum. The patient is instructed to bite on

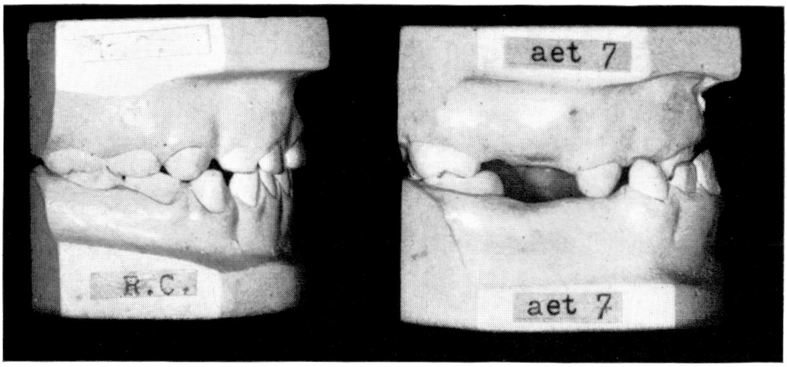

A B

Fig. 63.—A, Model at 5 years before loss of all deciduous molars. B, Model at 7 years showing pseudo-Class III due to overclosure in a mild Skeletal 3 case. *See* Chapter XII.

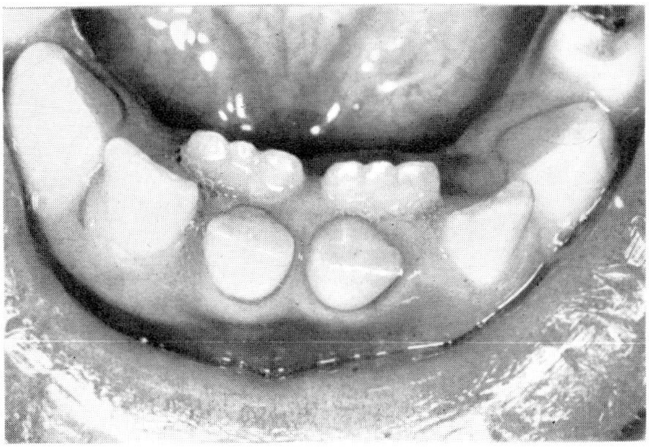

Fig. 64.—Common lingual eruption of lower incisors which causes the parents concern. Provided there is sufficient space these teeth move into good position when the deciduous incisors are shed.

the wooden spatula or spoon and to exert pressure intermittently for a quarter of an hour every day, preferably in the mornings. The tooth should be correctly alined in two to three weeks (*Fig.* 66). If this is not successful, a simple plate bearing a recurved spring can be used. There is rarely need to prop open the bite to achieve this simple tooth movement.

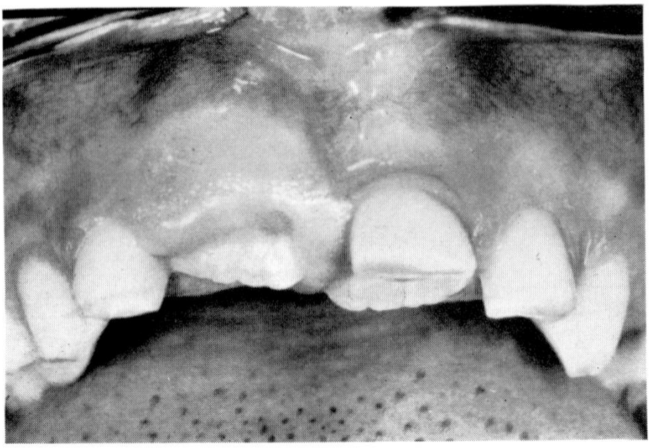

Fig. 65.—Prolonged retention of the deciduous incisors may deflect the upper permanent incisor palatally. Removal of the deciduous incisor at this time will prevent the incisor being locked inside the bite if there is room for it in the arch.

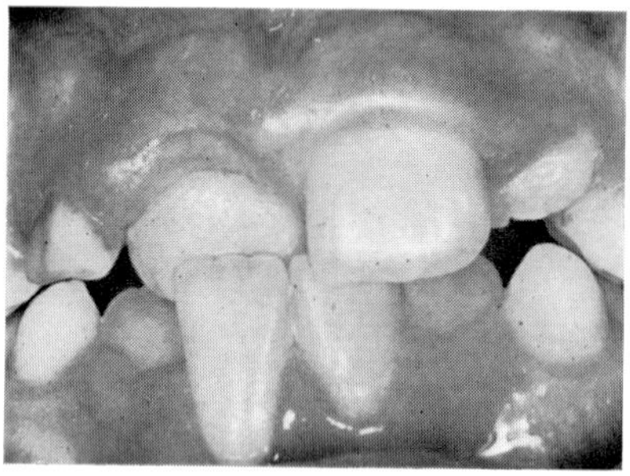

A

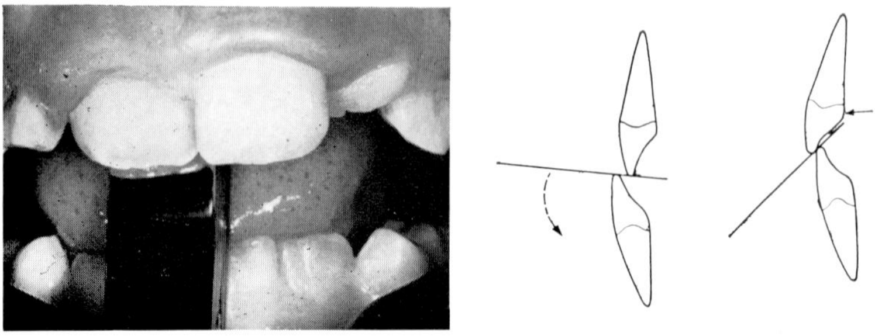

B

Fig. 66.—A, Shows example of inlocked 1| where use of spatula or spoon handle as a lever will correct its position. B, Shows method of using spoon handle as lever.

Sucking Habits.—The sucking of a finger and thumb or the lower lip is not uncommon in the infant and of no clinical importance. The mouth is a primitive area of exploration and the child derives comfort and pleasure from these habits. Considerable malformations of the deciduous dentition may be produced by persistent sucking and will reflect the way in which the force is exerted, but many children give up the habit before eruption of the permanent dentition.

Many articles have been written on the variation of these habits and have rather overemphasized the role of sucking habits in the aetiology of malocclusion.

A sucking habit is only one of the factors which may deflect the permanent incisors from their path of eruption.

The intervention of a habit prevents a true assessment of the underlying malocclusion, and it has been a common error to attribute most of the abnormal positioning of the teeth to the habit alone. Finger- and thumb-sucking may increase an overjet and open bite already present, and often produce an asymmetrical effect.

The error in tooth position caused by the habit may disappear when it is given up (*Fig.* 67). There are certain exceptions to this—if the upper incisors are held out by the lower lip they will not improve without active treatment. The tongue tends to thrust into an open bite created by a thumb or finger as a secondary effect, but it will not maintain an open bite if it is functioning normally. However, a certain type of oromuscular behaviour with persistent tongue to lower lip contact is associated with an open bite. In such cases where a sucking habit is an added factor the open bite will fail to close completely when the habit ceases.

Thus it may be said that where the morphology of the jaws and soft tissues is favourable an anterior open bite will tend to close, but where the morphology is unfavourable, the cessation of a sucking habit may well leave a persistent tongue action which will maintain the open bite.

Some clinicians state that a Class II, division 1 malocclusion can be caused entirely by a sucking habit. They suggest that the upper incisors are proclined and that the upper arch is narrowed by the excessive activity of the cheeks. The narrowness of the upper arch prevents a more forward positioning of the lower arch. This theory is based on the improvement in anteroposterior occlusion which may result from simple upper arch expansion and cessation of the habit (*see Fig.* 68). (However, note that the occlusal adjustment is rarely complete.)

Another explanation is that because the incisors are proclined there follows a unilateral or bilateral forward drift of the upper cheek teeth according to the particular habit, thus producing a Class II cheek tooth relationship. This is only an occlusal abnormality and *it is quite certain that a Skeletal 2 relationship cannot be caused by a habit.*

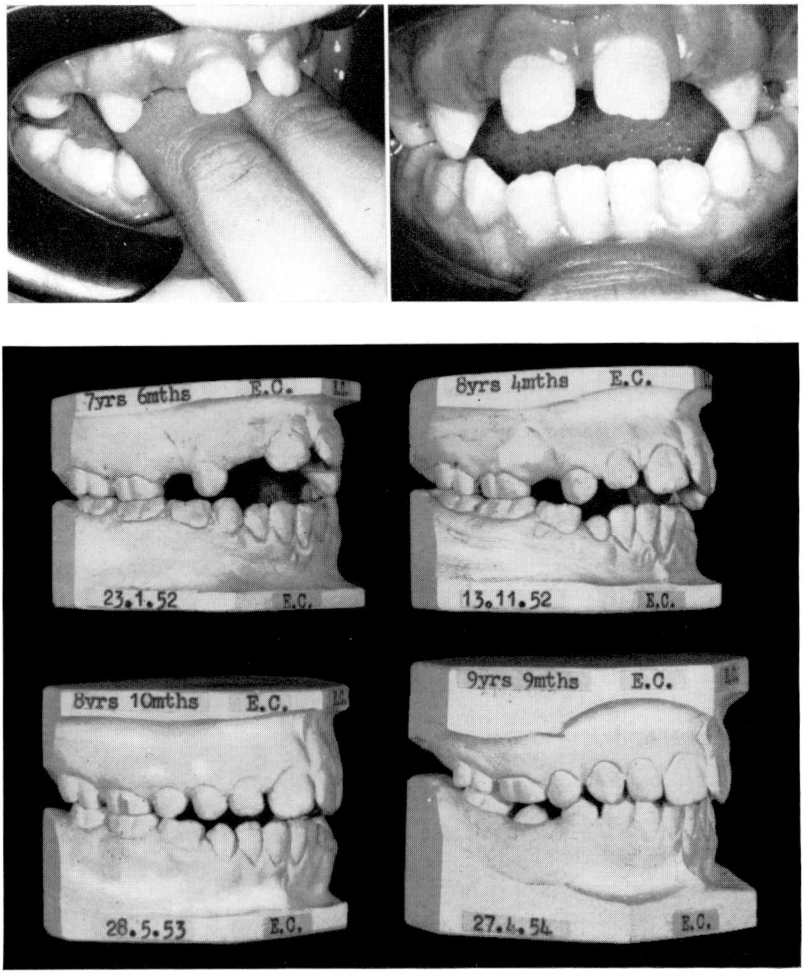

Fig. 67.—Open bite due to finger-sucking. Models showing improvement after the habit had been discouraged with a plate.

It is desirable to make an attempt to inhibit the habit when the permanent teeth begin to erupt. Some children will respond to a gentle talk on the subject; in others, the fitting of a simple appliance as *part of the general treatment plan* is effective as a deterrent.

The clinical problems associated particularly with Class II, division 1 and anterior open bite will be dealt with more fully in later chapters dealing with treatment.

Few children persist in the habit to the point of their behaviour being worthy of psychological investigation. However, drastic measures to break the habit are undesirable as the child may develop other more obnoxious habits. Lip sucking as a variation of digit sucking is usually confined to children with a tendency to Skeletal 2 relationship—the lower lip falling naturally under the upper incisor teeth.

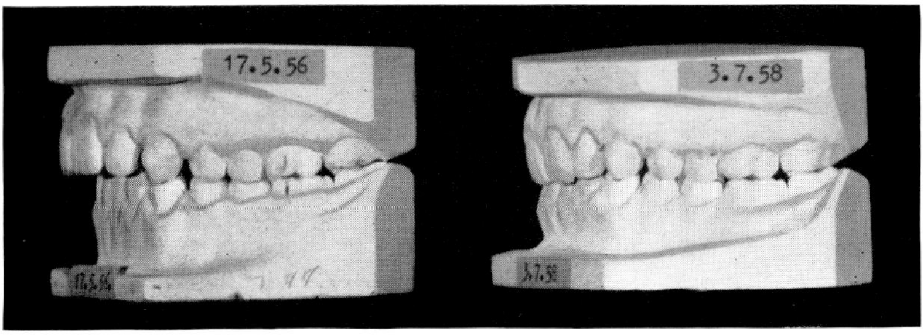

Fig. 68.—Self-correction of overjet and open bite after expansion of the upper arch in a case of thumb-sucking. To inhibit the habit a simple saddle plate was used without a labial bow.

Note this is fundamentally a Class II, division 2 type of case, so that the lip activity favours a return to retroclined incisors and did not perpetuate the incisor position. There has been some slight improvement in anteroposterior relationship of the cheek teeth.

Tongue-sucking as such is rare. It should not be confused with the lolling tongue of the child with true macroglossia, where the tongue is really too large for the size of the mouth, or those cases of tongue–lip contact which have been mentioned previously.

The problems created by sucking habits should not be magnified, but in persistent cases they are a real obstacle to treatment. Parents must be discouraged from nagging the child, and preventive measures should not be instituted too early.

Many appliances have been described which offer active mechanical deterrents to a sucking habit—being shaped and fashioned in such a way that it is uncomfortable or painful to continue with the habit. The authors feel that in view of the efficacy of simple apparatus these comparatively savage methods should not be employed.

The Labial Fraenum.—The upper labial fraenum has been cited as the primary cause of persistent diastema between the upper central incisors and many fraena have been removed unnecessarily. The present-day view is that the fraenum is rarely the primary cause of

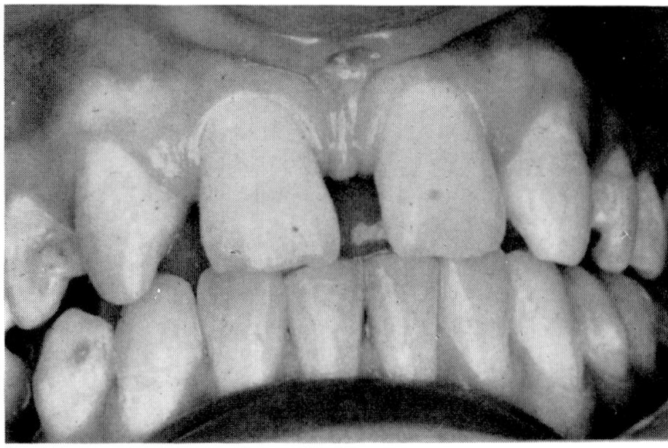

Fig. 69.—Missing $\underline{2}|$. Diastema not caused by the fraenum but rather by the absence of a tooth.

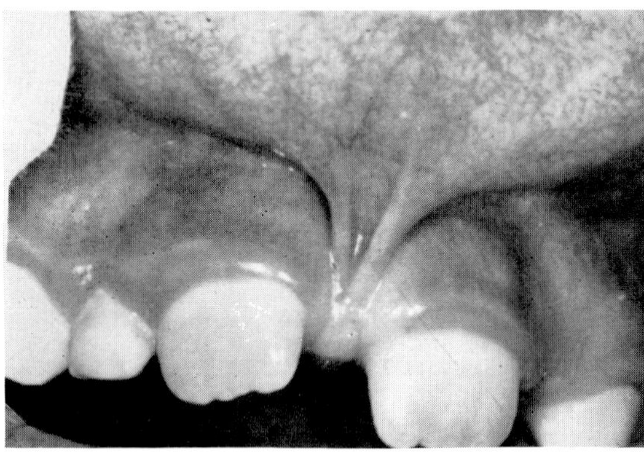

Fig. 70.—Thick fibrous palatal attachment of upper fraenum, blanching of tissues on traction. There is an indication for fraenectomy here.

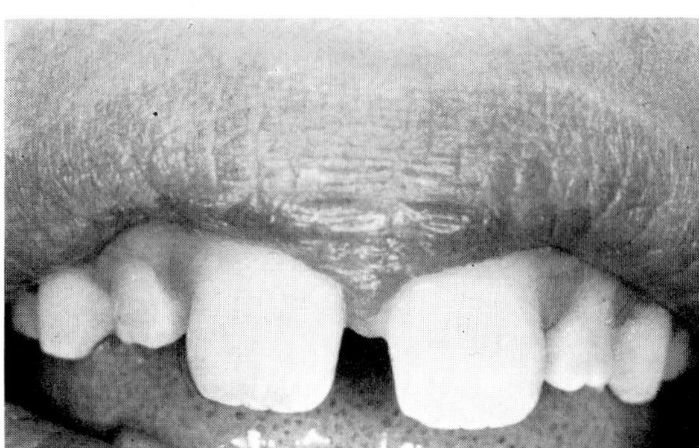

Fig. 71.—Large, thick, fleshy fraenum not aesthetically pleasing, although not primarily responsible for diastema.

the separation of central incisors and when there is a fleshy fraenum attached between the incisors, it does not necessarily prevent them from coming together naturally in a normal-sized arch.

A central diastema may be quite natural up to the time of eruption of the permanent canines, but it also may be due to:—

1. Missing upper teeth, particularly lateral incisors in a normal-sized or large arch (*Fig.* 69).

2. Extractions in large arches.

3. Small teeth in relation to the size of the arch. (Diastemata occur in families and there is often no enlargement of the labial fraenum.)

4. Proclined incisors due to a sucking habit. Also in Class II, division 1 they are over the lower lip and in some Class III cases they may spread forwards to remain anterior to the lower incisors.

5. A supernumerary tooth in the midline between the roots of the incisors.

6. Where there is apical crowding the crowns of the central incisors may be splayed and a space appear at the incisor edge.

Therefore the indications for fraenectomy are few. It is only performed in those cases where the fraenum is binding the lip down tightly fostering stagnation in the upper incisor region (*Figs.* 70 and 72 A), or where it is unaesthetic, showing as an ugly fold of mucous membrane (*Fig.* 71). *Fig.* 72 shows a case before and after fraenectomy. Details of the surgical procedure for fraenectomy are given in the APPENDIX.

Trauma.—Direct trauma to the permanent incisors or indirect trauma via the deciduous teeth has been discussed in Chapter V. Accidents to the incisors are very common and early treatment with continued observation is desirable.

Trauma to deciduous incisors may produce a degree of dilaceration which prevents the permanent incisor from erupting and it has to be removed surgically (*Fig.* 73). It is certainly desirable to remove the tooth early and to control the drift of the lateral incisor in order to prevent a considerable tilt of its crown as in *Fig.* 74.

Direct damage to one or more permanent incisors may also cause them to be lost despite all efforts. A decision has to be made as to whether the incisor space is to be maintained or allowed to close. The speed at which the space will naturally close depends on the arch size and the age of the patient.

The indications for a denture as a single incisor space maintainer are:—

1. In the older patient when there is no crowding. This particularly applies to large arches in normal relationship where there is little natural tendency for the space to close.

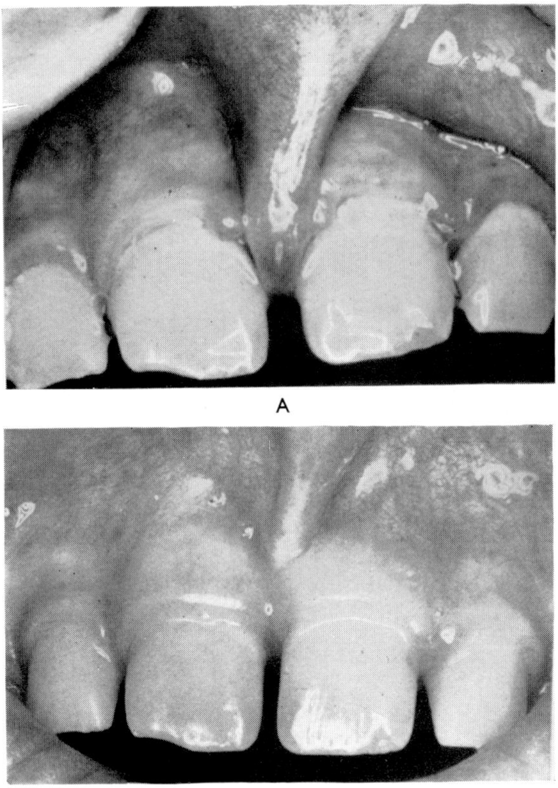

A

B

Fig. 72.—A, Thick fraenum binding down the upper lip and fostering stagnation around the upper incisors. B, Same case after fraenectomy and local gingival trimming.

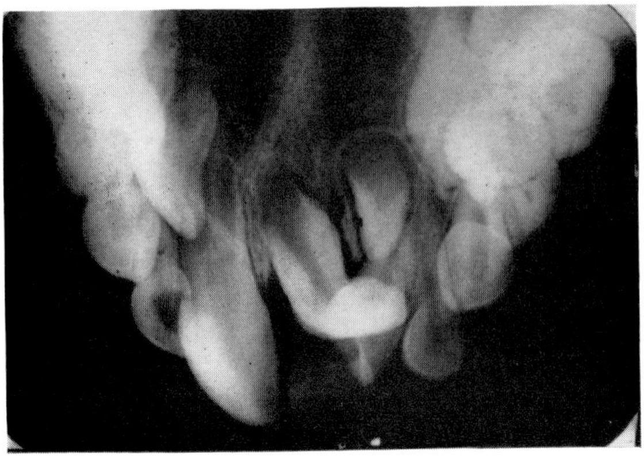

Fig. 73.—X-ray showing dilaceration of central incisor.

2. In Class III cases in the upper incisor area. The space can later be filled with a bridge or a spoon denture.

The indications for allowing space closure and controlling drift are:—

1. Where the extraction or loss of a tooth has occurred early, in the patient who has a small arch with potential crowding elsewhere in the arch. In this case the apex of the lateral incisor will tend to move round with very little tilt (*Fig.* 75).

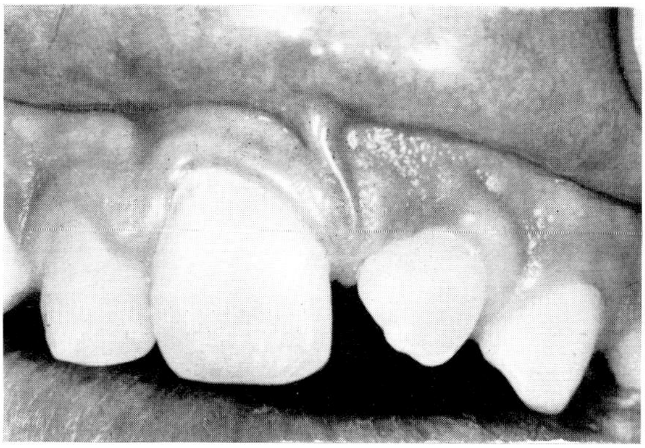

Fig. 74.—Delayed eruption of dilacerated central incisor. |2 has tilted mesially and the presence of |1 is obstructing movement of apex. |2 has to be uprighted before crowning to simulate |1.

2. In Class II, division 1 cases the space can be utilized to retract the three remaining upper incisors, whereas if the space was maintained extraction farther back in the upper arch would have to be considered.

Where the space is allowed to close or the lateral incisor is actively moved into the space of the central incisor there may be some movement of the centre line. Due consideration must be given to this from an aesthetic point of view. The lateral incisor can sometimes be crowned to simulate the other central incisor which has been lost. Although minor degrees of tilting can be masked by the placing of a crown, marked tilting makes jacket crown preparation, for this purpose, impossible. A localized fixed appliance may be used to control the position of the apex whilst moving the lateral incisor (*Fig.* 76).

Where the lateral incisor is large it is possible to allow the space to close and to reduce the length of the remaining central incisor (*Fig.* 77).

Traumatic loss of one or more lower incisors is not quite as common, but may result from a fall or following the use of gags in the mouth during general anaesthesia when the teeth are newly erupted.

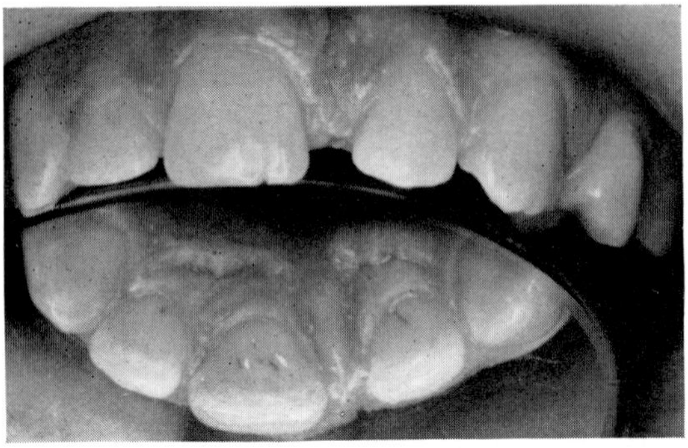

A

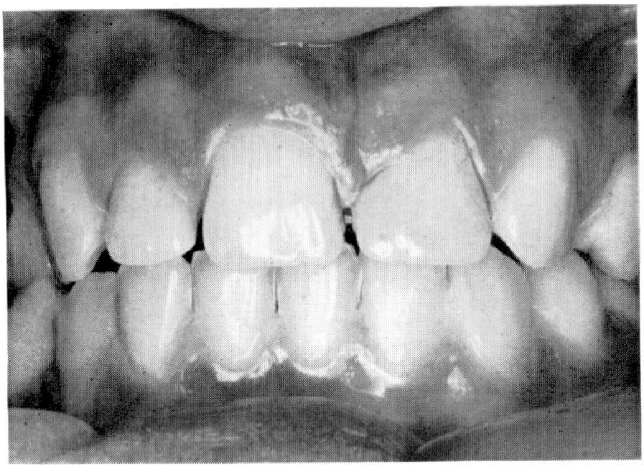

B

Fig. 75.—A, Lateral incisor encouraged to drift around the arch after early loss of |1. The arch is slightly crowded, favouring natural drift. B, |2 has been repositioned between 1|3 and jacket crown placed to simulate |1. (*By kind permission of Professor Herbert.*)

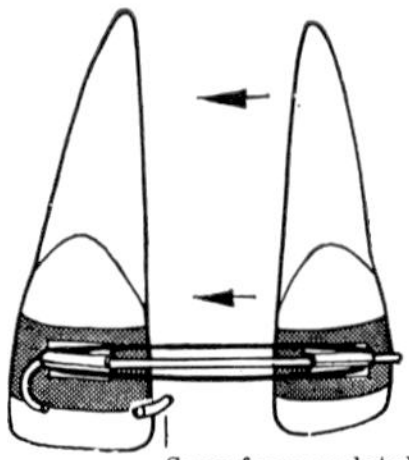

Fig. 76.—Appliance which can be used to approximate two central incisors or to approximate a lateral incisor to a central, if the central is held by a palatal spur from a plate. The tubes prevent tilting and the recurved portion prevents the bow tilting down. Traction in this case is applied by elastic bands.

Lower incisor spaces close rapidly, and except in Class II cases do not cause undue trouble. In Class I and Class II cases, compensating

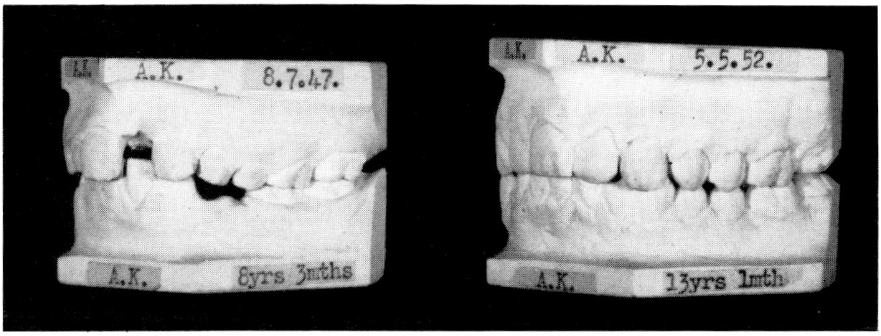

Fig. 77.—Case where |1 was knocked out at 8 years. Natural drift has allowed |2 to move up to 1|. |2 is a large tooth and by reducing the length of 1| a reasonable result is obtained, despite a slight shift of the interdental centre line.

upper extractions are necessary to prevent secondary collapse in the upper arch. It is not often a practical policy to try to hold a lower incisor space by artificial means.

BIBLIOGRAPHY

LUNDSTRÖM, A. (1959), 'How much can we hope to reduce the Incidence of Malocclusion through Prophylactic Measures?', *Dent. Practit.*, **9**, 129.

TULLEY, W. J. (1967), 'Prevention in Orthodontics within the Scope of the School Programme', *Int. Dent. J.*, **17**, 368.

CHAPTER VIII

MISSING TEETH AND EXTRACTIONS: THEIR IMPLICATIONS IN TREATMENT PLANNING

THIS chapter deals with the problems created by: (1) The congenital absence of teeth; (2) The enforced extraction of teeth due to dental caries; (3) The extraction of teeth as a deliberate measure. A full complement of teeth is not essential for facial harmony or functional efficiency. The aim of treatment is to produce a balance between the size of the dental arches and the amount of dental tissue which can be supported in good alinement.

A study of the results of unavoidable extractions due to caries has taught us what to expect in widely differing circumstances and the effects of missing and extracted teeth have to be considered as they affect an otherwise ideal dentition, and as they affect various forms of malocclusion.

Missing teeth and enforced extraction of teeth may require certain measures to minimize the ill effects. Other effects may be turned to advantage, resulting in decongestion of crowded arches and improvements in incisor relationship.

When considering any form of treatment which involves extraction of teeth, it is essential to observe the following facts:—

1. Are all the teeth present or developing?
2. Are all the unerupted teeth in normal developmental position?
3. Are there any teeth which are likely to give rise to symptoms through caries, injury, or congenital abnormalities?

CONGENITAL ABSENCE OF TEETH

In Chapter V it has been pointed out that there is a familial tendency for certain permanent teeth to be missing or to be excessively small. The upper lateral incisors are quite commonly missing, as are the lower second premolars. Lower third molars and lower incisors are less frequently missing. If the absence of teeth is noted early, the plan of treatment can be adjusted accordingly.

Missing Upper Laterals.—Upper lateral incisors may either be missing from the arch completely or they may be small and rudimentary. In some cases (*Fig.* 78) the tooth may be missing on one side and rudimentary on the other. When both are missing from *large* arches the central incisors will be spaced and the canines may erupt mesial to their predecessors (*Fig.* 79 A). It may be necessary to place theer

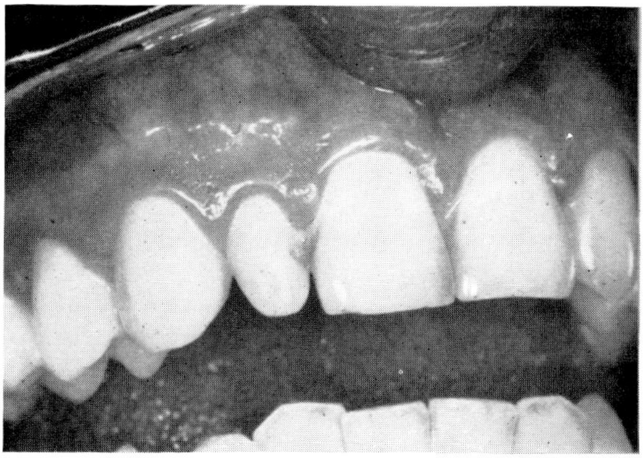

Fig. 78.—Rudimentary peg-shaped 2|, |2 missing with |3 next to |1.

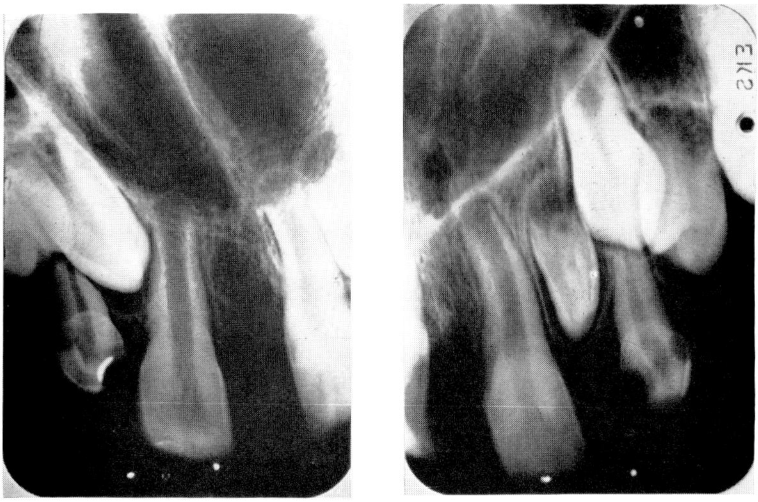

A B

Fig. 79.—A, Radiograph showing missing 2|, 3| erupting next to 1|. B, Radiograph to show abnormal form of erupting 'peg-shaped' lateral incisor. In such cases the pulp becomes infected and abscess formation frequently occurs soon after the tooth erupts.

missing teeth later with a denture or a bridge, in which case the deciduous canines should be removed so that they do not guide the permanent canines mesially. Spaced central incisors may have to be approximated and preparation made to receive pontics between the canine and the central incisor. Where upper laterals are missing in *crowded* arches, the permanent canines will erupt next to the centrals without spacing. The result is not aesthetically pleasing unless the tip of the canine can be reduced. The particular requirements of each individual case have to be considered. Where the upper laterals are missing in a case with a Class III tendency the lack of dental tissue in the front of the upper arch may tip the balance against establishing an incisor overbite.

Where there is unilateral absence of an upper lateral incisor the principal concern from an aesthetic point of view is to maintain the centre line in its correct position. This may call for the use of apparatus if the deciduous lateral incisor is lost early. Whether the space should be maintained for a pontic or whether the canine should be approximated to the central will have to be decided in each individual case bearing in mind the points mentioned above.

There are particular problems associated with the presence of rudimentary conical teeth in the lateral incisor positions. Not infrequently, these teeth are malformed and show evidence of an invagination at the tip (*Fig.* 79 B). In such a case the long-term prognosis is not good, so that in crowded arches consideration should be given to their removal rather than extraction of other teeth with a better prognosis. Conical teeth have a smaller mesiodistal diameter than their normal counterparts and, therefore, their presence upsets the delicate balance which normally exists between the size of the teeth in the opposing arches, and normally fosters a correct interdigitation of teeth. Sometimes the full mesiodistal diameter can be restored with a jacket crown, but this procedure has not been found to be universally successful where the teeth are very small.

Missing Lower Premolars.—The fact that lower second premolars and, less frequently, the upper premolars, may be missing makes it essential to take routine orthodontic radiographs before contemplating therapeutic extraction of permanent teeth (*Fig.* 80). In a Class I case with crowding, the absence of lower premolars is an advantage in that extractions of permanent teeth can be confined to the upper dental arch. In such cases it is as well to remove the lower second deciduous molars at the same time as the upper premolars. Likewise in cases tending towards a Class III malocclusion, missing lower second premolars may obviate the need for the extraction of permanent teeth in the lower arch. Where lower second premolars are absent in Class II, division 1 cases, an extraction in the upper arch as part of the general treatment plan is nearly always necessitated, unless the lower deciduous molars show every sign of long survival.

Missing Lower Third Molars.—Lower third molars are absent in some cases. This should be borne in mind if the extraction of other cheek teeth is contemplated.

Partial Anodontia.—In the rare instances where several teeth are missing, some orthodontic preparation of the mouth may be required

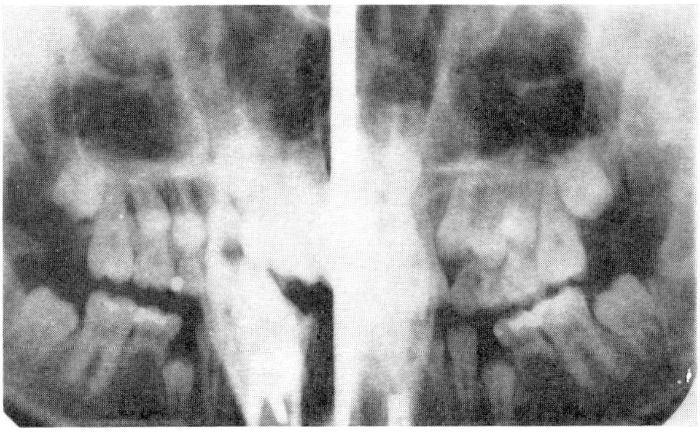

Fig. 80.—Radiographs to show missing $\overline{5|5}$.

to make the spaces available in the right region for a denture. The absence of upper central incisors and upper canines is extremely rare.

ENFORCED EXTRACTIONS

Such is the caries problem in the British Isles that a high percentage of first permanent molars have a very poor prognosis by the age of 8 years and deciduous molars also suffer a high caries experience at an early age.

Reference has already been made in Chapter V to the effects produced by the enforced extractions of single posterior teeth. Adverse tilting of the adjacent teeth has been described and the effects on the centre line, overbite, and overjet will depend on the varying situation. In view of this, careful consideration has to be given to the form of the developing occlusion whenever an extraction is indicated because of the quality of the teeth.

One of the most difficult factors to determine is whether extraction of sound or symptomless teeth should be undertaken in opposing quadrants and on the opposite side of the same arch (referred to as 'compensating' and 'balancing' extractions).

Enforced Extraction of First Permanent Molars.—

a. When the Occlusion is Normal.—In the early mixed dentition when the occlusion is developing normally on large and well-related jaws, the enforced extraction of one *upper* first permanent molar can often be accepted as its effects will be minimal. The enforced extraction of a single first permanent molar in the *lower* arch will have little effect on the incisor relationship but there may be a disturbance of precise cuspal relationship of the canines and premolars. In this case some authorities would advocate the extraction of the first upper permanent molar on the same side, provided that radiographs have shown that all the successional teeth are developing normally. This will ensure the correct cuspal interdigitation of the permanent teeth. The extraction of first permanent molars on the opposite side need not be considered unless they are of exceptionally poor quality.

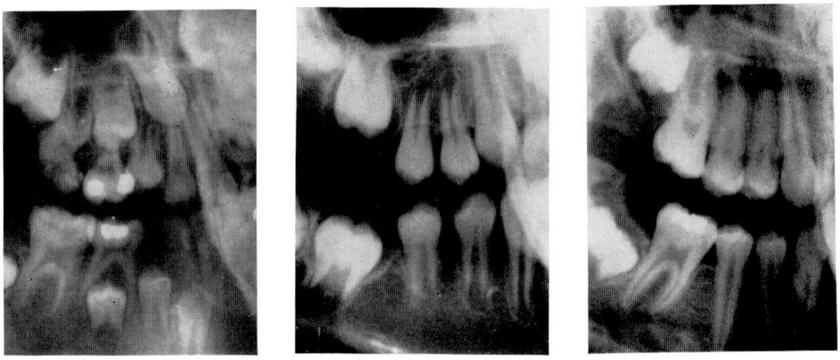

A B C

Fig. 81.—Radiographs to show the movements of teeth following the extraction of $\frac{6|6}{6|6}$. A, $8\frac{1}{2}$ years; B, $10\frac{1}{2}$ years; C, 15 years.

Note that the upper canine is accommodated in the arch and the second molars have moved into good position.

In the later mixed dentition and in the permanent dentition, the enforced extraction of one *upper* first permanent molar will have little adverse effect. The extraction of a single *lower* first permanent molar is likely to allow tilting of the teeth adjacent to the extraction site, but there will be little effect on the incisor relationship and a compensating extraction in the upper arch is less desirable. It may be necessary to maintain the space in the lower arch if it is exceptionally large and fill this space artificially later.

b. When the Occlusion is Abnormal.—

General principles: When there is an enforced extraction of one or more first permanent molars in the presence of malocclusion, the affected teeth rarely coincide with the plan of treatment which would otherwise have been considered in this case. Loss of these teeth makes appliances less readily controlled and space created by their extraction may be lost without relief of crowding in the incisor region.

i. *Class I Malocclusion*:—

Slight Crowding.—Where there is slight crowding in the early mixed dentition, the enforced extraction of one or both lower first permanent molars would indicate the extraction of upper first permanent molars where these teeth are also of poor quality. This is the type of procedure envisaged by John Hunter as early as 1750.

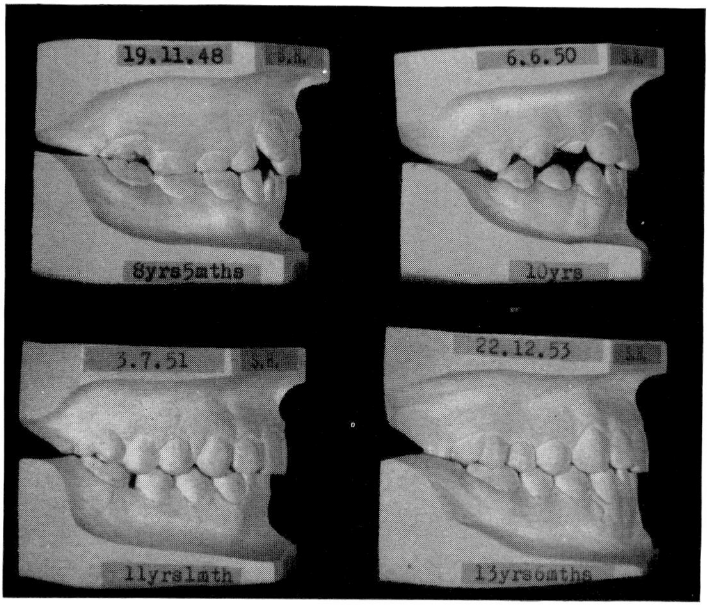

Fig. 82*a*.—Class I malocclusion treated by extraction of $\frac{6|6}{6|6}$ at 8 years 6 months. Note that the premolars erupt distal to their normal position allowing an improvement in the incisor alinement. There is minimal disturbance of the neighbouring teeth with no tilting or rotation of $\frac{7|7}{7|7}$ and all contact points are good. (*See also* p. 104.)

Wilkinson popularized this form of treatment in 1942 and made rather extravagant claims for its beneficial effect on the caries rate and relief of crowding. It must only be considered as a treatment of expediency. However, where the crowding is slight, a satisfactory result can be obtained. The premolars erupt in a relatively more distal position and certainly allow some improvement in the incisor and canine regions (*Figs.* 81 and 82).

It is important not to delay extraction of first permanent molars much after the age of 8–9 years and an early decision has to be made concerning the possibility of conserving them. Severe tilting of the erupted lower second molars may occur when the first molars are extracted after the age of 11 years (*Fig*. 83). Excessive drifting of lower second premolars is found when the arches are not crowded enough to

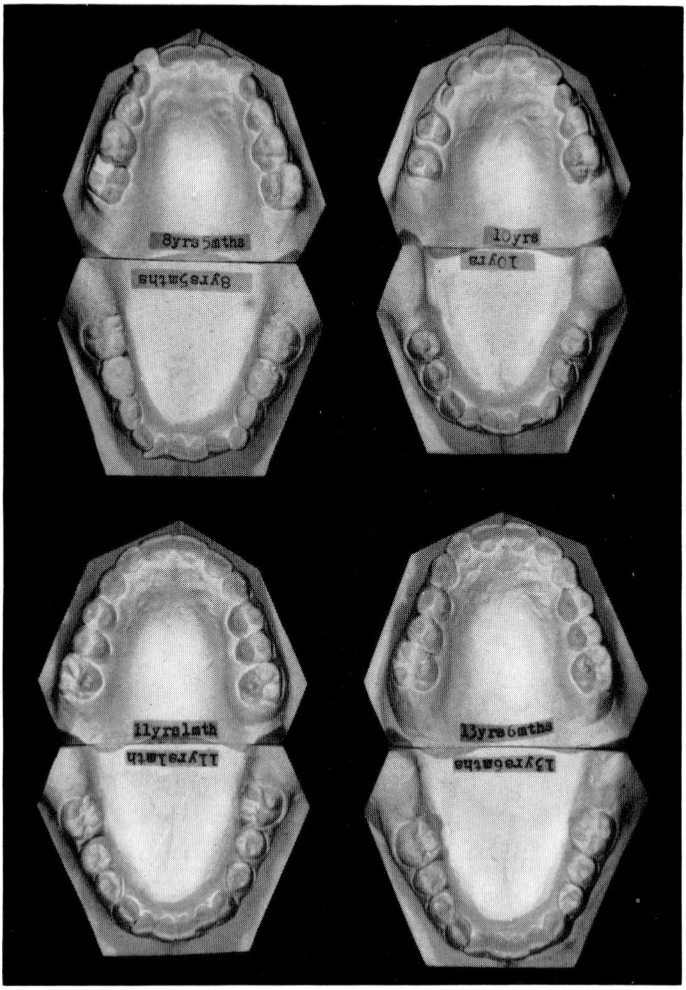

Fig. 82*b*.—The treatment of a Class I malocclusion (*continued from p*. 103). $\frac{6|6}{6|6}$ extracted at 8 years. No active treatment.

warrant extraction of any teeth (*Fig*. 83). It occurs when the lower second premolars show signs of escaping from the embrace of the second deciduous molars and when they are already rotated in their crypts. *Fig*. 84 shows an unfavourable position of the lower second premolar where drift and rotation of this tooth were foreshadowed and occurred following extraction of the first molar. Contrary to many authorities, the extraction of all carious first molars does not have to be delayed if

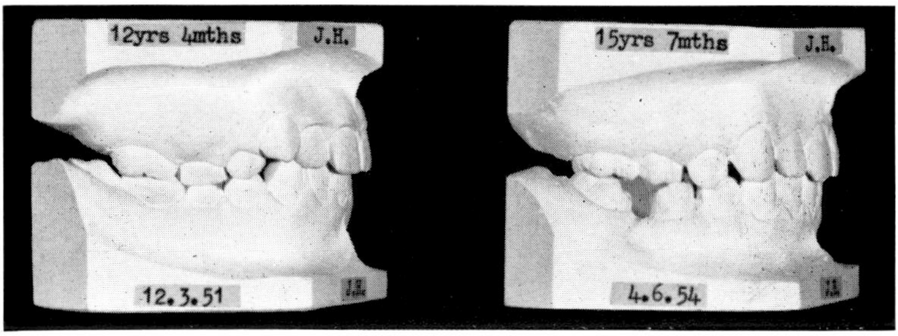

Fig. 83.—Case treated by late extraction of $\frac{6|6}{6|6}$ at 12½ years. Some space became available in the upper arch as $\underline{7|7}$ were delayed in eruption. Thus $\underline{3|3}$ were accommodated. *Note* marked tilting of $\overline{7|7}$ which occurs with the late extraction of $\overline{6|6}$.

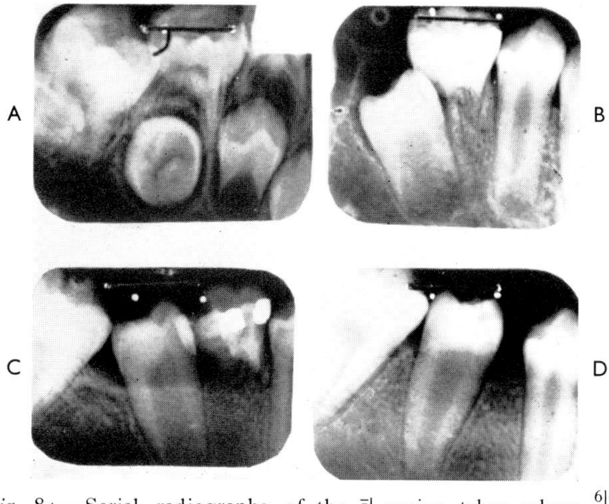

Fig. 84.—Serial radiographs of the $\overline{5}|$ region taken where $\frac{6|6}{6|6}$ were extracted showing: A, That $\overline{5}|$ was displaced in its developmental position; B, That it absorbed the distal root of $\overline{E}|$ after $\overline{6}|$ had been extracted; C, That it erupted distal to $\overline{E}|$; D, That after extraction of $\overline{E}|$ the space began to close, but $\overline{5}|$ was markedly rotated. Rotation of $\overline{5}|$ in its crypt is not uncommon. It is not caused by the extraction of $\overline{6}|$, but the break in continuity of the arch does not favour self-correction. Therefore, in such cases the extraction of 6's is not advocated except where it is unavoidable because of caries.

the deciduous teeth have been lost prematurely and there is potential mild crowding in both arches, provided there is a *normal overbite and overjet* (*Fig.* 85).

Where the overbite is reduced and there is a Class III tendency, removal of the only occluding cheek teeth may allow a postural pre-normal incisor relationship to develop—*see* p. 69.

Where only the upper first permanent molars are carious, it is unwise to extract the lower first permanent molars. In the lower arch, crowding can be treated with planned extractions of more suitable teeth with the use of apparatus at a later date.

Class I Marked Crowding.—Where crowding is severe in the premolar regions, the extraction of lower first molars will have little

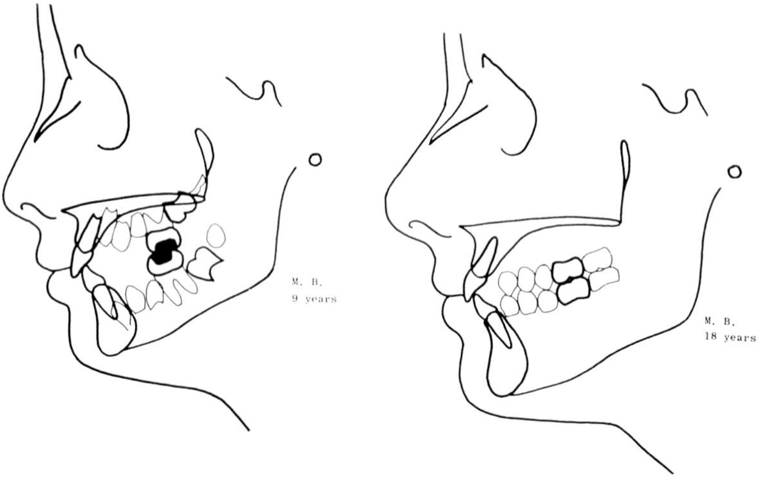

Fig. 85.—Tracings of lateral radiographs at 9 and 18 years. Case treated by extraction of $\frac{6|6}{6|6}$. Note no disturbance of overjet or overbite. 7's and 8's erupted in good position.

effect on the incisor relationship, and will provide significant decongestion of the lower arch with little or no tilting of the neighbouring teeth. Enforced extraction of one lower molar can, under these circumstances, be satisfactorily balanced by the extraction of the molar on the opposite side. It would be unwise, however, to compensate for these extractions by removing the upper first permanent molars unless forced to do so, as the upper second permanent molars will erupt prematurely so far mesially that little or no space will be made available for the alinement of teeth farther forward in the upper arch. In such cases, the planned extraction of upper premolars at a later date is preferable. Alternatively, if the upper molars are of relatively poor quality but can be preserved for a limited period of time, they should not be removed until the upper second permanent molars have erupted. These can then be engaged in apparatus and held back whilst teeth farther forward are moved distally into the extraction spaces. When it is not possible to conserve the upper first permanent molars even for a short period of time, apparatus should be used to move the remaining buccal teeth distally (*Fig.* 86).

ii. *Class II Malocclusion*:—

In all Class II cases the enforced extraction of a lower first permanent molar where there is little or no lower arch crowding may complicate treatment. No extraction should be considered in the contra-lateral quadrant where the forced extraction is on one side only, but the need for upper arch extractions in a plan of orthodontic treatment is reinforced.

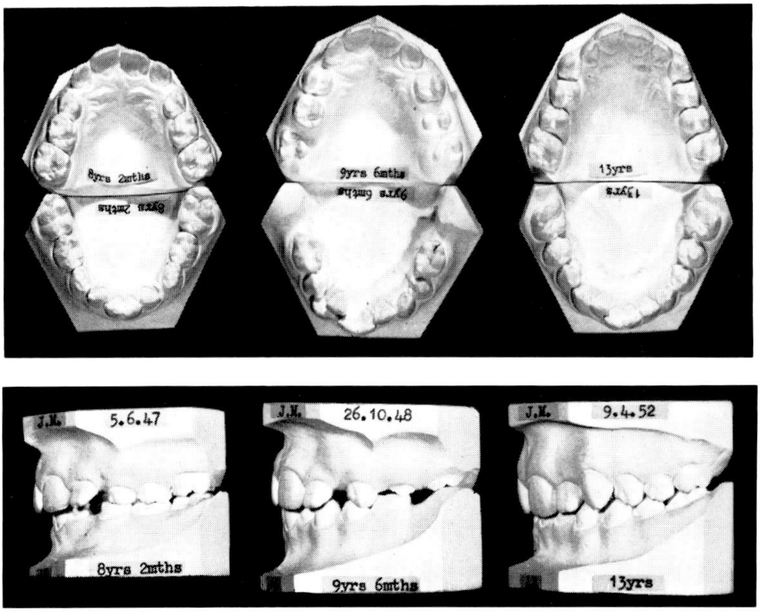

Fig. 86.—Class I case treated by extraction of $\frac{6|6}{6|6}$ at $8\frac{1}{2}$ years. $\frac{C|C}{C|C}$ were exfoliated. Note eruption of premolars distal to their normal position. An appliance was used to move $\underline{54|45}$ distally before the forward drift of $\underline{7|7}$ was complete in order to accommodate $\underline{3|3}$.

Where all four first permanent molars are in a very poor state and have to be removed, then intermaxillary traction can sometimes be applied satisfactorily with a monobloc in the absence of posterior teeth for banding or clasping (*see* Chapter XI).

When it is only the upper first permanent molars which are at risk, every effort should be made to preserve them until the second molars erupt, so that these teeth are not permitted to move forward prior to their eruption. If allowed to do so, they will have obliterated all the space which extraction could have made available for the retraction of anterior teeth.

iii. *Class III Malocclusion*:—

In Class III malocclusions with a Skeletal 3 dental base relationship, the early extraction of the upper first molars will hamper appliance

A

B

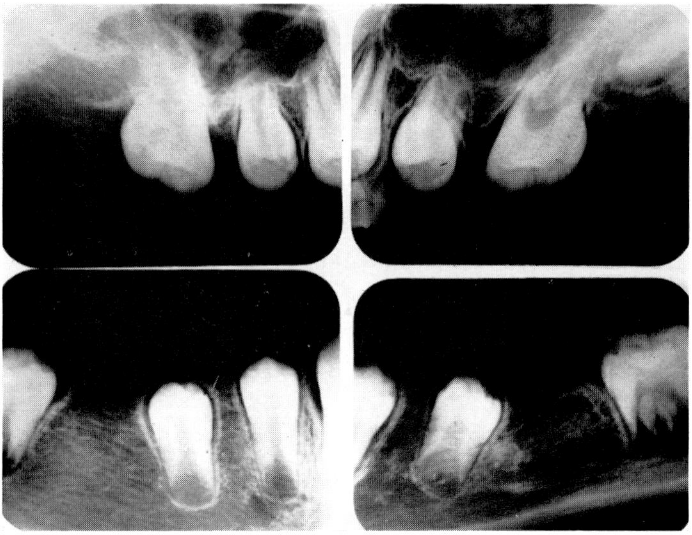

Fig. 87.—Radiograph to show the effect of enforced extraction of $\frac{6|6}{6|6}$ at the age of 8 years (A). In a small upper arch $\underline{7|7}$ have moved rapidly forward (B). In a large lower arch there has been a relative distal drift of $\overline{5|5}$ and there will be residual spacing.

therapy which is designed to move forward the upper incisors. Where possible extractions should be delayed until the incisor relationship has been corrected. Enforced early extraction of lower first molars may have some helpful effect on the lower incisor position if the arch is small, but if the arch is large there will be marked distal drifting and rotation of premolars with little effect on the incisors (*Fig.* 87).

Enforced Extraction of Deciduous Molars.—

General Principles.—Enforced extraction of deciduous molars is an unfortunate necessity in certain cases.

There is little justification for the extraction of other *second* deciduous molars as a therapeutic measure when one or more have to be extracted. They merely allow posterior teeth to drift forward without any benefit. There may be more justification for compensating and balancing extractions where one or more *first* deciduous molars have to be extracted. This is a controversial subject and each case has to be judged on its merits. The following points can only give general guidance.

Normal Occlusion: In cases where there is an excellent occlusion and where the size of the dental bases is more than adequate and there is a normal incisor relationship, the enforced extraction of one or more first deciduous molars should not be followed routinely by the extraction of the remaining first deciduous molars.

Class I—Mild Crowding in Mixed Dentition: The enforced extraction of one *lower* first deciduous molar is an indication for the extraction of the remaining first deciduous molars where this will allow the incisors to move into better alinement without mechanical aid. It will also prevent movement of the centre line. This is a modification of the planned 'serial extraction' technique described on p. 112. A later planned removal of four permanent teeth will be necessary under these circumstances.

If one *upper* first deciduous molar has to be extracted, the one on the opposite side of the arch can well be removed rather than conserved, where incisor alinement will naturally improve. This will also maintain the centre line. If, under these circumstances, the lower first deciduous molars are sound teeth, they should not be extracted and crowding in this arch can be dealt with by planned extraction of permanent teeth later.

Class I—Marked Crowding: The enforced extraction of one *lower* first deciduous molar should not be balanced by any other extractions which are not clinically necessary because of caries. It is obvious that permanent teeth will have to be extracted later, but the circumstances will only be worsened if the space is lost by forward drift of posterior teeth without any benefit to the incisor segment.

Class II: In Class II cases with any degree of overjet, the enforced extraction of one *lower* first deciduous molar should certainly *not* be followed by any compensating extractions. Likewise, any enforced extraction of a single upper first deciduous molar should not be made symmetrical as little natural improvement can be gained by this and mechanical treatment of the malocclusion will have to be considered at a later date.

Class III: In a case with mild Class III tendency with reduced overbite, the enforced extraction of one lower first deciduous molar can well be balanced by the extraction of that on the opposite side of the lower arch. Where there is a slight shortage of space this may help to improve the incisor relationship slightly with the need for follow-up extractions in the permanent dentition. If one upper first deciduous molar has to be extracted no balancing extraction should be undertaken merely to correct the centre line but consideration will have to be given to extraction of both lower first deciduous molars.

In a true Class III malocclusion enforced extraction of one or both *lower* first deciduous molars will have little effect on the arch if it is extremely large. The enforced extraction of one *upper* first deciduous molar should be confined to that side only and compensating extractions in the lower arch will be of little value.

PLANNED EXTRACTIONS

Apart from those cases where teeth are congenitally missing or have to be extracted due to caries, treatment of crowding has to be considered when the teeth are all present and sound.

Axel Lundström, in his paper 'Malocclusion of the Teeth regarded as a Problem in connection with the Apical Base', was among the first to point out that the size of the dental bases has a predetermined limit in each individual. Rix and others have shown that the size of the dental arches developing on these bases is influenced by the shape, size, and function of the surrounding soft tissues (*see* Chapter V).

In most of the ethnic groups found in the British Isles the 'dental bases' are extremely short anteroposteriorly and crowding of the teeth is very common. This crowding may be found in the incisor region, it may be localized to the premolar and canine region following premature loss of deciduous cheek teeth, or it may be present in both regions. Those dentitions which appear to be developing quite normally until the early teens often show a degree of incisor irregularity at the time of the eruption of second and third molars.

Angle, in the early editions of his book, *Malocclusion of the Teeth*, advocated the extraction of teeth in the treatment of crowding although later he opposed it emphatically. Chapman, a pupil of Angle, made a large contribution to the knowledge of orthodontics in the British Isles and stated clearly that extraction or non-extraction are not essentially alternative treatment methods for a particular case. Either the dental arches will ultimately accommodate all the teeth in good alinement or they will not, according to the size of the apical base in relation to tooth size. There are many experienced clinicians who wished they had extracted teeth in more cases which showed incipient signs of crowding. The lateral expansion or anteroposterior expansion of upper and lower dental arches merely to gain space is no longer tenable (*Fig.* 88).

The general principles involved in the treatment of crowding are described here. The treatment of crowding superimposed on underlying malrelationships of the dental arches will be dealt with in more detail in later chapters.

Extractions in the Treatment of Crowding in the Mixed Dentition.—Crowding of the permanent incisors may have been

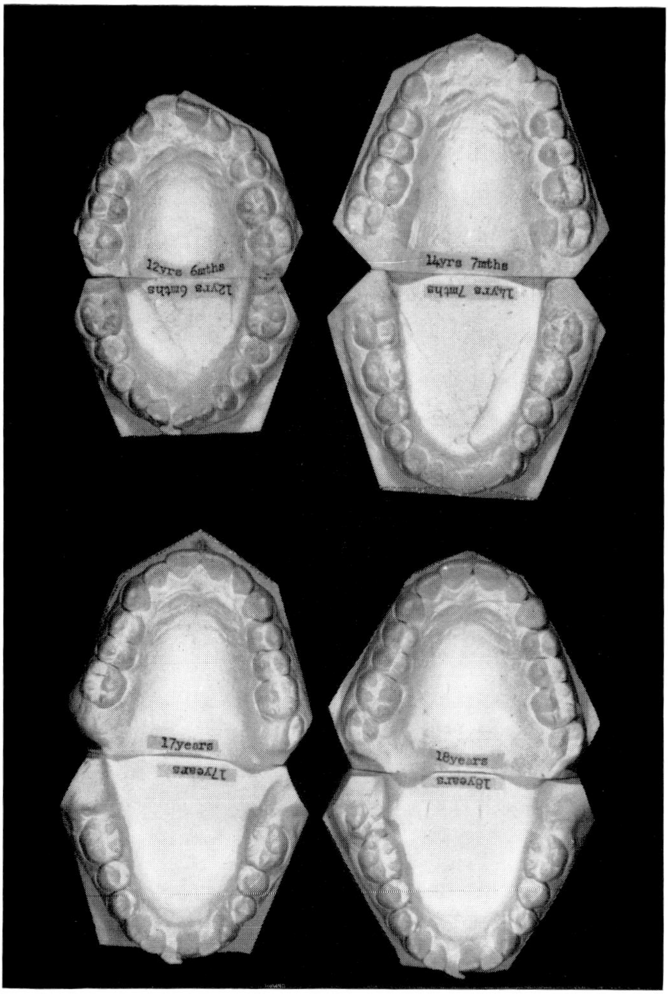

Fig. 88.—Case treated by expansion of upper and lower arches and intermaxillary traction. Because of the change in arch relationship the upper arch has not relapsed, but the lower arch has relapsed completely despite extraction of $\frac{7|7}{7|7}$, showing the futility of expanding both arches laterally.

foreshadowed in the deciduous dentition by actual crowding or lack of spacing, but there is no infallible method of forecasting. There may be an appearance of slight crowding of the permanent incisors at 7–8 years of age which can improve naturally, but any marked crowding at this age will not be self-correcting with growth, and a reduction in the number of teeth will be required.

SERIAL EXTRACTIONS.—Serial extraction is the term applied to a planned reduction of the deciduous dentition followed by a planned reduction in the permanent dentition. This is not a new procedure. Palsson in 1956 reported that the first reference to it was in *An Essay on Diseases of the Teeth* by Robert Bunon, published in 1743. He was later followed by Hunter, Fox, Bell, and in more recent years by Chapman, Duyzings, Haupl, Kjellgren, Hotz, and Dewel.

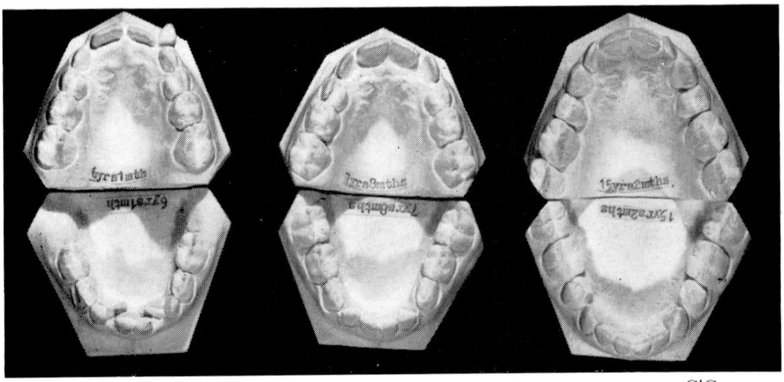

Fig. 89.—Occlusal view of case treated by serial extraction. $\frac{C|C}{C|C}$ extracted at 7 years. $\frac{4|4}{4|4}$ extracted at 10 years 6 months. Note movement of $\frac{2|2}{2|2}$ without an appliance to occupy $\frac{C|C}{C|C}$ space and later $\frac{3|3}{3|3}$ erupt to occupy the premolar spaces.

The process of serial extraction is usually started in the early mixed dentition (*Fig.* 89). When crowding is present it is usually in the incisor region although some degree of relief may have been obtained by early enforced extraction of deciduous molars in one or more quadrants. Extraction of all four deciduous canines or the remaining first deciduous molars may temporarily provide space for the alinement of the permanent incisors. This comes about by the drift of the lateral incisors into the space previously occupied by the deciduous canine. At a later stage, permanent teeth will have to be extracted in order to relieve the crowding which has deliberately been transferred to the permanent canine region.

This form of treatment must never be undertaken lightly and only after a full appraisal has been made. There are relatively few cases where the lateral incisors improve in alinement without help from an appliance. Forward movement of the buccal segments may not allow sufficient space for the natural alinement of the permanent canines after extraction of the first premolars. The main disadvantage is that if a serial extraction case requires appliance therapy, it has to be given at an early age to aline the incisors and to hold back the buccal segments. In most cases it is better to wait, and treat the malocclusion when the first premolars erupt and can be extracted. Further elaboration of the principles are discussed under the various headings.

Serial Extraction in Class I Malocclusion.—Where the arch relationship is Class I and there is crowding in both arches, the extraction of all the deciduous canines or first deciduous molars provides space temporarily in the vicinity of the incisors. Rotation or overlapping of the incisors will not be entirely self-correcting and, as mentioned above, appliances will be necessary in most instances. If sufficient space can be created for the permanent canine by the extraction of the first premolars, the canines will fall back into the arch. However, the lower canines quite commonly erupt before the first premolars and may not readily aline themselves. Some authorities have suggested that the first deciduous molars should be extracted just prior to their natural loss to promote early emergence of the first premolar, but if the first deciduous molar is extracted too early, scar tissue may deter the eruption of the first premolar. The earlier the premolars can be extracted the better, but only in rare instances is their surgical removal desirable.

Fig. 90 shows a case where the extractions alone have allowed natural alinement of the incisors and eruption of the canines into good position. An ideal result of this kind encourages undue optimism. *Natural alinement does not always occur, and unless appliances can be used, the early extraction of deciduous canines may only complicate the treatment.*

Serial Extractions in Class II Arch Relationship.—It is better not to consider serial extraction technique in Class II malocclusions. Where there is only a tendency to a Class II relationship with an overbite deeper than normal, it was suggested at one time that extractions might be 'staggered', the upper extractions being carried out six months in advance of the lower. The effect of lower arch extractions on the overbite is now in doubt, and this practice has been discontinued. Problems of very deep overbite where crowding occurs in both arches always present a difficult problem and serial extractions should be avoided.

Serial Extractions in Class III Arch Relationship.—There is little place for this form of treatment in cases with true Class III arch relationship. If the lower arch is mildly crowded there are some cases where extractions of lower deciduous canines followed by lower first premolars may be desirable, but this will be discussed in detail in Chapter XII.

Extractions in the Treatment of Crowding in the Permanent Dentition.—With the tendency to avoid serial extractions except in those cases where premature extractions of the first deciduous molars was a clinical necessity, the treatment of crowding ideally commences in the early permanent dentition at the time of eruption of the first

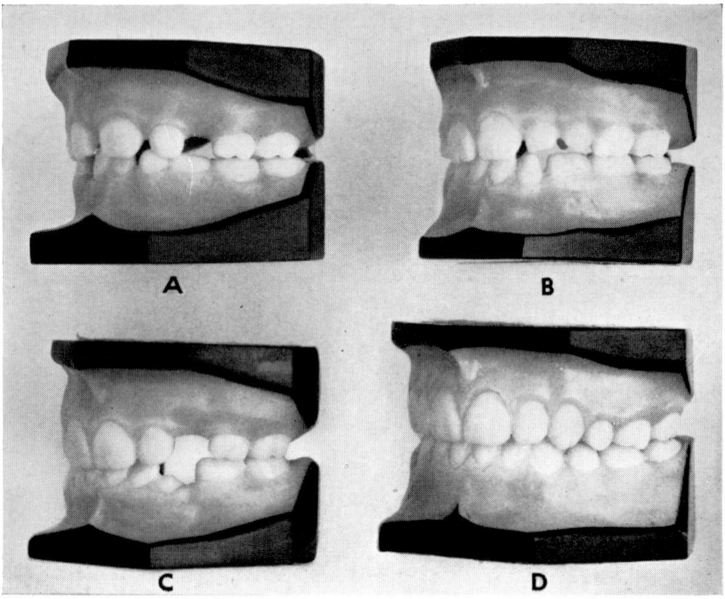

Fig. 90.—Case treated by serial extraction. A, Before treatment at 8 years. No space available for $\underline{2|2}$. $\overline{2|2}$ are lingually displaced. B, At 8½ years after $\frac{C|C}{C|C}$ have been extracted. Note $\underline{|4}$ erupts next to $\underline{|2}$. C, After extraction of $\frac{4|4}{4|4}$. D, At 14 years after $\frac{3|3}{3|3}$ have moved into space occupied by extracted premolars.

premolars. The choice of teeth to be extracted (other factors being equal) depends on the degree of crowding and the site of crowding.

Incisor Crowding.—Severe incisor crowding with normal arch relationship is best dealt with by extraction of the first premolar in the upper and lower arches (*Fig.* 91). Appliances are usually required to retract the upper and lower canines so that they are correctly related, and to aline incisors (*see* Chapter X).

It is not always possible to allow natural alinement of the canines because forward movement of the buccal segments may not allow sufficient space for incisor alinement.

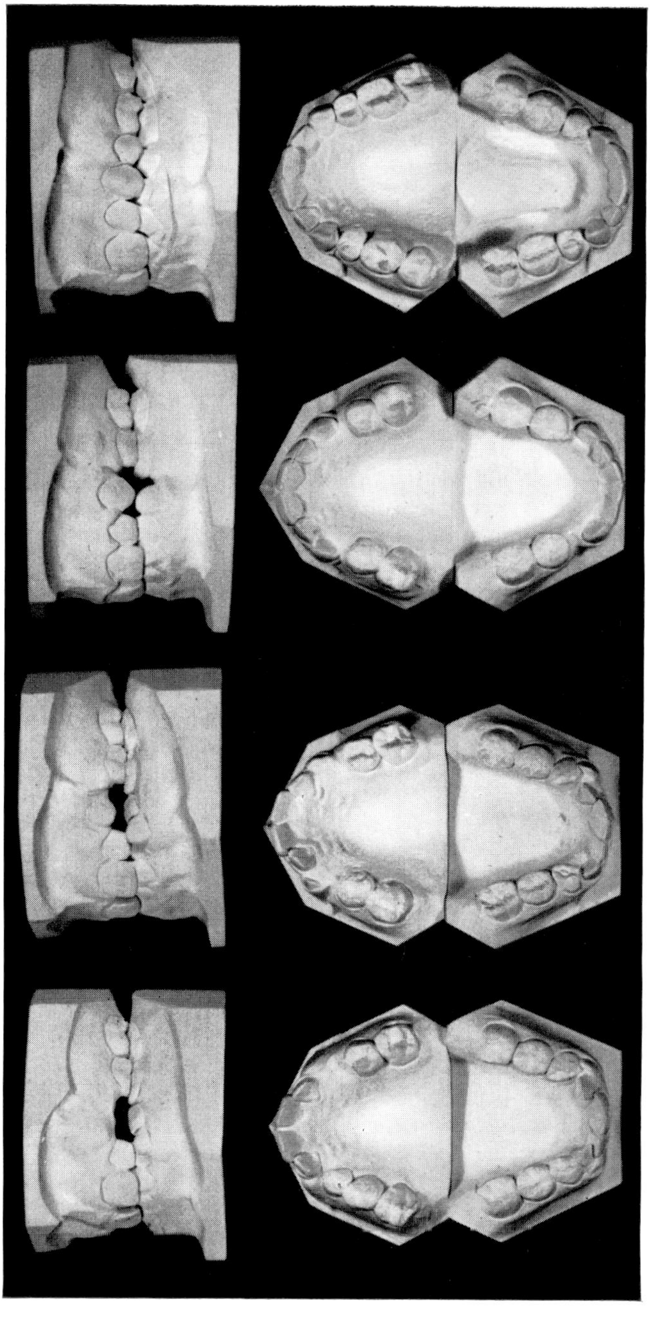

Fig. 91.—Class I malocclusion with incisor crowding and outlocked $\frac{3|3}{3|3}$. Treated by extraction of $\frac{4|4}{4|4}$ and upper and lower appliances to complete alinement.

The practice of extracting *second premolars* in order to obtain sufficient space for incisor alinement is undesirable as the contact points established between the first molar and the first premolar are often poor. Therefore the extraction of *second premolars* is usually

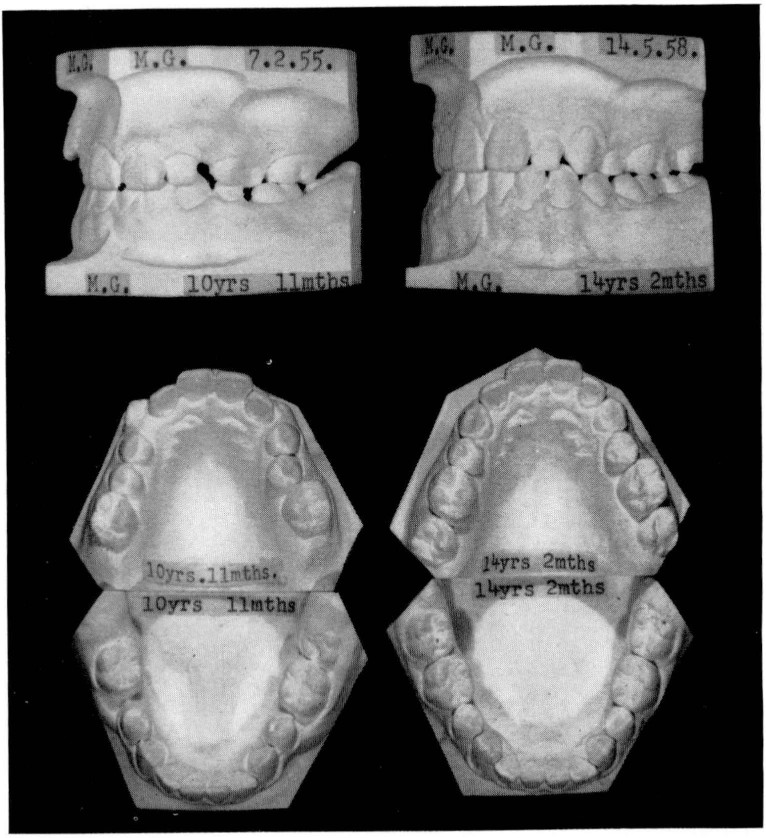

Fig. 92.—Class I malocclusion with Skeletal 3 tendencies. $\underline{3|3}$ out-locked and $\overline{5|5}$ crowded lingually. Treated by extraction of $\frac{4|4}{5|5}$ without appliances. Note a marked decrease in the overbite following the upper extractions.

confined to those cases where their quality is extremely poor or they are already displaced from the arch (*Fig.* 92).

The extraction of the *first molars* has already been discussed and it has been emphasized that they are never the teeth of choice unless their quality dictates their extraction (*Figs.* 93 and 94).

The extraction of *second molars* is too remote from the site of the incisor crowding to be particularly useful. Cryer has shown that their extraction may prevent some deterioration in incisor alinement which is already visible at 12 years of age, but the extraction of second molars produces no marked improvement in already established crowding in

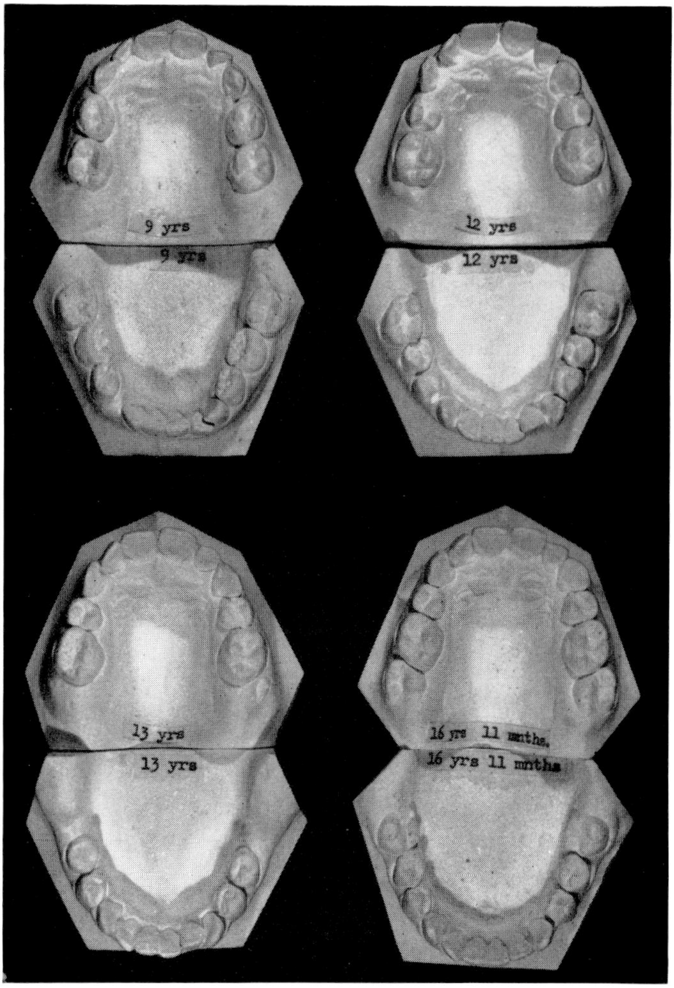

Fig. 93.—Class I malocclusion. Early loss of $\underline{D|D}$. Treated by extraction of $\underline{4|4}$ at 10 years. Carious $\overline{6|6}$ extracted at $12\frac{1}{2}$ years, too late for natural alinement of $\overline{7|7}$ which have tilted badly.

the incisor region. This deterioration is an expression of arch crowding and may or may not be related to the eruption of the third molars. Without recourse to appliances, the extraction of second molars produces little improvement in incisor alinement when they are already imbricated (*Fig*. 95).

The Extraction of Anterior Teeth.—From time to time it becomes necessary to extract anterior teeth from crowded arches. The reasons for doing this are as follows: (1) Because of caries, injury, or structural defects of the tooth; (2) Because the patient is unable to attend for appliance therapy for one reason or another when the tooth is so

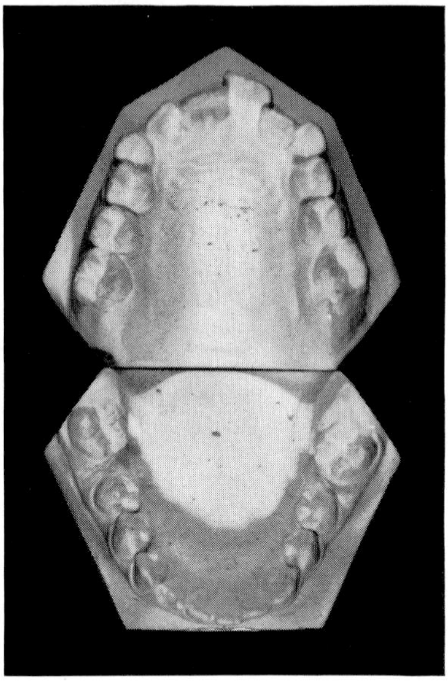

Fig. 94.—$\frac{6|6}{6|6}$ extracted because of caries at 11 years of age. Note forward drift of $\underline{7|7}$ to contact $\underline{5|5}$ without improvement in incisor alinement. $\overline{7|7}$ have tilted markedly.

displaced that there is not a reasonable chance of bringing it into good alinement.

The Upper Canine.—It may be necessary to remove a canine which has been grossly displaced buccally or palatally. It may be undertaken in a case as shown in *Fig*. 96, where the first premolar is in contact with the lateral incisor and does not show its palatal cusp. The decision to extract a canine depends mainly on the position of its apex. If its apex is in good position and there is a good chance of it erupting into the palate or high buccally, it may be moved into the arch, provided space can be obtained for it. The problem of the unerupted displaced canine which requires surgical exposure will be dealt with in the APPENDIX.

The Upper Lateral Incisor.—Extraction of a sound upper lateral incisor may be considered under exceptional circumstances, e.g., where the canine is in contact with the central incisor and the lateral incisor is completely locked inside the bite. The upper canines do not appear aesthetically pleasing next to the central incisors, but they

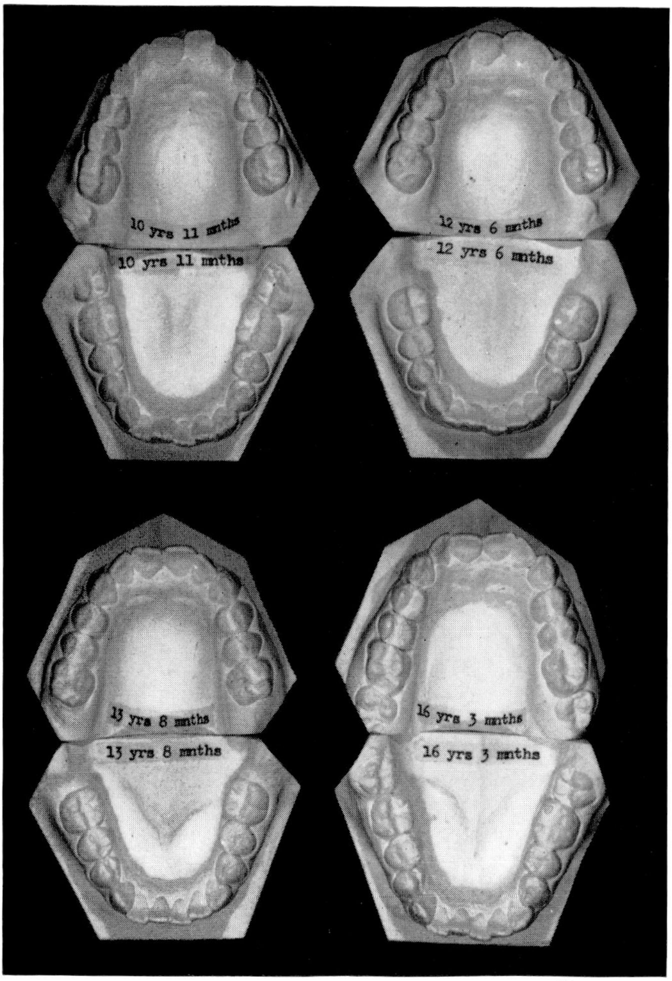

Fig. 95.—Class I malocclusion treated by extraction of $\frac{7|7}{7|7}$ at 12 years of age. No apparatus. The incisors show slight initial improvement but relapse after eruption of $\frac{8|8}{8|8}$.

may be stoned to reduce their length. Some lateral incisors, particularly the conical type, have invaginated crowns and become infected through the cingulum pits. This makes it desirable to extract such teeth rather than sound premolars, particularly if they are grossly displaced.

The Upper Central Incisor.—Upper central incisors are prone to fracture. If such a tooth has a *very* poor prognosis it may be better to remove this tooth rather than two upper premolars, and to aline the remaining incisors, arranging for the lateral incisor to have a jacket crown, shaped to simulate a central, if it can be moved into a satisfactory position (*see* Chapter VII).

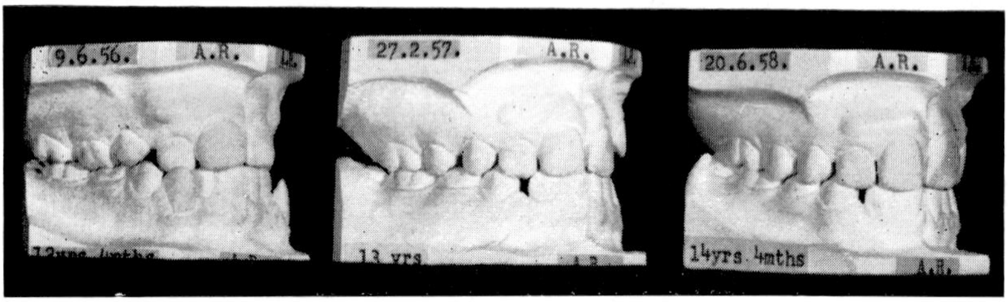

Fig. 96.—Case treated by extraction of $\frac{3|4}{3|4}$. Note upper $\underline{3|}$ completely outlocked and $\underline{4|}$ in contact with $\underline{2|}$ and not showing palatal cusp.

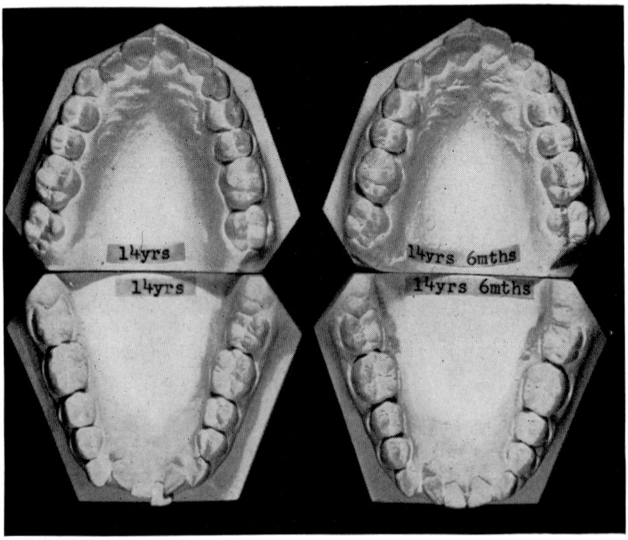

Fig. 97.—Extraction of outstanding $|\overline{1}$. Note that remaining lower incisors are still crowded and there has been secondary deterioration of upper incisor alinement.

The Lower Incisors.—Imbrication of lower incisors is a common feature, and the treatment of this condition is not easy, particularly in Class II cases. It is often tempting to remove a lower incisor from a crowded arch, but this will usually cause some narrowing of the arch in the canine region, resulting in crowding of the three remaining incisors (*Fig.* 97). Where the upper incisors are closely applied to the lower, deterioration in alinement of upper incisors will follow, and where the incisors are not closely applied originally, there will be an increase in overjet. However, exceptions may be made in cases with

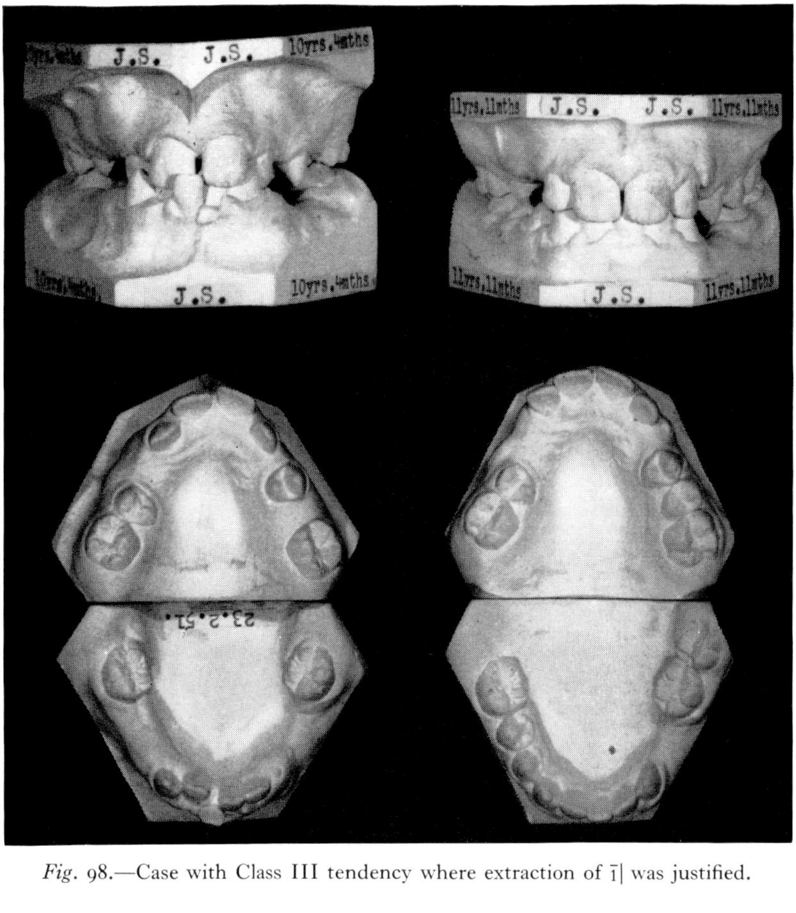

Fig. 98.—Case with Class III tendency where extraction of $\overline{1}|$ was justified.

Class III tendency where some minor reduction in the perimeter of the lower arch is desirable or where a lower incisor is completely outlocked and the remaining incisors are in good position (*Fig.* 98).

Crowding in the Premolar and Canine Region.—Crowding presenting in this region is frequently but not invariably exaggerated by the early loss of deciduous molars. (*See* Chapter V.) Where the deciduous canine or the first deciduous molar has been lost early, the permanent canine is usually displaced buccally, but in the lower arch the lower canine may be in the arch and the lower first premolar may be displaced buccally. Crowding in this region is most commonly treated by the extraction of the first premolar, other things being equal. The problem of the unerupted canine will be discussed in detail on p. 252.

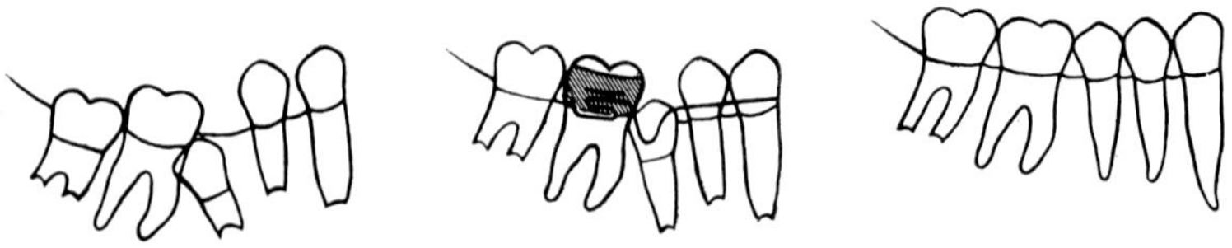

A, Where there is space in the arch a fixed lingual bow has tilted $\overline{6}|$ distally and allowed $\overline{5}|$ to erupt without further assistance.

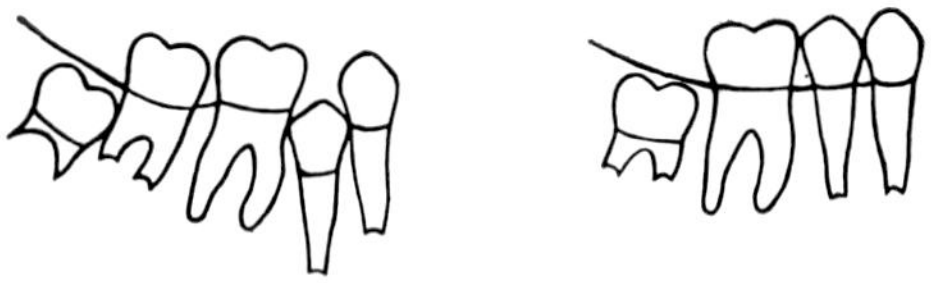

B, Extraction of $\overline{7}|$ where $\overline{6}|$ is a sound tooth. Partial impaction of $\overline{5}|$ required no active distal movement of $\overline{6}|$, but it may require active distal movement in some cases.

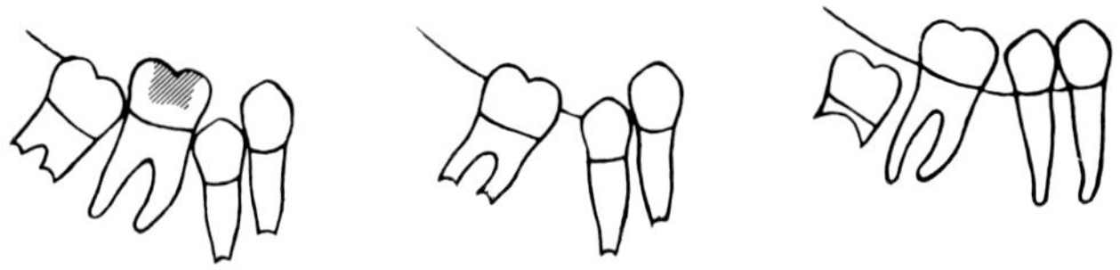

C, Extraction of carious $\overline{6}|$ allows $\overline{5}|$ to erupt. If this is later than 11 years $\overline{7}|$ may tilt excessively, but in this case it is quite acceptable.

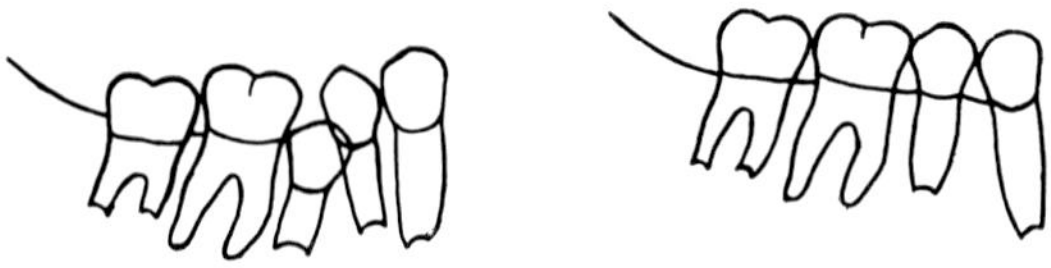

D, Where $\overline{6}|$ is a sound tooth and $\overline{5}|$ is tilted mesially, the extraction of $\overline{4}|$ will allow it to erupt. A retainer may be required to hold the space if the $\overline{5}|$ is slow to erupt.

Fig. 99.—Serial X-ray tracings showing the vertical impaction of $\overline{5}|$ and illustrating alternative methods of treatment and the resulting eruption.

Where the second deciduous molar has been lost early, the second premolar is commonly displaced palatally in the upper arch and lingually in the lower. Occasionally it impacts vertically between the first molar and the first premolar. The second premolar is a tooth which finds its way into the mouth, if at all possible, and some mild degrees of impaction may be overcome by the eruptive forces of the tooth at the expense of the alinement of the anterior teeth. Where it is completely impacted it may have to be removed surgically but minor degrees of impaction can be relieved by extraction of an adjacent tooth (*Figs.* 99 and 100).

If the first molar is heavily filled or carious it has to be extracted, but the result is not perfect owing to the tilt of the second molar. Where the lower second premolar is tilted mesially the lower first

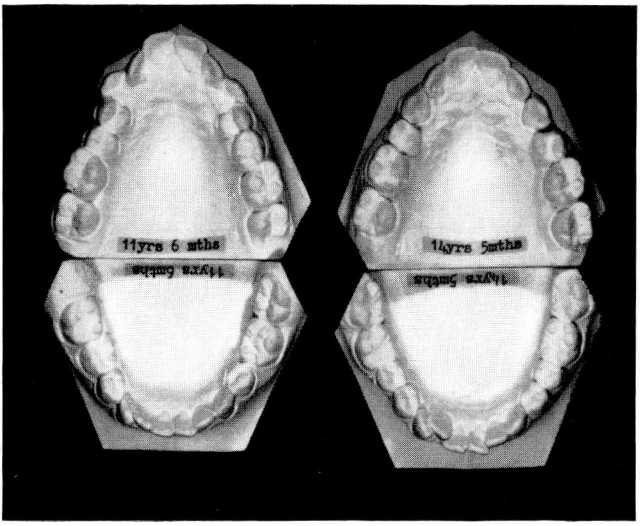

Fig. 100.—Case treated by extraction of $\underline{4|4}$. Despite loss of space $\overline{|5}$ has forced its way into the arch at the expense of lower incisor alinement.

premolar may be extracted. The variations of the treatment of this local impaction are shown in *Fig.* 99.

Crowding in the Molar Region.—This is mainly confined to the impaction of the third permanent molar, although on occasions both the first and second molars may be impacted. As impaction of the first and second molars is rather rare, this is dealt with in the APPENDIX.

At one time the extraction of second molars was advocated as a means of disimpacting the lower third molar, but at the present time this is a somewhat controversial issue as a good position of the third molar cannot be guaranteed. *Fig.* 101 shows an excellent result.

Cryer analysed 66 cases of second molar extractions and concluded that only in 35 per cent was the position of the third molar really good. However, in carefully selected cases, extraction of second molars can be recommended if: (1) The extraction is carried out at about the time the crown of the third molar is fully formed, before there is any root formation which could be between 12 to 14 years of age; (2) the third molar angulation was not more than 30° to the long axis of the second molar; (3) where the first permanent molar has a good prognosis. *Figs.* 102–104 show some of the illustrations from Cryer's paper with analysis of results.

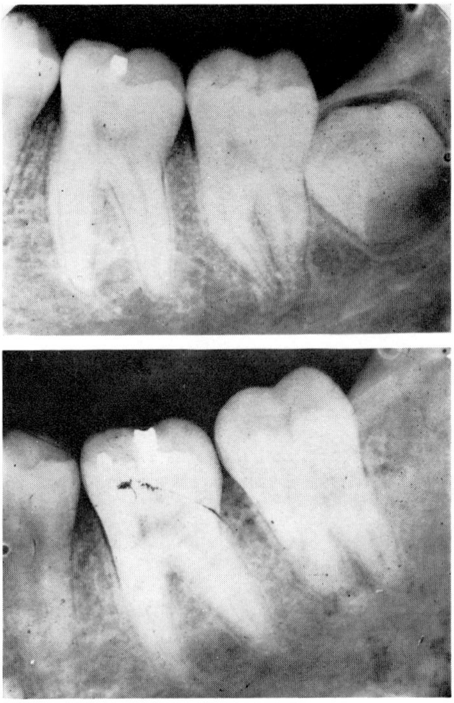

Fig. 101.—Impacted third molar at the age of 14 erupting into good position following the extraction of the second molar to prevent deterioration of lower incisor alinement. (*By courtesy of R. E. Rix and the 'Dental Practitioner'.*)

There is support for the early removal of the third molar through a lateral approach which involves trepanation through the buccal plate when the crown is formed, leaving a well-positioned second molar in place.

This approach to the treatment of crowded arches cannot be applied to all racial groups, as there are widely differing growth patterns. This accounts for international differences of opinion on the subject. The fact that expansion of both upper and lower dental arches may produce a stable end-result in some cases does not invalidate the general statements already made. In the British Isles, particularly, arch expansion is not a treatment which can be applied as a general rule when both arches are crowded, the dental bases potentially small and short, and where the muscular environment of the dentition is restricting adequate centrifugal development.

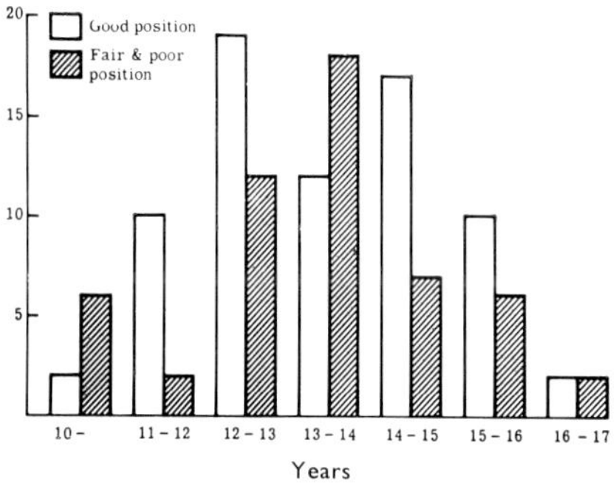

Fig. 102.—Relationship between age at the time of lower second molar extractions and final position of lower third molars. (*By courtesy of B. S. Cryer and the 'Dental Practitioner'.*)

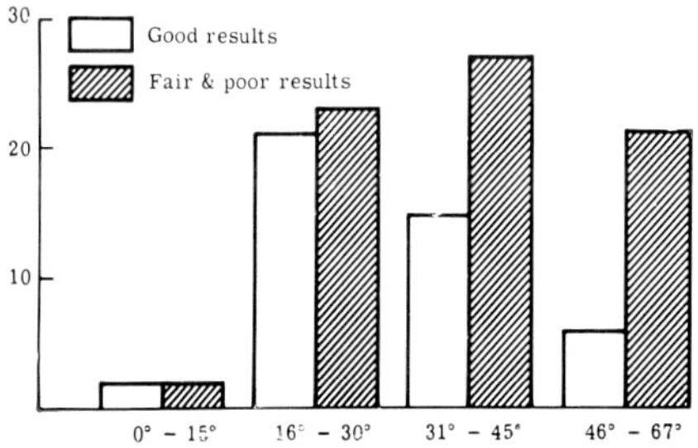

Fig. 103.—Analysis of results of extracting lower second molars in relationship to the angulation between the lower third molar and the long axis of the second molar. (*By courtesy of B. S. Cryer and the 'Dental Practitioner'.*)

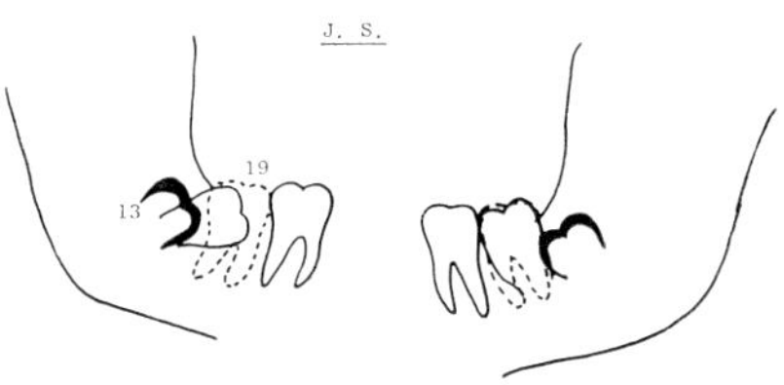

Fig. 104.—Tracings from radiographs superimposed on 6|6. Position of $\overline{8|8}$ at the time of extraction of $\overline{7|7}$ shown by heavy outline. Broken line shows position of $\overline{7|7}$. Continuous line shows final position of $\overline{8|8}$. (*By courtesy of B. S. Cryer and the 'Dental Practitioner'.*)

The Use of Extractions to affect the Incisor Relationship.—It has been explained that the extraction of cheek teeth may affect the overbite either favourably or adversely. The practical applications have been discussed on pp. 68–69 and the change in attitude should be noted.

In the treatment of Class II and Class III malocclusions where there is a fundamental error in dental base relationship, extractions may be employed to attempt to shorten one dental arch relative to the other, in order to improve the incisor relationship. In Class III cases, although lower extractions may offer the opportunity for the retraction of lower incisors, the size of the lower jaw and the position and action of the

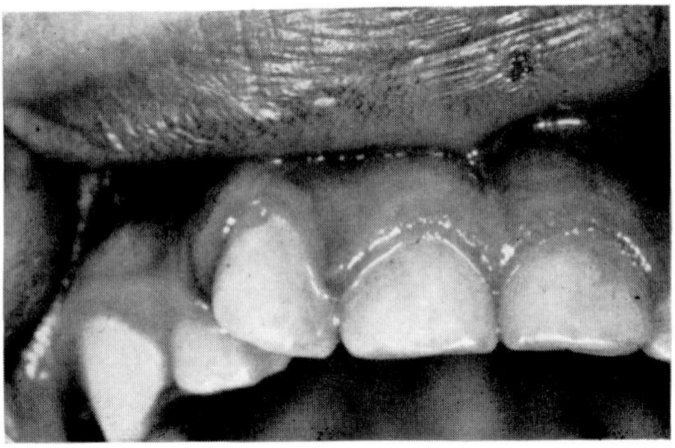

Fig. 105.—Supplemental lateral incisor.

tongue may prevent any material improvement in the incisor relationship.

It is convenient at this stage to consider the problems created by extra teeth as in nearly every case they have to be extracted, or extractions are required elsewhere in the arch.

Extra Teeth.—Supernumerary teeth are not as common as missing teeth. They may occur anywhere in the jaws as aberrant developments of the dental formative organ. Those which resemble teeth of the normal series are called supplemental teeth and the tooth most frequently duplicated in this way is the upper lateral incisor (*Fig.* 105). In such a case the most displaced tooth is extracted. An upper lateral incisor may have a coronal invagination as distinct from a simple cingulum pit. This predisposes the pulp to infection soon after the tooth erupts. It is advisable not to extract one supplemental lateral until both have been carefully examined and radiographed for evidence of abnormal crown structure.

Apart from these supplemental teeth, supernumerary teeth are of two main types—either simple conical teeth or tubercular and resembling

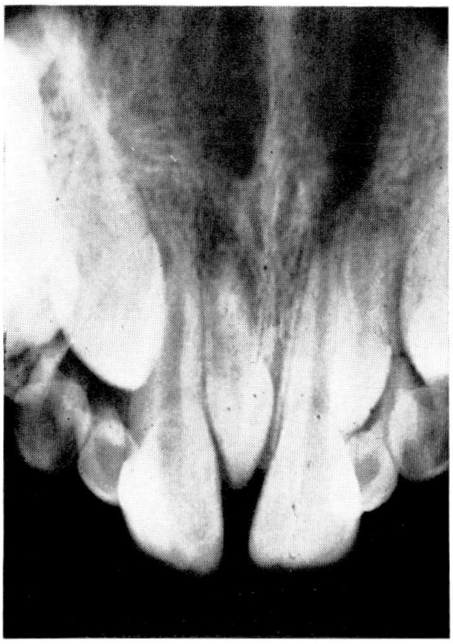

A

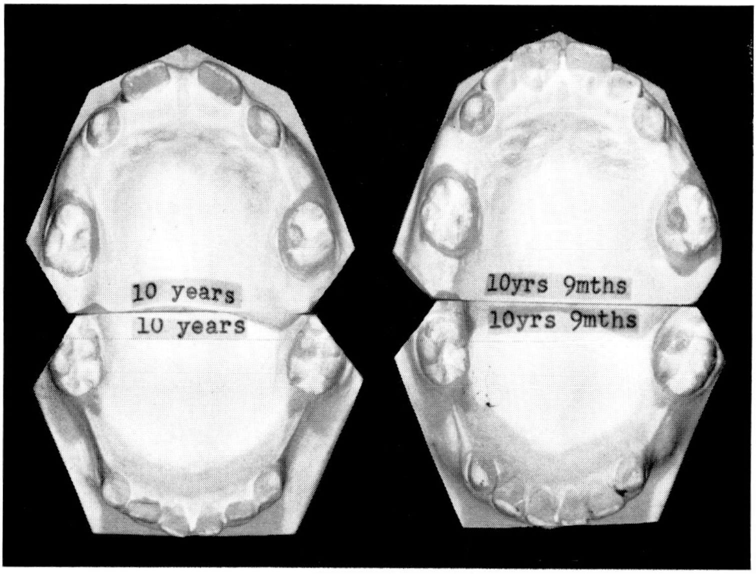

B

Fig. 106.—A, Conical supernumerary in the midline causing separation of the incisors. B, Diastema closing after midline supernumerary has been removed and lateral incisors have erupted.

a lower second premolar. They are most likely to occur in the upper incisor region, particularly on the palatal side. They are found singly in the midline (*Fig.* 106), in pairs (*Fig.* 107), or in larger groups. They may be upright, inverted, or horizontal, and either completely obstruct incisor eruption or cause deflexion. Occasionally they erupt without causing any derangement of the incisors, and can then be extracted. Where there is obvious interference with incisor eruption they should be removed surgically. (*See* APPENDIX.)

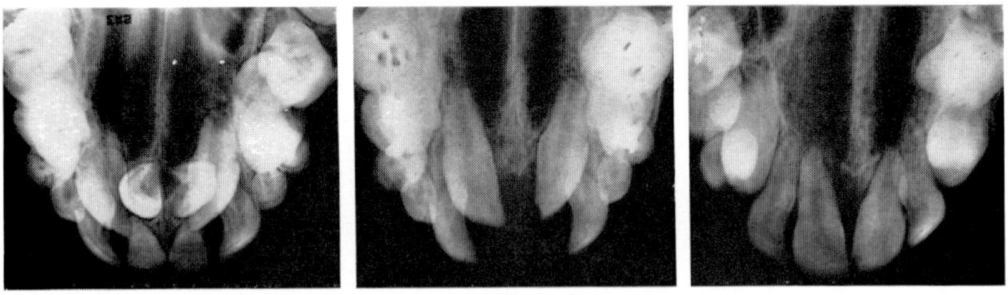

A

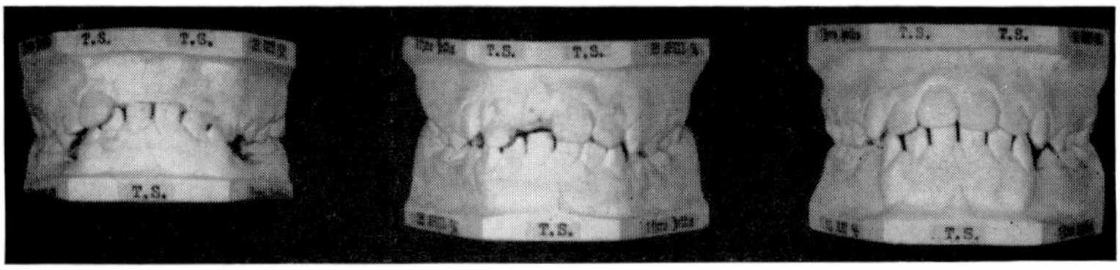

B

Fig. 107.—A, Series of radiographs of tuberculated supernumeraries palatal to 1|1 preventing their eruption, showing eruption of incisors after surgical removal of the supernumerary. B, Models to show the same sequence. 4|4 had to be extracted to create sufficient space.

Where a supernumerary tooth is noticed in a routine orthodontic radiograph with no derangement of the dentition and no other symptoms, it should be left alone. It is also undesirable to operate for the removal of supernumerary teeth before 6 or 7 years of age, as the area is full of developing teeth which may be subluxed. It is undesirable to wait too long, because, once the incisor apices are well formed, they are slower to erupt when the obstruction is removed.

Fig. 107 shows a series illustrating the eruption of the incisors after the removal of two supernumeraries. Where there is delayed eruption, the upper lateral incisors may move around the arch and encroach on the available space. This space may have to be regained by extraction of two premolar teeth and the distal movement of upper canines and lateral incisors (*Fig.* 107 B).

There are three standard ways of assessing the position of supernumeraries:—

1. Clinical examination: displacement of the crowns of erupted incisors gives some indication of where the supernumerary teeth are lying.

2. Stereoscopic radiographs may be taken with two occlusal films by moving the tube from the position of the pupil of the eye on one side to the pupil on the other side. A stereoscope will give depth to the picture.

3. A 'vertex occlusal' radiograph taken through the long axis of the incisors gives an indication as to whether supernumeraries are palatally or labially placed, and a true lateral picture of the incisor region will indicate their depth.

(Further details of the methods of location of buried teeth will be given in the APPENDIX.)

This chapter has dealt with general problems in relation to the extraction of teeth. Given the right circumstances, improvement can be made by extraction therapy alone, but considerable experience is required to forecast the natural drift of other teeth in the arch in the years following extraction. It would be wrong, therefore, to stress treatment by extraction alone as many cases require some active treatment with appliances. This will be dealt with in the following chapters.

BIBLIOGRAPHY

ANGLE, E. H. (1900), *Malocclusion of the Teeth*, 6th ed. Philadelphia: S. S. White Dental Manufacturing Co.

BALLARD, C. F., and WALTHER, D. P. (1953), 'Some Cases to illustrate the Relationship between Aetiology, Prognosis and Treatment Planning in Orthodontics', *Dent. Rec.*, **73**, 669.

BRODIE, A. G. (1944), 'Does Scientific Investigation Support the Extraction of Teeth in Orthodontic Therapy?', *Amer. J. Orthodont.*, **30**, 444.

CHAPMAN, H. (1950), 'Tooth Extraction as an Orthodontic Measure', *Int. Dent. J., Lond.*, **1**, 101.

CRYER, B. S. (1965), 'Lower Arch Changes during the Early Teens', *Trans. europ. orthod. Soc.*, 87.

— — (1967), 'Third Molar Eruption and the Effect of Extraction of Adjacent Teeth', *Dent. Practit.*, **17**, 405.

DEWEL, B. F. (1954), 'Serial Extraction in Orthodontics: Indications, Objectives, and Treatment Procedures', *Amer. J. Orthodont.*, **40**, 906.

— — (1959), 'A Clinical Analysis of Serial Extraction in Orthodontic Treatment', *Ibid.*, **45**, 424.

— — (1969), 'Prerequisites in Serial Extraction', *Amer. J. Orthodont.*, **55**, 633.

FOX, J. (1803), *The Natural History of the Human Teeth.* London: Thomas Cox.

HUNTER, J. (1771), *The Natural History of the Human Teeth, explaining their Structure, Use, Formation, Growth and Diseases.* London: J. Johnson.

KJELLGREN, B. (1948), 'Serial Extraction as a Corrective Procedure in Dental Orthopædic Therapy', *Trans. europ. orthod. Soc.*, 134.

LUNDSTRÖM, A. F. (1925), 'Malocclusion of the Teeth regarded as a Problem in connection with the Apical Base', *Int. J. Orthod.*, **11**, 591.

PRINGLE, K. E. (1938), 'The Relation between Incisor Overlap and the Extraction of Upper Temporary Teeth', *Trans. Brit. Soc. Orthodont.*, 95.

Rix, R. E. (1953), 'Some Observations on the Environment of the Incisors', *Dent. Rec.*, **73**, 427.

Smith, D. I. (1957), 'The Eruption of Third Molars following Extraction of Second Molars', *Trans. Brit. Soc. Orthodont.*, 55.

Tulley, W. J. (1959), 'The Role of Extractions in Orthodontic Treatment', *Brit. dent. J.*, **107**, 199.

Tweed, C. H. (1944), 'Indications for the Extraction of Teeth in Orthodontic Procedure', *Amer. J. Orthodont.*, **30**, 405.

Wilkinson, A. A. (1942), 'The Early Extraction of the First Permanent Molar as the Best Method of Preserving the Dentition as a Whole', *Trans. Brit. Soc. Orthodont.*, 13.

CHAPTER IX

GENERAL PRINCIPLES OF APPLIANCE THERAPY

THIS chapter deals specifically with the basic design and component parts of removable appliances. Illustrations of complete appliances will be given in the chapters dealing with the treatment of particular malocclusions.

Tooth Movement.—It has been known for centuries that when pressure is applied to the crown of a tooth it will move away from this pressure. This was the principle adopted by Celcus in 25 B.C. when he is reported to have used leverage to move a tooth over the bite.

Teeth may be tipped, rotated, moved along their long axes, or moved bodily. The forces are transmitted by the periodontal ligament to the alveolar bone and the architecture of the tooth socket is modified by resorption of bone in areas of pressure and deposition of new bone in areas of tension. The classic histological experiments of Oppenheim and Schwarz deserve special mention and more recently Reitan has published a very comprehensive study of histological reactions to tooth movement.

These reactions may be summarized as follows: In areas of both pressure and tension, the periodontal tissues show a mild degree of hyperaemia in excess of that seen with the normal physiological migration of teeth. This hyperaemia encourages an increased cellular activity with the production of osteoclasts, osteoblasts, and fibroblasts.

Where the periodontal fibres are inserted into the laminated bone, the bone is rearranged in spicules at right-angles to the root surface. In areas of pressure, osteoclastic activity can be seen on the surface of these bony spicules adjacent to the tooth. Osteoblastic activity produces new bone in areas where tension is transmitted (*Fig.* 108). This remodelling of the bony wall of the socket occurs with the laying down of bundle bone which is eventually remodelled as true laminated cortical bone when the teeth take up their final position. Fibroblasts produce new fibres in the periodontal ligament when rearrangement of the non-elastic collagen bundles is required. Reitan has stated that when a tooth is moved slowly by intermittent pressures osteoid tissue is laid down. Some authorities have argued that intermittent pressure of this kind, with cessation in movement over a period of time, fosters production of a tissue which is resistant to resorption.

Where excessive force is used, but not of a sufficient degree to produce pain or haemorrhage, 'hyalinization' of the periodontal tissues may occur producing 'cell-free zones'. Resorption of the bone fails to occur unless there is undermining resorption in an adjacent area.

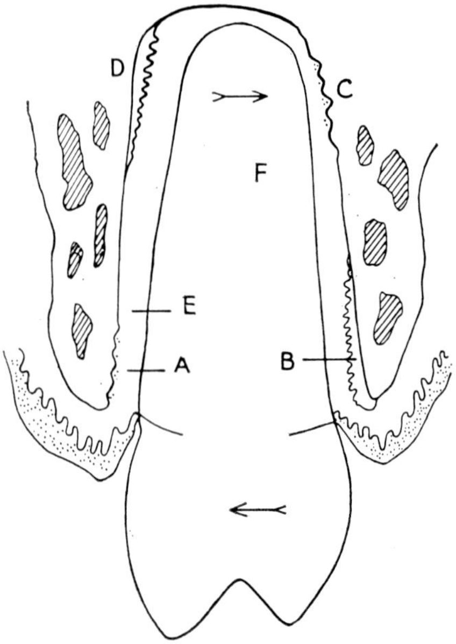

Fig. 108.—The fulcrum during physiological tipping of a tooth is located at F. Initial tissue changes after orthodontic movement are first observed in the cervical region. A, Resorption on the pressure side; B, Apposition on the tension side. In a tooth movement of some duration secondary pressure and tension sides will be found at C and D. If the tipping movement is continued, a new pressure area will be located approximately at E, following elimination of bone substance by resorption in the marginal region. (*By courtesy of K. Reitan and 'Current Orthodontics'*.)

Although cementoblasts may be produced by the metaplasia of cells in the periodontal tissues, the cementum covering the root surface is more resistant to resorption than the bony socket; only rarely is there root resorption with normal orthodontic procedures and then the reparative process is rapid.

Where tipping movements are applied to the crown of the tooth the axis around which this occurs is in the region of the apical third of the root, as illustrated in *Fig.* 108. The more gentle the force, the nearer the apex is the axis of rotation.

When teeth are rotated, Reitan has shown that the tooth must be held in position for a prolonged period as torsional forces are set up in the periodontal tissues and remain in the marginal free fibres for a considerable period of time. The subject of retention following orthodontic tooth movement is dealt with on p. 275 (*see* APPENDIX).

Bodily movement of teeth can be produced by some forms of fixed apparatus. There is naturally a much greater resistance to the movement and greater danger of producing apical resorption. Apical resorption has been described as one of the 'scars of orthodontic treatment'. It is most likely to occur where teeth have been moved into a position where they are not in equilibrium with the various forces acting upon them and are subjected to continuous 'jiggling'.

The use of bite planes may retard the eruption of teeth by transmitting occlusal forces along their long axes. Active forces are rarely applied to depress teeth in their sockets or to elongate them. Elongation may lead to disturbance in the vascular supply.

The investigations which have been carried out indicate that pressure exerted on a tooth should not exceed the capillary blood-pressure, otherwise damage with local haemorrhage in the periodontal tissues may result in the tooth becoming painful and loose. Practically speaking, a pressure of 20–25 g. (1 oz.) can be applied to a single-rooted tooth.

Schwarz described four degrees of force:—

1. A force which is too gentle or of too short a duration to produce any movement.

2. The ideal force, one which produces tooth movement without damage.

3. The force which exceeds the capillary blood-pressure and could produce damage; but this is reversible if the pressure is withdrawn.

4. A force which produces irreversible damage to the periodontal tissues. This may be followed by strangulation of the apical vessels and death of the pulp.

There are still differences of opinion as to whether forces used to move teeth should be continuous and light or of a stronger degree with periods of rest. From the clinical point of view, both principles are used in various forms of appliance therapy and no hard-and-fast rule can be made, provided the forces exerted at any time are not excessive and there are no unduly prolonged resting periods.

The Use of Apparatus.—Each appliance should be designed to achieve a specific purpose as efficiently and as simply as possible. Certain limits are imposed by the tolerance of the child who will have to wear it.

When a removable appliance is first fitted the child should be given practice in removing and in inserting it in front of a mirror.

Most children appreciate an explanation of its function and this will often help them to care for it properly. Instruction should be given in cleaning the plate, particularly after meals. Unless specific instructions are given to the contrary, removable appliances should be worn full time, day and night.

PRINCIPLES OF DESIGN OF APPLIANCES

1. Anchorage.
2. Means of retention.
3. The activating mechanism.

ANCHORAGE

This is the term used for the buttress from which forces may be applied to move a tooth or group of teeth. The movement of the malposed teeth depends on two things: first, that the force exerted is sufficient to effect the movement; and, secondly, that the anchorage is sufficient to resist this force either entirely or to a required extent.

According to Newton's third law of motion, 'To every action there is an equal and opposite reaction'. Thus the resistance to movement of anchorage is rarely absolute—it is relative. The aim in most cases is to secure anchorage in which the resistance to movement is as high as possible, so that if a force is applied from it to some other body of less resistance, almost all the movement resulting will be with the latter.

Anchorage should not be confused with clasping or devices used to retain the plate in the mouth. It may be classified in the following ways:—

Intramaxillary Anchorage.—This is where teeth in one arch are used as an anchorage for traction to move teeth in the same arch.

Intermaxillary Anchorage.—This is where teeth in one arch are used as anchorage for traction to be applied to teeth in the opposing arch.

Extra-oral Anchorage.—This is where the neck region or the occipital region carry forms of 'harness' from which traction is applied to an intra-oral appliance. A combination of all these types of anchorage may be used.

Simple Anchorage.—This is where a large tooth is used as anchorage to move a smaller tooth and both are free to tilt. Most forms of anchorage, however, are *compound.* In this instance a number of teeth and other structures such as the fit of the plate into the palate are compounded together to form a greater resistance, but the teeth are still free to tilt.

'Stationary' Anchorage.—This is the term used to describe a compound anchorage which is so designed that the teeth can only move bodily, so that the name is a relative misnomer. This type of anchorage can only be obtained by multiband techniques such as the edgewise appliance.

In certain instances reciprocal movement of teeth is required. Examples of this are when upper central incisors are to be approximated. This might be described as *simple reciprocal anchorage*. A more elaborate example is when the upper arch is being expanded and two segments are being moved apart. At one time intermaxillary traction was cited as an example of reciprocal effect, e.g., upper arch being retracted and the lower arch advanced. This is a disadvantage as far as the lower arch is concerned.

Reinforcement of Anchorage.—There are various ways in which the resistance provided by the anchor teeth could be increased. The most positive method is by using a headcap or neck strap which is attached to an intra-oral device (*see Fig.* 129). Removable appliances or a combination of fixed and removable appliances allow contact of acrylic with the mucosa of the palate or lingual sulcus. An inclined plane on an upper appliance combined with a well-positioned labial arch allows the biting force to be delivered in such a way that the upper incisor segment is less likely to tilt forward (*see Fig.* 135).

For the reasons stated above, traction applied to the opposing arch to reinforce anchorage is not very satisfactory as the reciprocal effects may be undesirable, e.g., lower incisors may be moved forward out of balance with the soft-tissue forces acting on them.

MEANS OF RETENTION OF REMOVABLE APPLIANCES

There are many forms of clasp which have been used to retain removable appliances with varying degrees of success. The clasp which has become universally accepted is that described by Adams and this is the only form of clasp which will be described in detail.

Adams Crib.—*Fig.* 109 illustrates the Adams crib, which is probably the most efficient and most commonly used clasp. It depends upon the engagement of the U-loops into undercut areas on the mesio-buccal and distobuccal aspects of the crown of the tooth. The loops are insinuated into the crevice between the crown of the tooth and the interdental papillæ, to lie at the gingival margin.

It is capable of many modifications, as in *Fig.* 110, to provide only one loop for engagement, or the addition of hooks and tubes for use with elastic traction. Where necessary, these attachments may be

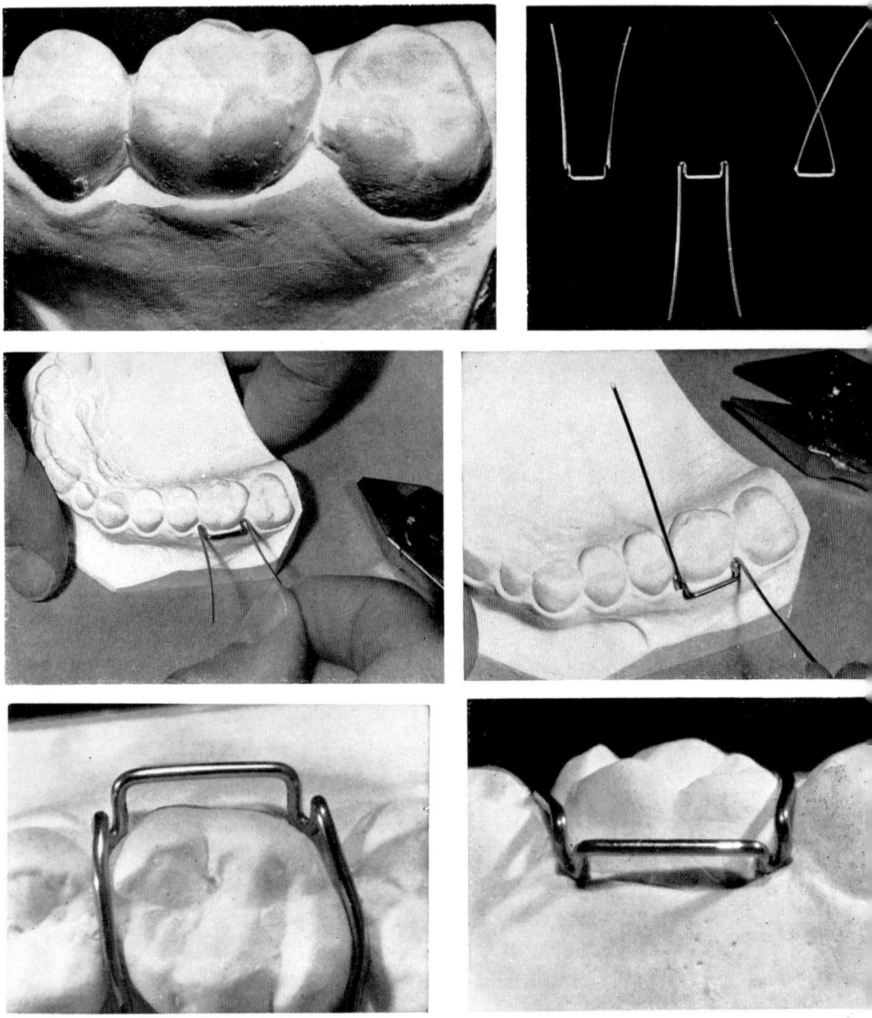

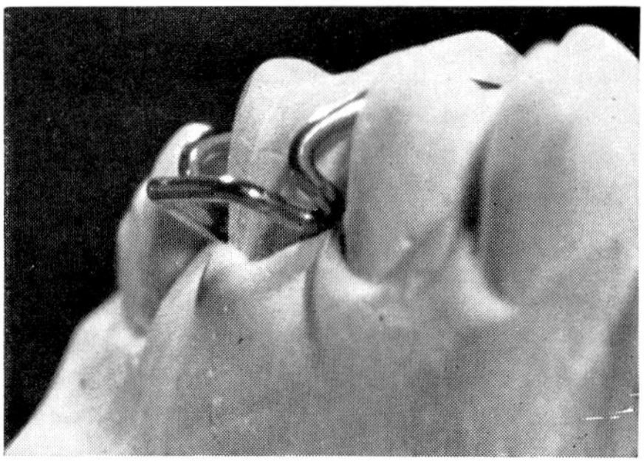

Fig. 109.—The Adams crib showing stag in the construction. The important poi to note are: (*a*) The arrowheads should insinuated in the undercut area on the mes and distal of each tooth. (*b*) The arrowhea should not touch the adjoining teeth and shaped to follow the gum margins. (*c*) T bridge between the arrowheads should straight and stand away from the tooth enable the area to be self-cleansing. (*d*) T recurved portion of wire passing interdenta should not stick out into the cheek, whi is a common fault. (*By courtesy of C. Adams.*)

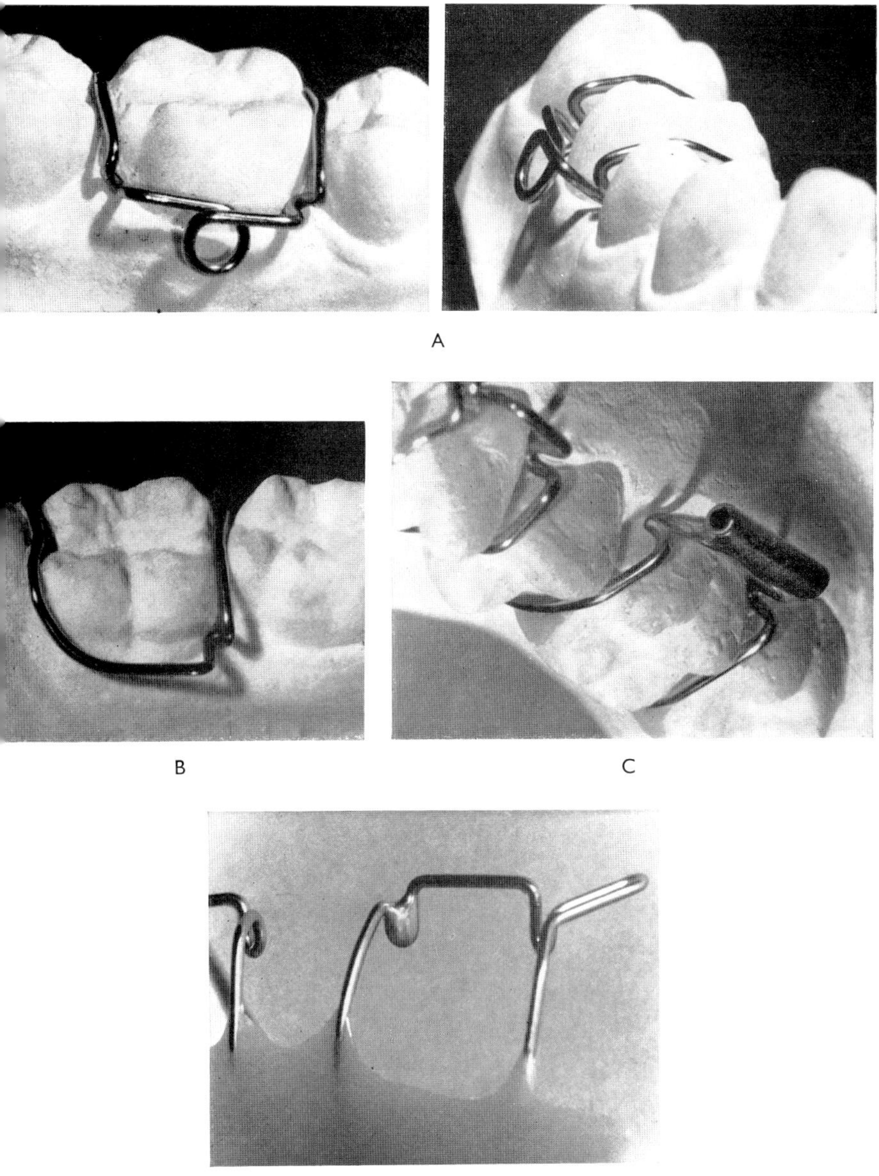

Fig. 110.—Modifications of the Adams crib. A, Showing the bridge portion of the clasp incorporating a loop for attachment of elastics. B, Single arrowhead where the tooth is partially erupted. C, Attachment of tube to bridge by soldering to take a freely sliding arch. D, Soldered repair of an arrowhead and modification of the clasp to form a hook for elastic attachment. (*By courtesy of C. P. Adams.*)

satisfactorily soldered to the bridge and the U-loops may be repaired by soldering.

On permanent molar teeth the crib is usually constructed in 0·7-mm. stainless-steel wire, whilst on premolar teeth or deciduous molar teeth it is usually constructed in 0·6-mm. wire.

Clasps for Anterior Teeth.—These may contribute little to the stability of an appliance in themselves, but can assist where most of the retention is provided elsewhere.

A simple low labial bow in 0·7-mm. wire may assist in stabilizing an appliance.

A simple free-ending clasp on an incisor will assist in stabilization of an appliance near the point of application of pressure—e.g., where one incisor is being 'moved over the bite'. The Adams crib can be adapted to be used on anterior teeth where necessary.

THE ACTIVATING MECHANISM

Teeth may be moved by several basic mechanisms with fixed or removable appliances:—

1. Springs—depending upon the elastic return of a spring-tempered wire towards its undeformed state.

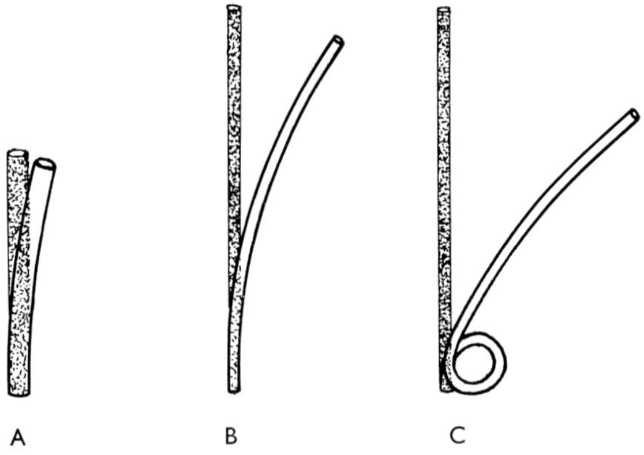

Fig. 111.—The effectiveness of a spring is increased by using a finer gauge wire and reasonable length. Compare (A) with (B) in a long wire. C, Insertion of a coil is the same as increasing the total length.

2. Rubber bands—depending upon the return of elastic rubber to its unextended state.

3. Wedging appliances using expansion screws.

4. Appliances which rely on occlusal forces and other muscular activities for their function.

1. Springs.—The material in common use is stainless steel of a spring-hard temper. Springs are designed to exert a gentle pressure over as great a range as possible. They should be constructed of fine-gauge wire and should be as long as space will permit. The gauge of wire used should also be able to stand up to normal handling by the patient—generally it is 0·45–0·6 mm. in diameter for protected palatal or lingual springs, but long unprotected buccal springs should be constructed in 0·7-mm. round wire.

The length of a spring is strictly limited in the mouth by the amount of space available, particularly in a lower removable appliance. The

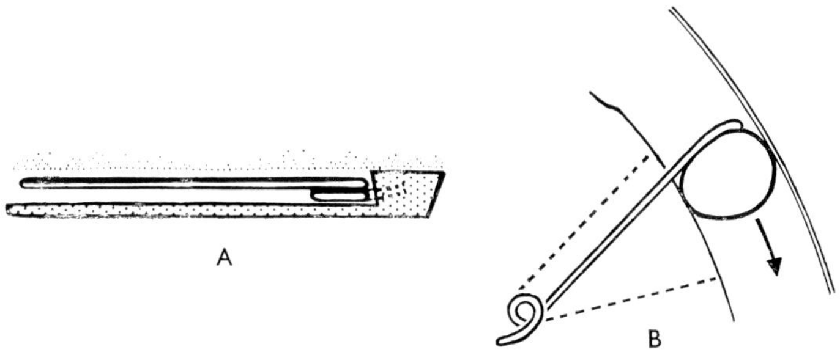

Fig. 112.—Springs may be 'boxed in' so that they are protected by acrylic on the appliance. A, The free arm should lie nearer the soft tissues to facilitate adjustment. B, The area between the dotted line is filled in with plaster during the 'wax up' stage to allow the spring freedom of movement. Note also the length of spring and position. The tooth movement is controlled by the acrylic and the labial bow. The point of contact of the spring with the tooth can be adjusted.

effective length of a spring can be increased by incorporating a coil as in *Fig.* 111. The way in which the coil is wound is shown not to be critical by Bass and Stephens, but it is desirable that the free arm of the spring should lie nearer the soft tissues than the acrylic to facilitate adjustment. *Fig.* 112 illustrates the importance of the correct siting of a spring. The free end of the spring will move through a curve, and it must be placed so that this end is in constant contact with the tooth throughout its activity and will move the tooth in the desired direction. However, a tooth does not necessarily move in the same arc as the free end of the spring—it depends upon the point of application, which can be altered.

There are many types of springs in common use, but the undermentioned will achieve most of the required tooth movements.

Springs for Use on Removable Appliances.—*Fig.* 112 illustrates a spring which may be used to move a tooth around the line of the arch—e.g., moving a canine or premolar tooth distally.

Fig. 113 illustrates a spring with a recurved end designed to move a tooth labially or buccally. The movement is the resultant of movements induced by each separate part. Adjustment of the recurved portion makes it possible to change the point of application.

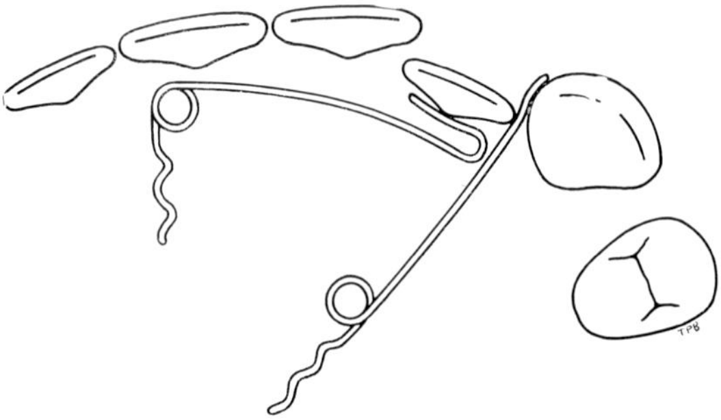

Fig. 113.—Recurved finger spring to push a tooth buccally or labially. The arm should be as long as possible and the recurved portion enables adjustment to be made in direction.

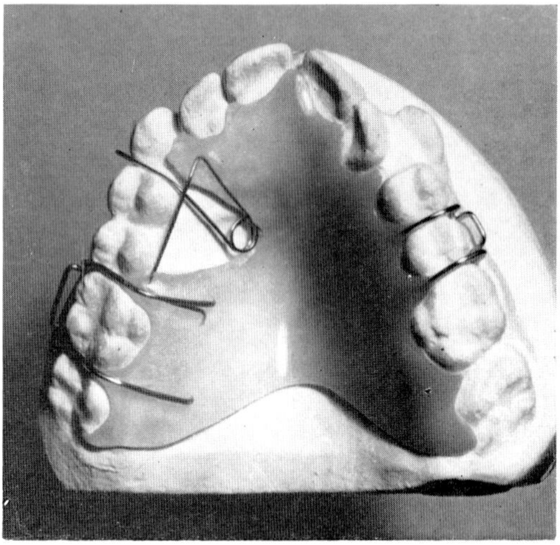

Fig. 114.—Use of guide wire instead of acrylic to protect palatal finger spring. (*By courtesy of C. P. Adams.*)

Most springs need to be stabilized either by boxing under a shelf of the acrylic of the plate or by the provision of guide wires. When a spring is to be 'boxed in' it should be plastered out before the plate is waxed, so that acrylic will not interfere with the movement of the spring through the full range of its activity (*Fig.* 112). When guide wires are used as in *Fig.* 114 they should be placed so that they will exert their effect throughout the active range of the spring.

Fig. 115 illustrates an 'S' spring to move a group of upper incisors labially. This is a long and rather mobile spring and is used to exert pressure against the sloping palatal surfaces of the upper anterior teeth. A constant point of application is given by providing an oblique overlying guide wire where the spring is not 'boxed in'. Where this type of spring is 'boxed in' the free end should be recurved so that as the anterior teeth are moved forward the free end of the spring is still

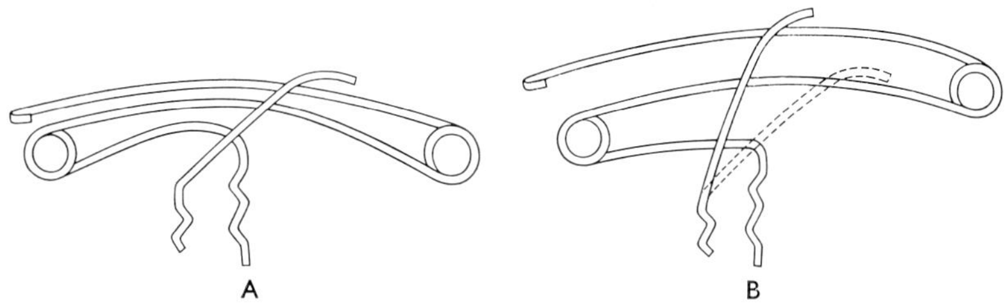

Fig. 115.—A, 'S' spring in 0·7-mm. wire for labial movement of incisors protected by 0·8-mm. guard wire (spring inactive). B, Spring activated to show adjustment of guard wire to cover spring as the incisors are advanced.

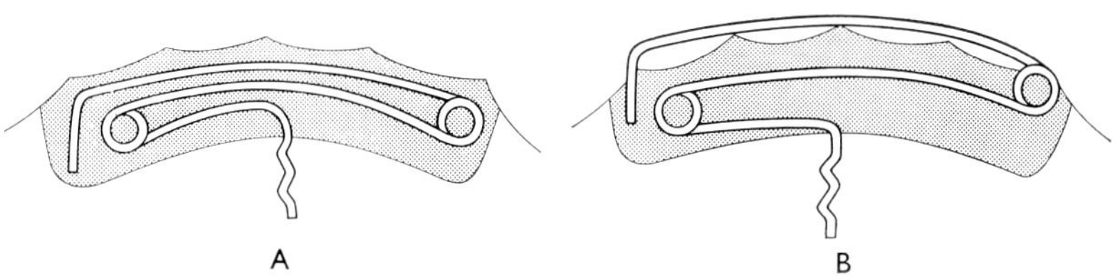

Fig. 116.—A, 'S' spring boxed in under the acrylic of the appliance with recurved end to the spring, constructed in 0·7-mm. wire (spring inactive). B, Activated spring. As the spring emerges from under the acrylic it is still controlled by the recurved end.

contained under the shelf of acrylic and prevented from riding down the sloping surface (*Fig.* 116). This is less effective than the overlying guide wires.

Fig. 117 A, B, C illustrates buccal springs for use where a canine tooth is so placed that a spring from the palatal or lingual aspect would not engage satisfactorily. This is rather a long spring wire and therefore should be constructed in 0·7-mm. stainless-steel wire. Care should be taken to avoid muscle attachments in the buccal sulcus and it is inadvisable to take the curve of the spring too near the mucosal deflexion as it is likely to produce ulceration.

Fig. 117 D illustrates a further type of buccal spring in which the active wire is 0·5-mm. stainless steel. Stability is given to this fine wire in its long run from its attachment into the acrylic of the plate by including the proximal portion within stainless-steel tubing. Such a spring is useful in the upper or the lower arch. It should be sited so that the free end does not slip off the tooth to be moved.

Low Labial Bow.—The labial arch wire constructed in 0·7-mm. stainless steel with one take-up loop is used in a variety of ways. It may be mainly as a retaining device or as a means of reinforcing anchorage in conjunction with a bite plane as illustrated in *Fig.* 135 or as a framework to which auxiliary springs may be attached. It should lie at the junction of the incisal and middle third of the crown, but

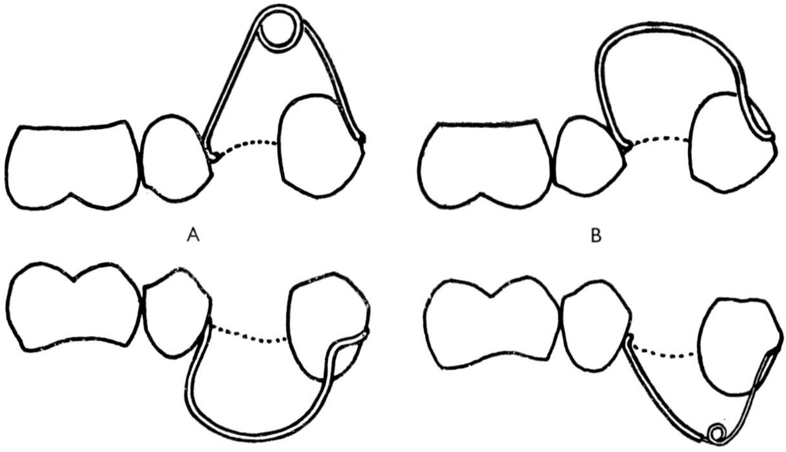

Fig. 117.—Buccal canine retractors: A, Buccal retractor with coil in 0·7-mm. wire. B, 'Fly-over' type of buccal retractor in 0·7-mm. wire. Note that the end is flattened to fit interdentally and some palatal movement can be obtained by allowing the spring to contact the buccal surfaces of the tooth. C, 'Fly-over' retractor used in lower arch. D, Buccal retractor with active portions in 0·5-mm. wire supported by tube into sulcus.

in some cases where anchorage is being reinforced by inclined plane it should be placed nearer the incisal edge. Take-up loops are used to permit some adjustment, but care should be taken to ensure that they are not too large and impinge on the mucosa.

The use of this type of rigid arch is not a very practical way of retracting anterior teeth. Frequent adjustments are required as the force is exerted for a short space of time and then the arch is inactive.

In some cases the take-up loop can be made in a reverse direction to prevent interference with other structures on the appliance. *Fig.* 118 shows that this type of bow can be divided in the midline to retract incisor teeth using the two free ends. The long arms are easily distorted by misuse. If they are constructed to overlap, however, a sleeve of welded tape could be made to prevent this displacement.

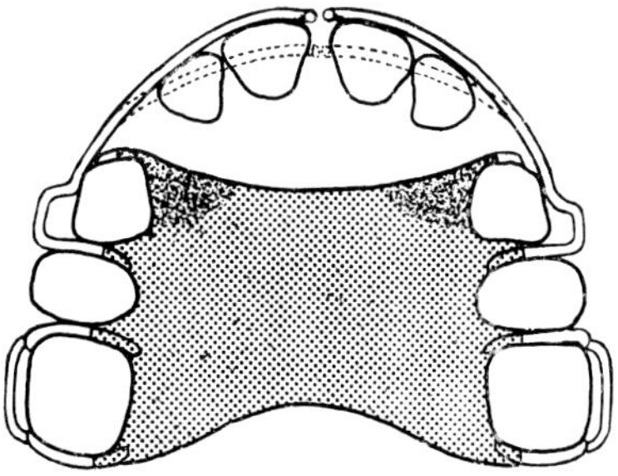

A

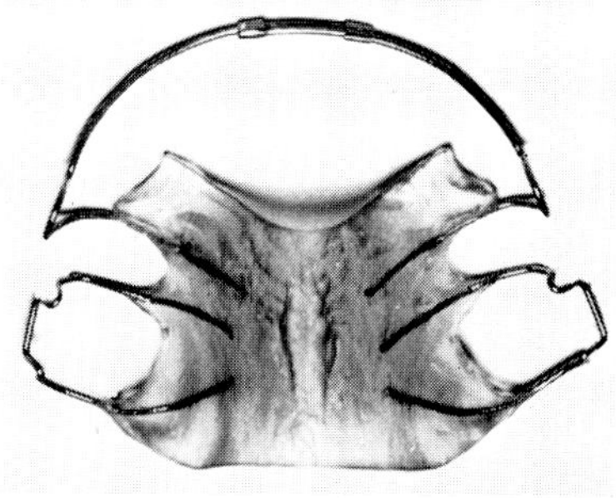

B

Fig. 118.—Divided labial bow constructed in 0·7-mm. or 0·8-mm. wire, divided in the midline and used as two free ending arms. A, Dotted line shows how free ending arms are adjusted; B, Shows stainless-steel wrapping embracing the two free ending arms to prevent displacement.

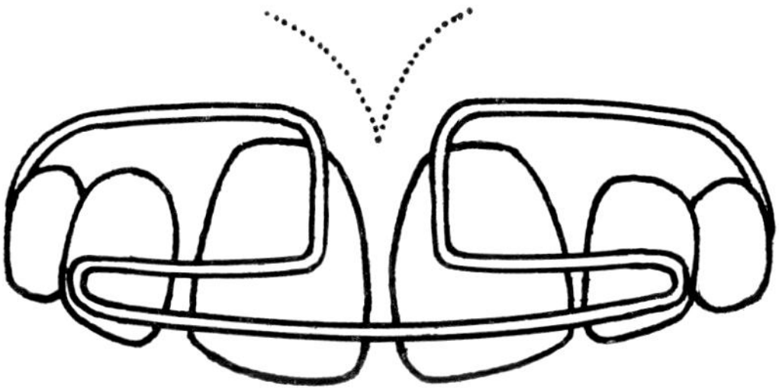

A

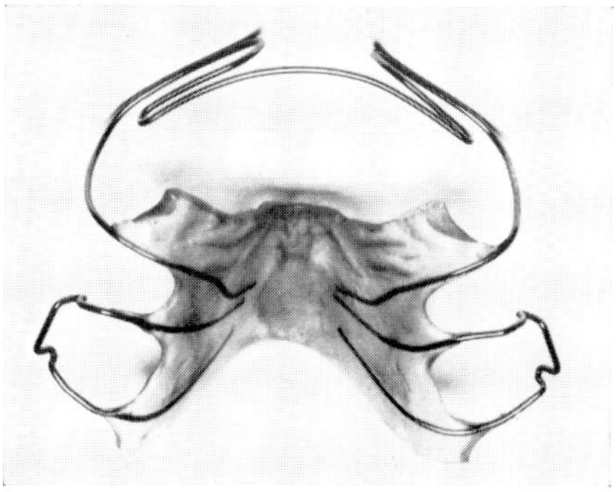

B

Fig. 119.—A, Labial bow for active retraction of incisors. (*Diagrammatic after Mills.*) B, Modified form of Mills retractor in 0·7-mm. wire.

Mills has described a form of labial arch in a 0·7-mm. wire with large loops as shown in *Fig.* 119. Because of the greater length of wire, this form of bow can be used for active retraction of incisors without continuous adjustment but it is liable to distortion by the patient.

High Labial Bow.—Figs. 121, 123 illustrate this framework in 0·8-mm. or 0·9-mm. wire to which many auxiliary springs may be attached. To facilitate this it is desirable that it should be constructed with well-defined angles.

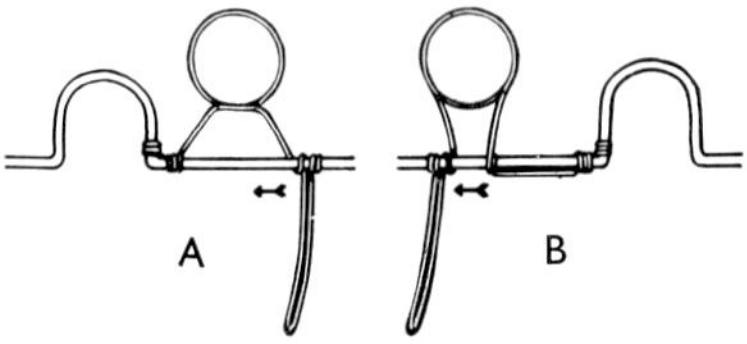

Fig. 120.—Auxiliary travelling spring wound on labial bow in 0·3-mm. wire to: A, Move a tooth distally; B, Move a tooth mesially. (*Figs.* 120, 121 *by courtesy of R. E. Rix* (1938), '*British Dental Journal*'.)

Auxiliary Springs.—Various methods may be used to attach auxiliary springs to an arch wire. The simplest is to wind coils around the arch wire at a sharp angle. However, a tube attachment can be most useful where a welder is available. Direct welding and soldering require a very careful technique.

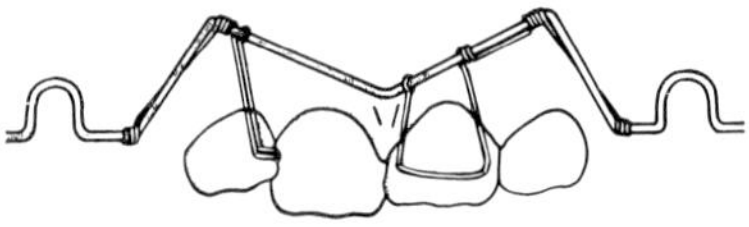

Fig. 121.—'Golf club' spring in 0·3–0·4-mm. wire wound on a high labial bow, also a local apron spring to retract an outstanding incisor.

These springs are constructed of fine-gauge wires, 0·3–0·4 mm., to act from the support of either a high labial or low labial bow. They have the advantage that they can provide gentle pressure and that new springs can be added to an existing appliance. They can, however, be more readily damaged than a heavy gauge wire.

Fig. 120 illustrates a travelling spring wound on to a low labial bow which may be used to move a tooth around the arch. As shown, it may be designed to either push or pull. This type of spring can be added to an existing appliance on occasions.

Fig. 121 illustrates the 'golf club' spring which is attached to a high labial bow and can be used to move anterior teeth around the arch.

Fig. 122 illustrates 'self-straightening wires' wound on to a low labial bow and used to retract upper incisor teeth in particular. With careful adjustment this form of apparatus works very gently over a fairly extensive period of time. The long spring arms are rather liable to distortion and where the incisors are proclined the springs tend to slide on to and damage the gingivae.

Figs. 121 and 123 illustrate methods of retracting incisor teeth by attaching auxiliary apron springs of 0·3–0·4-mm. wire to a high labial

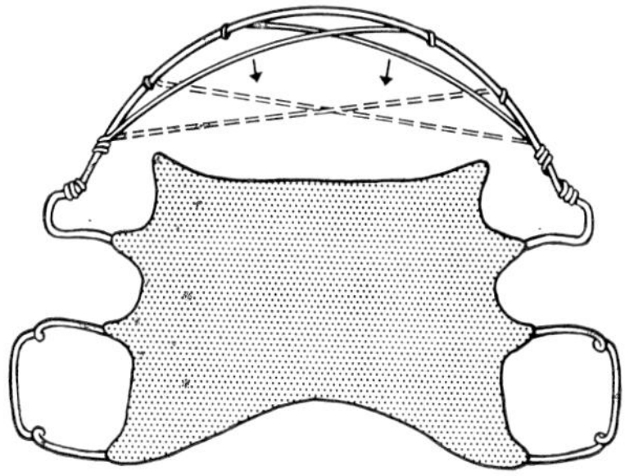

Fig. 122.—Attachment of fine self-straightening 0·3-mm. wire to a labial bow to retract incisors. One end is fixed and the other freely sliding.

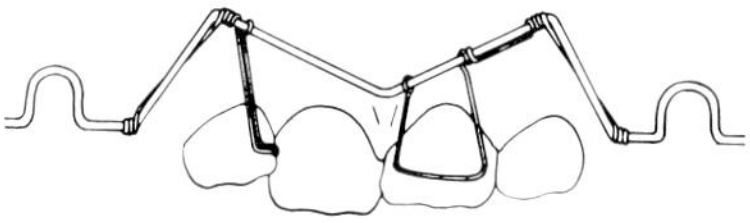

A

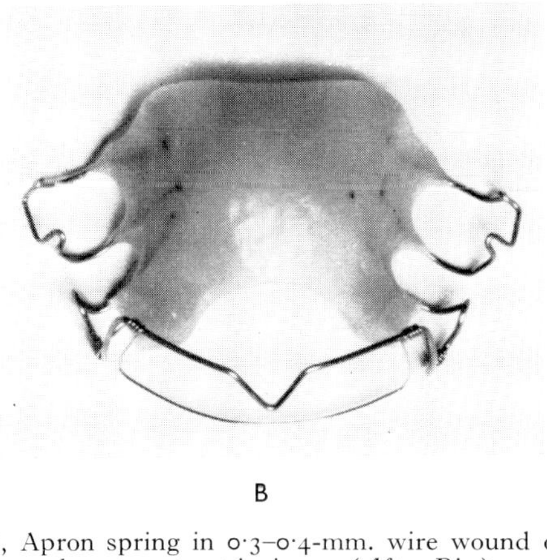

B

Fig. 123.—A, B, Apron spring in 0·3–0·4-mm. wire wound on high labial bow to retract incisors. (*After Rix.*)

bow. Such aprons, if wound in fine wire, can be constructed to act on individual teeth or a group of teeth. These are relatively inconspicuous, but the length of the fine wire renders it liable to distortion. It is possible to use a heavy-gauge flap apron—0·7 mm.—which is activated by 0·3–0·35-mm. springs.

Fig. 124 illustrates a 'T' spring used in conjunction with a band and hook for effecting rotation of incisor teeth.

Rotation of a single tooth can also be obtained by using a 'whip' (*Fig.* 125). This is a small auxiliary spring attached to a band and can

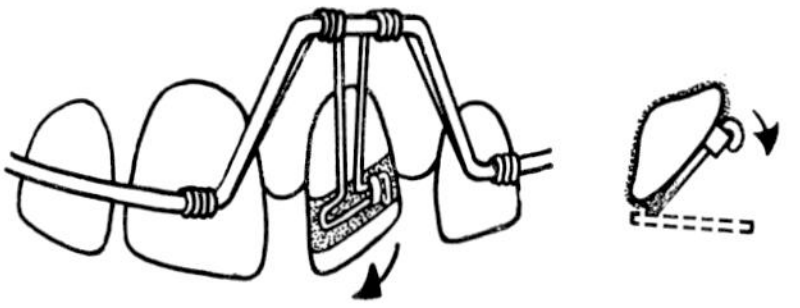

Fig. 124.—'T' spring from high labial bow in a 0·3-mm. wire incisor. The tooth is banded and has a hook soldered or welded on to the instanding corner. Torque is applied to fix arm of 'T' under hook. (*After Rix.*)

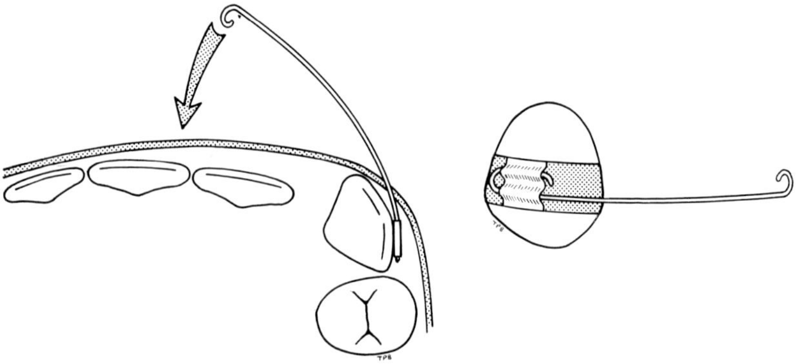

Fig. 125.—The 'whip' appliance incorporating a band on the canine in 0·35-mm. wire which is hooked under the labial bow of the removable appliance. As the wire attempts to straighten, the desired rotational movements occur. (*After Smythe and Friel.*)

be used in the incisor, canine, or premolar regions. The end is adapted to clip over the labial arch of a removable appliance and in returning to its undeformed state a torquing effect is produced. It is surprising how patients will tolerate this type of spring, but it is to be used with caution because it is liable to be extremely traumatic if the removable appliance is broken for any reason. It may produce undesirable root torquing effects. However, it does ensure that the patient wears the appliance most of the time.

2. Elastics.—These have the disadvantage that their range of activity is not as readily controlled as that of spring wires. Anterior teeth may be retracted by using an elastic band attached to hooks on a removable appliance.

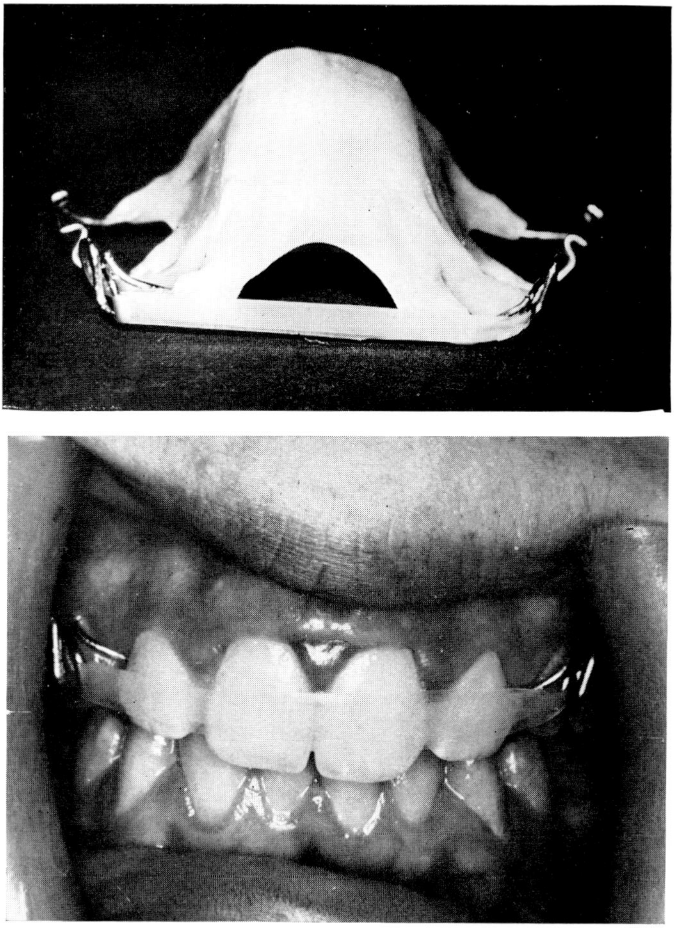

A

B

Fig. 126.—A, Rubber band cut from Paul's tubing attached to adjustable buccal hooks as described by Walther. B, Note trauma to interdental papilla where the elastic has slipped up. It should be adjusted to lie about $\frac{1}{2}$ in. from the incisal edge.

Walther has described the use of thin latex elastic bands cut from varying widths of Paul's tubing (surgical drain). This can be stretched between two buccal hooks as shown in *Fig.* 126. This material is commonly supplied in widths from $\frac{1}{2}$ in. up to $1\frac{1}{2}$ in. and sections of

$\frac{1}{8}$ in. can be cut. It has the great advantage of being almost invisible and is popular with the older patients who are not keen to show the labial arch wire and it is easily replaceable by the patient. It lies against the labial surface of the tooth and is less liable to 'ride up' than other forms of elastic band, but if the incisors are markedly proclined it is better to initiate their movement by some other form of retractor. The elastic may be controlled by a spur carried between the central incisor teeth to prevent it from moving gingivally.

Elastics may be used to give continuous traction to a labial bow which is freely sliding in tubes attached to a plate. The main difficulty with such an appliance is associated with the divergence of the tubes, which tends to foster 'binding' of the arch wire passing through them.

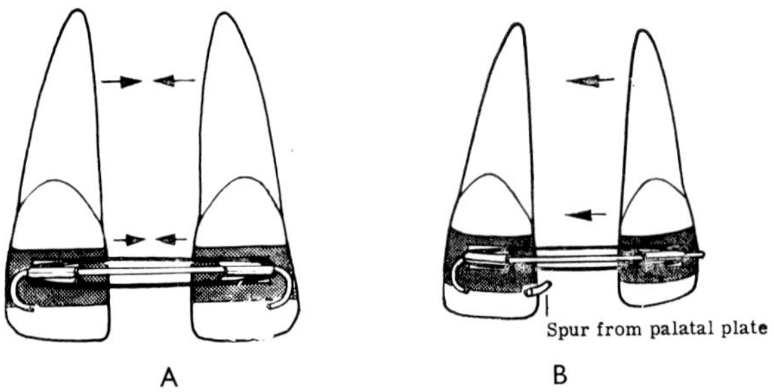

Fig. 127.—A, Local fixed appliance to approximate central incisors. Small arch in 0·7-mm. wire travelling in tubes soldered to bands and bent towards the incisal edge to prevent tilting. Traction applied by elastic. B, Central incisor controlled by spur from plate. Lateral incisor moved mesially and controlled by arch.

Elastic traction for the closure of a median diastema using a local fixed appliance is illustrated in *Fig.* 127 A. Such an appliance moves the teeth together in parallel, and a plate with a spur may be used to reinforce anchorage where all the movement is required in one tooth—as for example where a lateral incisor is being moved into the position of a missing central prior to crowning (*Fig.* 127 B).

With well-stabilized upper and lower appliances intermaxillary elastic traction may be employed either to produce changes in arch relationship or to reinforce anchorage whilst anterior teeth are retracted.

Both upper and lower appliances are well clasped so that they are adequately retained against the pull of the elastics, and designed so that they do not tip.

Traction using elastics from extra-oral anchorage can be utilized with removable appliances.

Fig. 128 A illustrates a method of using $\frac{1}{2}$-in. elastics attached to acrylic 'cheek rests' from which wire arms pass into the mouth to secure attachment to a labial bow or hooks attached to a removable appliance.

It is desirable that the direction of pull should be upwards and backwards to assist in stabilizing the appliance.

Fig. 128 B also illustrates methods of attaching wire arms to the intra-oral appliance.

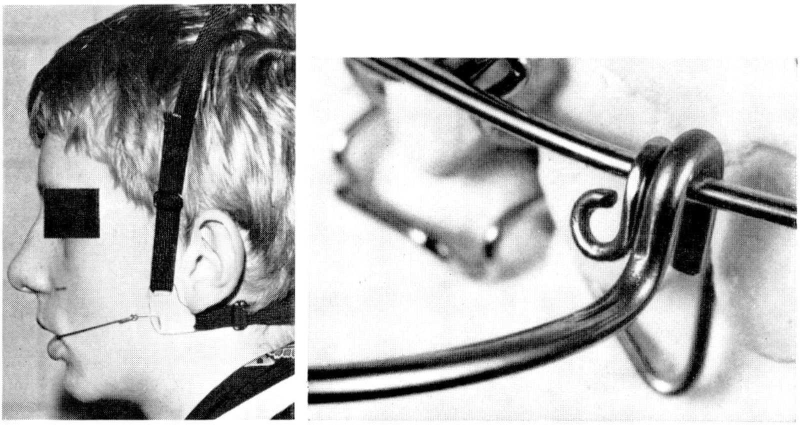

A B

Fig. 128.—A, Elastic headgear, the 'Northwestern' type, attached to intra-oral appliances by engaging hook on labial arch. B, Method of intra-oral attachment. (*By courtesy of C. P. Adams.*)

In *Fig.* 129 A the anchorage is provided by a cervical strap with hooks from which elastics pass to 'cow horns' attached to the intra-oral appliance (*Fig.* 129 B).

3. Wedging Appliances.—This is the term given to appliances whose shape or size is slightly altered from time to time so that, when fully inserted, pressure is exerted on a tooth or a group of teeth to move them in a desired direction. Expansion screws are usually the means of changing the size or shape.

Fig. 130 A, B, C illustrates a screw and shows how one can be cut down in size, where space is restricted, without a significant reduction in the stability.

An exhaustive investigation into orthodontic screws was carried out by Haynes, who examined various patterns, including those illustrated in *Fig.* 131.

Each of these screws moves 0·2 mm. per quarter-turn and it is suggested that activation should not exceed one quarter-turn per week. There is probably little to choose between the various types where

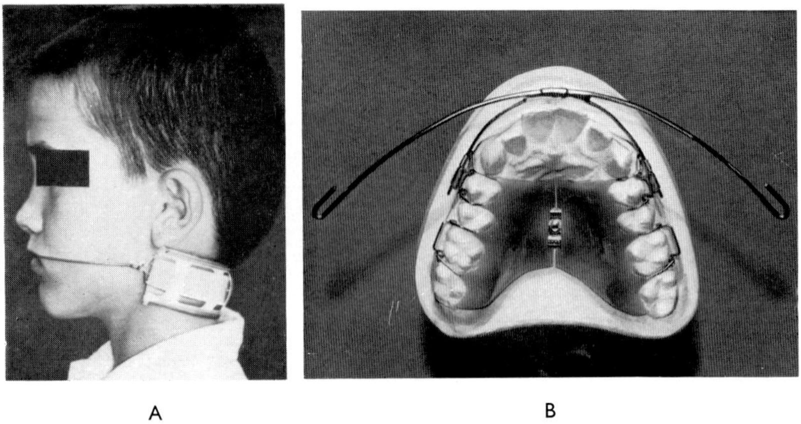

Fig. 129.—A, Cervical anchorage. 1-in. elastic cervical strap with adjusting buckle and hooks which can be attached to B, a cow-horn type of bow which is soldered to the intra-oral bow. This same type of bow can be used with webbing headgear and elastics. (*By courtesy of C. P. Adams.*)

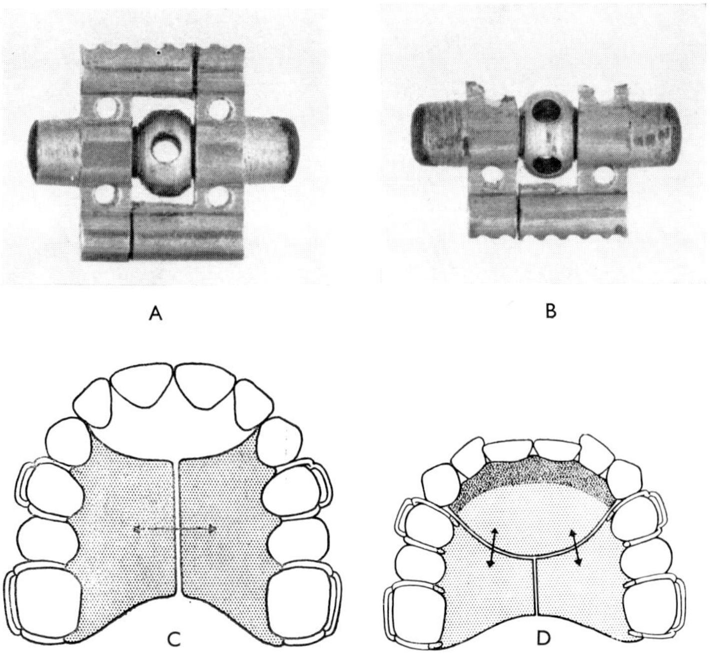

Fig. 130.—A, Glenross screw. B, Screw with one stabilizing arm removed to reduce bulk (rough edges assist retention in acrylic). (*By kind permission of Glenross Ltd., London.*) C, Siting of expansion screw in plate which is well clasped. D, Twin screws used to move buccal segments distally.

little expansion is required, but where a longer traverse is needed the screw remains stable for 6 mm. but its length precludes its use in a confined space.

Whenever screws are incorporated in an appliance it is advisable to carve an arrow into the surface of the acrylic to indicate the direction in which the screw should be turned.

In a simple upper expansion plate to produce lateral expansion of the upper dental arch, the screw is placed in the deepest part of the palate, usually in the centre, approximately between the premolar teeth. The appliance must be well clasped so that the full effect of the screw is transmitted to the dental arches. After each adjustment, the plate must be well thrust home and worn continuously.

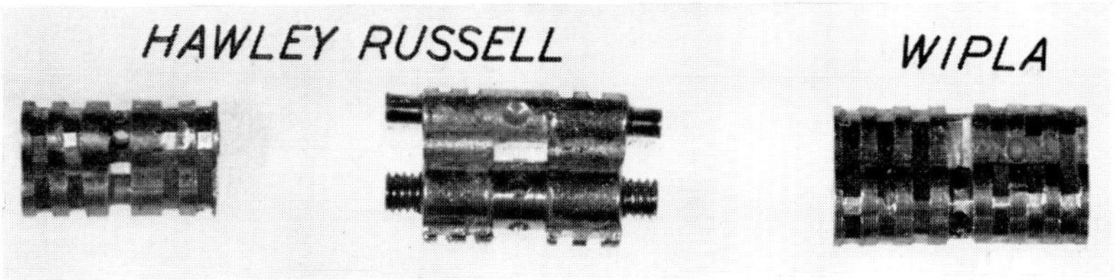

Fig. 131.—Some orthodontic screws which are available. (*By courtesy of S. Haynes and the 'Dental Practitioner'.*)

4. Appliances which rely on Muscular Activities for their Function.—These are sometimes referred to as 'functional appliances'. This is a term used to describe appliances which rely on the functional movements of the jaws, lips, or tongue for their activation. The origin of the term 'functional appliances' came from the European literature and suggested that these appliances brought about the stimulus to growth but there is no scientific proof of this. It is convenient to divide these appliances into those that act merely by virtue of forces of occlusion and the more elaborate type described in the literature under the heading of 'functional jaw orthopaedics'.

APPLIANCES WHICH ARE PRIMARILY ACTIVATED BY FORCES OF OCCLUSION.—

a. Displacement Appliances.—This is the term given to those appliances which are modified so that occlusal forces are necessary to bite them into position and, in so doing, induce a particular tooth movement.

Teeth may be moved by adding quick-curing plastic to the plate in a position where it will press on the palatal surface of the incisor. There is a biting surface so that in attempting to gain occlusion the plate will be 'bitten in'.

The same purpose can be achieved by inserting into the plate a rubber bung or a threaded rod which can be extended from time to time.

Such an appliance, though simple, tends to be uncomfortable and cumbersome and may be rather traumatic in action; the principle is still used on occasions but has been largely superseded.

b. Bite Planes.—The anterior part of an upper appliance may be thickened for three reasons:—

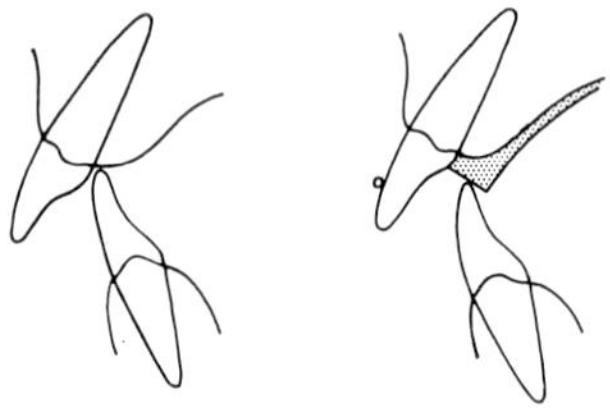

Fig. 132.—Anterior inclined bite plane used to reduce overbite and to reinforce anchorage.

i. As a stage in treatment leading to a reduction in overbite.
ii. To prop the bite temporarily and relieve occlusal interference during a particular tooth movement.
iii. To reinforce anchorage in the upper arch.

i. *Reducing overbite*: *Fig.* 132 illustrates a Class II, division 1 incisor relationship and the use of an anterior inclined biting surface.

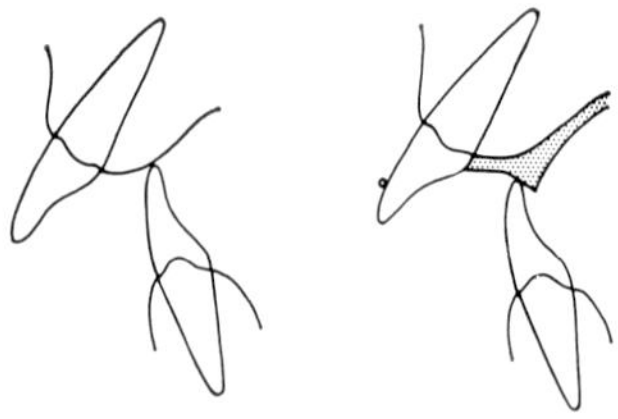

Fig. 133.—Type of bite plane when there is an extreme overjet to prevent undue bulkiness of the plate.

Such an appliance needs care in design, for if the incline is too bulky it will not be worn consistently. *Fig.* 133 illustrates a form of biting surface where there is a marked overjet.

If such an appliance is worn consistently, particularly at meal times, a differential rate of occlusal rise of the anterior and posterior teeth is induced, so that in effect the anterior teeth do not erupt further, whilst the posterior teeth erupt until they come into occlusion. It is probable that there is no actual depression of the lower incisors, but further eruption of these already over-erupted teeth is prevented.

Such an appliance does not effect a permanent reduction in overbite unless incisor positions can also be adjusted so that satisfactory contact is established between the tips of the lowers and the cingulae of the uppers.

ii. *Bite propping*: A flat anterior biting surface may be used as a temporary prop for the bite whilst an individual tooth movement is being carried out (*Fig.* 134). Occasionally the acrylic of the appliance may be carried over the occlusal surfaces of the posterior teeth. As a

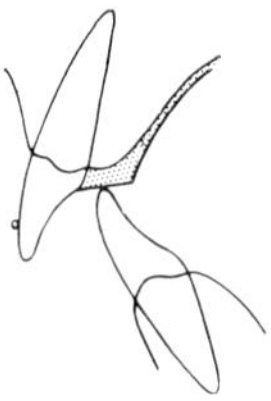

Fig. 134.—Flat anterior biting surface used as a temporary prop for the bite.

temporary measure during treatment it may lead to some depression of the posterior teeth, or over-eruption of the anterior teeth.

iii. *Anchorage reinforcement*: The use of an inclined plane to reinforce anchorage and to prevent forward thrust on the upper labial segment is questionable. If the labial bow is set near the incisal edge of the upper incisors and the plate fits closely to the cingulum as shown

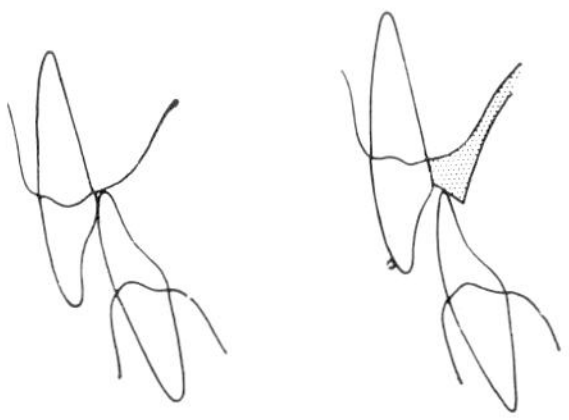

Fig. 135.—Very steep inclined plane used in cases of deep overbite and particularly to reinforce anchorage when teeth are being moved distally. Note position of labial bow.

in *Fig.* 135, this does seem to have a 'splinting' effect on the upper labial segment when teeth in the buccal segment are moved distally. The theory is that the incisors are gripped between the bow and the palatal acrylic and offer more resistance to forward movement as they could only move bodily. Although it has been said that the forces acting on the appliance when the lower incisors occlude with the appliance produce some distal component of thrust, there is no scientific evidence to support this. It is also questionable whether an anterior inclined bite plane produces any untoward proclination of lower incisors.

'FUNCTIONAL' APPLIANCES.—There are a number of appliances, some of which are quite complex. These are collectively referred to as 'activators' in the literature. In the authors' opinion these appliances act by harnessing certain muscle forces to produce tooth movement within the alveolar process and do not have any basic effect on skeletal development.

The Monobloc.—This is a combined upper and lower plate used as a loose interdental splint, and was first described by Robin. It has been modified in many ways by Haupl and Andresen and many others (*see* p. 210). The most important feature in construction is the wax bite. The position in which the bite is taken will depend upon the proposed function of the appliance. It is taken with the posterior teeth apart so that they are separated by a little more than the estimated freeway space or interocclusal clearance at rest. In Class II, division 1 malocclusion the mandible is postured forward to a normal cheek tooth relationship (*see* Chapter XI). *Fig.* 136 illustrates the construction.

The models are mounted backwards on a straight line articulator or in a plaster box 'articulator' with the wax bite to facilitate waxing up.

The lower model has all its lingual undercuts plastered out, and wax plates are constructed on both upper and lower models.

A labial bow in 0·8-mm. wire is constructed as shown and taken into the palatal section about half-way between the occlusal surfaces of the upper and lower teeth just distal to the upper canines.

Small wires may be incorporated in the plate to make a more precise contact mesial to the upper canines. The 'bloc' is waxed up so that half of the occlusal surfaces of the posterior teeth are covered. The models are removed from the articulator and cut down to facilitate embedding in a flask.

After processing and polishing the 'bloc' is tried in the mouth prior to any trimming.

It was originally thought that the appliance stimulated jaw growth by increasing muscular function—hence the term 'Activator'. Some authorities still believe that the mandible can take up a forward position and that a definite change takes place in the temporomandibular articulation. There is no scientific evidence for these beliefs, but the following explanations seem most likely:—

With the appliance fitting loosely in the mouth, the mandible is held in a forward position at rest. The muscles of mastication which produce elevation and retraction of the mandible are slightly stretched beyond their normal resting state. They are therefore in a constant

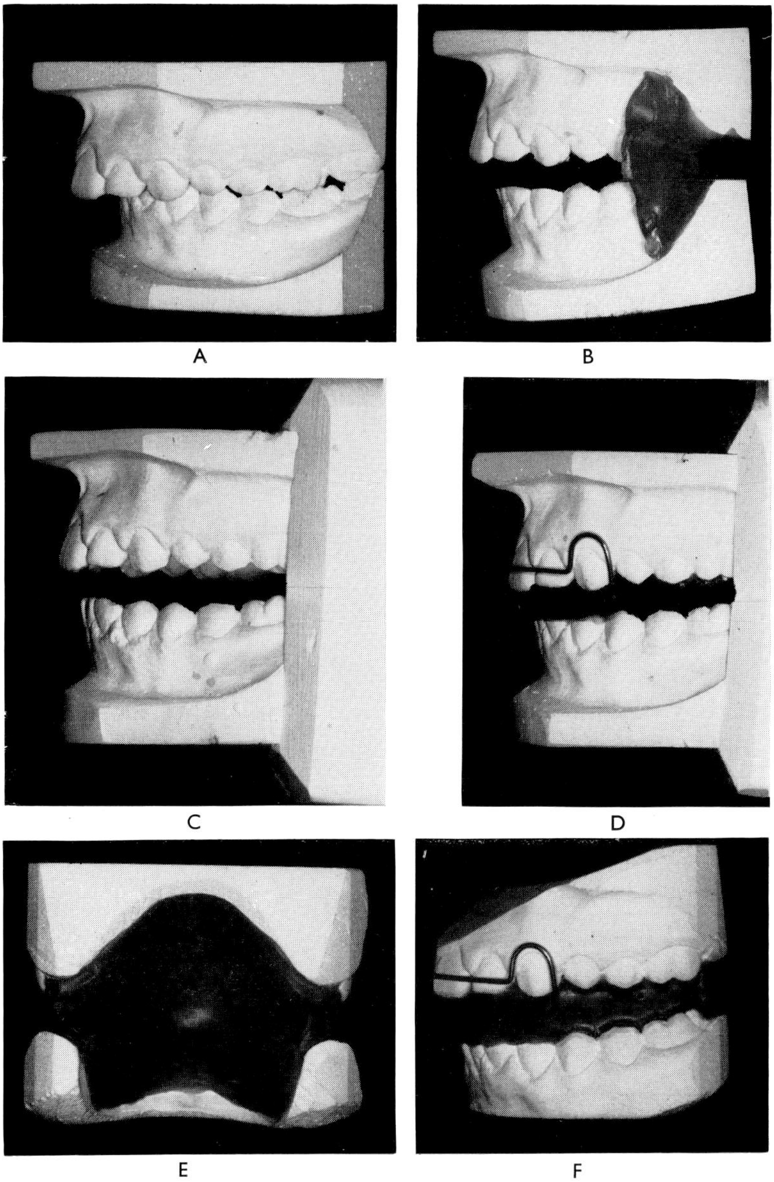

Fig. 136.—Processes in the construction of the 'Monobloc'. A, Models of Class II, division 1 malocclusion. B, Models articulated to forward working bite with posterior parts 'waxed out' prior to casting plaster-box articulator. C, Models without bite located in plaster articulator. D, Labial bow in 0·8–0·9-mm. wire after 'waxing up' of individual arches. E, Posterior view of completed 'wax up' stage with upper and lower elements fused. F, Models cut down for flasking.

state of activity, in addition to that normally required to maintain the resting posture of the mandible. Electromyographic records show increased motor unit activity.

Whenever the plate is bitten into place, during idle movements and swallowing, quite considerable forces act as the teeth clamp down on the appliance, and considerable muscle pull is exerted in an upward and backward direction. Thus the appliance acts as a complex bite plate allowing occlusal rise of cheek teeth but preventing lower incisors from continuous eruption.

The appliance is therefore producing an effect similar to inter-maxillary traction using elastic bands. A distal thrust is exerted on all upper teeth. There is a tendency for the lower arch to move reciprocally forward.

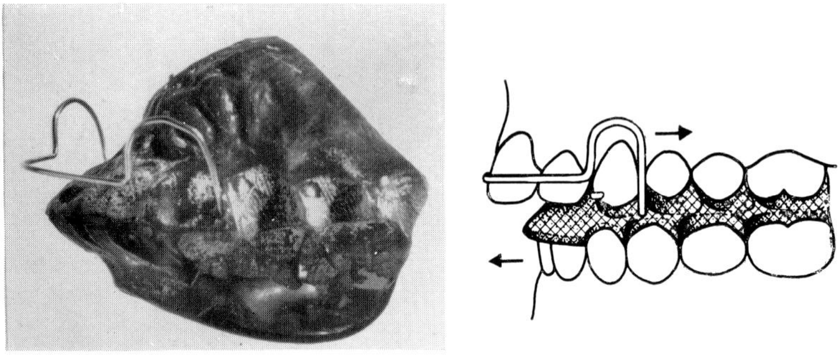

Fig. 137.—Shows how thrust is exerted on upper and lower teeth.

The distal drag on the upper arch with the buccal segments moving into a wider part of the arch is a movement which is highly desirable. The reciprocal forward movement of the lower arch can be minimized by splinting the lower incisor teeth together. This will be described in the details of appliance construction and design.

The upper arch is therefore moved distally and/or restrained from downward and forward development. A considerable amount of mandibular growth has been demonstrated by some authorities, but this can be found in cases which are untreated and should not be construed as being caused by the appliances.

Fig. 137 illustrates the forces exerted on upper and lower teeth in a Class II case, and it may be that much of the effect is a prevention of downward and forward movement of upper teeth with facial growth.

This appliance is worn principally during the night and for at least an hour before bedtime. Patients should be warned that it may come out during the night at first, but they should persevere.

It may cause some difficulty and embarrassment to breathing if there is a persistent nasal catarrh. Rix has shown that these appliances will work if a 'window' is cut in the anterior portion of the appliance and it is then more readily accepted by children who have some degree of upper respiratory obstruction (*Fig.* 138). Further details of the use of this appliance in the treatment of Class II, division 1 malocclusion will be found on p. 210.

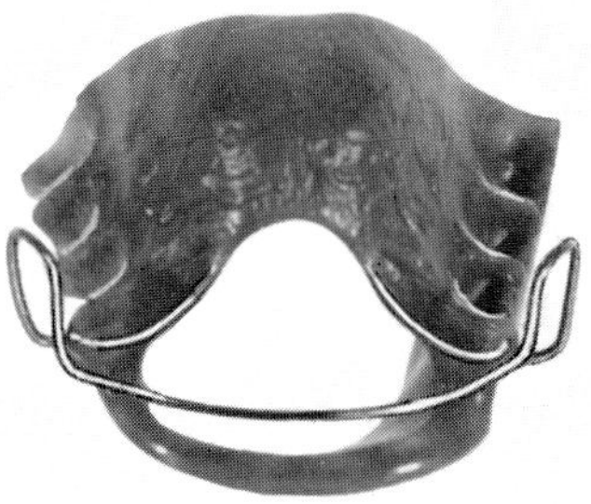

Fig. 138.—Half-moon shaped window. Base line formed by capping over the lower fronts, sides limited by boxed-in canine wires. Left side of bloc untrimmed. (*By courtesy of R. E. Rix and the 'Dental Practitioner'*.)

The Bimmler Appliance.—This is a form of monobloc or activator with a wire framework but with approximately the same features and method of function. Because it is less bulky it is intended for full-time wear. There are many modifications of this appliance with various adjustments to produce local tooth movement. Reference to details of such an appliance should be obtained from relevant texts.

The Frankel Appliance.—A more recent addition to the literature of functional jaw orthopaedics has been put forward by Dr. Frankel of Leipzig. The appliance is again constructed with a skeleton of stainless-steel wire with certain active and passive elements. It would appear to have some of the properties of the activator in treatment of horizontal muscle forces but, at the same time, it is intended to remove adverse pressures of lips, cheeks, and tongue by acrylic guards. The reader is referred to the BIBLIOGRAPHY for details.

The Propulsor.—This appliance has had a number of names given to it. It was first described by Muhlemann of Zürich and there is also another similar form of apparatus known as the 'Kinetor', used by Stockfish. There are a number of these appliances made to a forward working bite and containing labial and lingual elements which come under the general heading of FUNCTIONAL APPLIANCES. *See* BIBLIOGRAPHY.

The Oral Screen.—This simple appliance illustrated in *Fig.* 139 has been used for many years in the field of periodontology to fit into

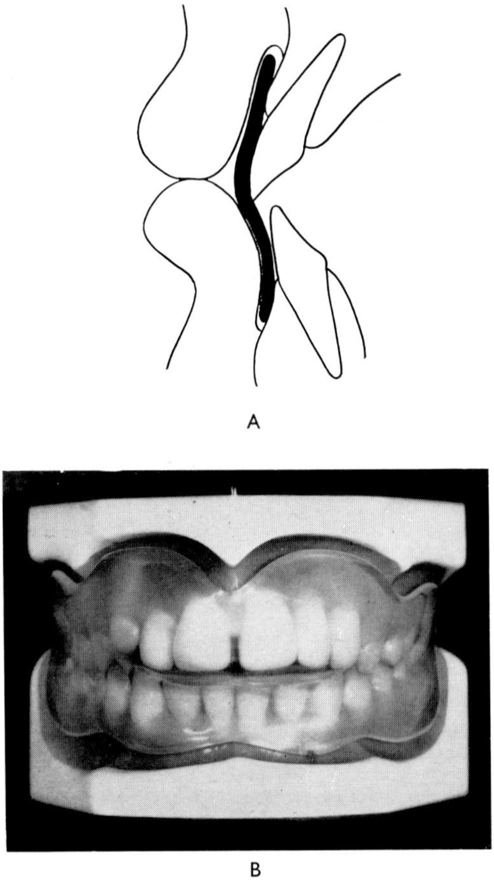

Fig. 139.—A, Diagram to show oral screen in place in labial sulcus. Pressure is exerted against labial surfaces of the upper incisors as the appliance is constructed on a model where the labial surfaces of these incisors have been scraped away. B, Oral screen mounted on models. (*After Walther.*)

the labial vestibule to protect exposed gingivae in those cases with lip incompetence. It has been used, however, by orthodontists as a retention device by applying local pressure to the upper incisors but, as will be seen in Chapter XI, once the upper incisors have been brought within the control of the lower lip, prolonged retention is unnecessary.

Some operators still use this appliance for active retraction of upper incisors where there is an increased overjet, but this should only take place as part of a full course of treatment, which may well have involved upper premolar extractions, and in the authors' opinion is rarely the appliance of choice. In order to obtain pressure on specific teeth the labial surfaces of the upper incisors have to be reduced on the plaster model prior to construction of the appliance.

Choice of Apparatus.—Most malocclusions can be treated satisfactorily with removable apparatus, and various forms of simple fixed appliance are described in the chapters on treatment.

In some orthodontic circles, there is a tendency to look upon removable appliance therapy as 'the easy way out'. However, subtle mechanical principles can be used to reinforce anchorage and a knowledge of the natural drift of teeth following extractions can produce results which, in the late teens, compare very favourably with those obtained by complex fixed apparatus. Probably the reason why removable appliances have been used to a greater extent in the British Isles and in some parts of Europe is because tooth movements required are primarily those of tilting teeth back into a specific position as the dental bases are often small and both in cases of crowding and Class II there has been a mesial movement of the crowns in relation to the apices.

To base one's entire armamentarium solely on removable apparatus would be as biased as those who maintain that all movements should be carried out with banded appliances. There are many excellent textbooks describing multi-banded techniques in detail and, therefore, this aspect has not been included here.

The advantages and disadvantages of removable and fixed appliances are now summarized:—

Advantages of Removable Appliances.—

1. Generally simple in construction.
2. Require little surgery time for fitting and adjustment.
3. Can be easily repaired and modified.
4. If the activating mechanism becomes disturbed the plate can be left out by the patient before there is any significant damage.
5. The plate can be removed for cleaning, enabling the teeth to be carefully brushed.
6. With careful design, the appliance need not be aesthetically displeasing.
7. Some forms of functional appliance need only be worn during the evening and at night-time.

8. They are capable of carrying out most tooth movements. Although these movements are of a tilting nature, with small apical bases this is the most common type of movement which is required to re-position teeth.

Disadvantages of Removable Appliances.—

1. The active co-operation of the patient is required if the appliance is to be worn regularly and properly replaced after cleaning.

2. However well-designed, they do occupy a certain amount of space. Separate upper and lower removable appliances are not well accepted.

3. It is very difficult to move teeth bodily or apply root torque.

Advantages of Fixed Appliances.—

1. They do not rely on the active co-operation of the patient.

2. Multiple tooth movement may be carried out with the same appliance.

3. They are particularly useful in the lower dental arch, being less bulky and more precise in their action on the lower incisors.

4. They may reduce the length of active treatment.

Disadvantages of Fixed Appliances.—

1. Multi-banded appliances require considerable surgery time for fitting and adjustment.

2. Repairs may be time-consuming.

3. If they become distorted, they can have untoward effects before the patient is able to return for adjustment.

4. They cannot be removed to enable the teeth and gingival tissues to be thoroughly cleaned.

BIBLIOGRAPHY

ADAMS, C. P. (1964), *The Design and Construction of Removable Orthodontic Appliances*, 3rd ed. Bristol: John Wright.

ANDRESEN, V., HAUPL, and PETRIK, L. (1953), *Funktionskieferorthopädie*. Munich: Barth.

BASS, T. P., and STEPHENS, C. D. (1970), 'Some Experiments with Orthodontic Springs', *Dent. Pract.*, in press.

BIMLER, H. P. (1956), 'Vom Wesen der funktionellen Therapie', *Fortschr. Kieferorthop.*, **17**, 138.

CASELEY, R. (1947), 'The Principles and Construction of an Oral Screen as a Functional Appliance', *Trans. Brit. Soc. Orthodont.*, 81.

DICKSON, G. C., GROSSMANN, W., and MILLS, J. R. E. (1965), 'Symposium on Functional Therapy', *Dent. Practit.*, **15**, 255.

ENDICOTT, C. L., PEDLEY, V. G., and GROSSMAN, W. (1947), 'Symposium on Practical and Theoretical Observations on the Norwegian System', *Ibid.*, 31.

ESCHLER, J. (1953), *Die funktionelle Orthopädie des Kausustems*. Munich: Carl Hanser Verlag.

FRANKEL, R. (1967), *Funktionskieferorthopädie und der Mundvorhof als apparative Basis*. Berlin: Verlag Volk und Gesundheit.

FRIEL, E. S. (1933), 'The Practical Application of Stainless Steel in the Construction of Fixed Orthodontic Appliances', *Dent. Rec.*, **53**, 322.

HAYNES, S. (1962), 'A Comparison of the Mechanics and Efficiency of 21 Orthodontic Screws', *Trans. Brit. Soc. Orthodont.*, 41.

HOTZ, R. (1961), *Orthodontie in der taglichen Praxis*. Berne and Stuttgart: Medizinischer Verlag H. Huber.

MCCALLIN, S. G. (1954), 'Retraction of Maxillary Teeth with Removable Appliances using Intermaxillary or Extra Oral Traction', *Dent. Rec.*, **74**, 36.

MCKEAG, H. T. A. (1935), 'The Teaching of Appliance Design in Orthodontia', *Trans. Brit. Soc. Orthodont.*, 260.

MILLS, J. R. E. (1956), 'Modifications of Standard Orthodontic Appliances', *Ibid.*, 131.

REITAN, K. (1951), 'The Initial Tissue Reaction Incident to Orthodontic Tooth Movement', *Acta odont. scan.*, Supplement 6.

— — (1958), 'Experiments on Rotation of Teeth and their Subsequent Retention', *Trans. europ. orthod. Soc.*, 124.

RIX, R. E. (1938), 'Some Useful Orthodontic Appliances', *Brit. dent. J.*, **64**, 13.

ROBIN, P. (1902), 'Demonstration pratique sur la construction et la mise en bouche d'un nouvel appareil de redressement', *Rev. Stomat., Paris*, **9**, 561.

CHAPTER X

TREATMENT OF ANGLE'S CLASS I MALOCCLUSIONS

THE term 'Class I malocclusion' embraces all occlusal abnormalities with the exception of those which have an abnormal anteroposterior arch relationship.

In this chapter it is proposed to deal strictly with Class I malocclusions with one or more of the following: (1) Crowding (outstanding, instanding, or rotated teeth). (2) Spacing. (3) Disturbances in radial relationship of the dental arches where there is an abnormal buccolingual relationship of the cheek teeth or labiolingual relationship of the incisors. (4) Abnormalities in the vertical relationship of the anterior teeth (open bite and deep overbite). (5) Disturbances in the vertical relationship of the posterior teeth (lateral open bite).

All these abnormalities may also be found where there is a Class II or Class III arch relationship, and the treatment of these cases will be dealt with in subsequent chapters.

1. CROWDING

It has been pointed out in Chapter VIII that where crowding occurs the dental bases may be too small to accommodate all the teeth. The soft tissues surrounding the dentition may also restrict the full development of the dental arches. Where there has been no premature loss of deciduous cheek teeth, the crowding is mainly confined to the incisor region.

Premature loss of deciduous cheek teeth may completely or partially relieve incisor crowding at the expense of premolar or canine alinement. Crowding is usually due to anteroposterior shortness of the dental base rather than lack of lateral development of the arches. **Lateral expansion of both upper and lower arches for the relief of crowding places teeth in an unstable relationship to their muscular environment and they will inevitably relapse.**

Extractions to relieve crowding in Class I cases have been fully described in Chapter VIII. The method of serial extractions, which entails a planned extraction of the deciduous canines followed by planned extractions in the permanent dentition, may lead to natural alinement of the incisors in some cases. Rotated, inlocked, and overlapping incisors are not self-correcting and the temporary space created by extractions may be lost by forward movement of posterior teeth. In these cases control by appliances is necessary.

In this chapter it is assumed that the need for symmetry and balancing of extractions is appreciated and the purely mechanical

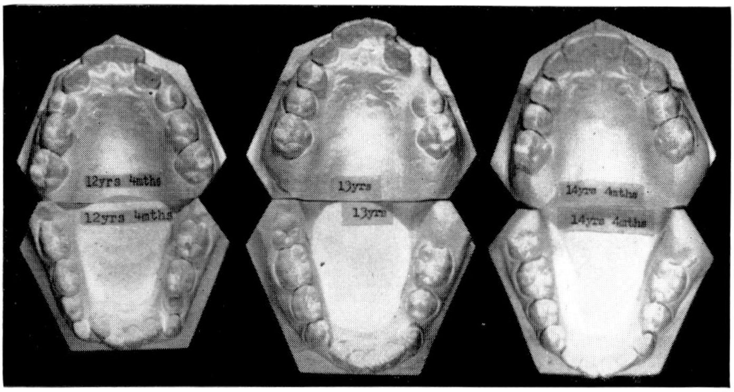

Fig. 140.—Models illustrating $|\underline{2}$ moved labially after extraction of $\left|\frac{4}{4}\right.$ and retraction of $\left|\frac{3}{3}\right.$.

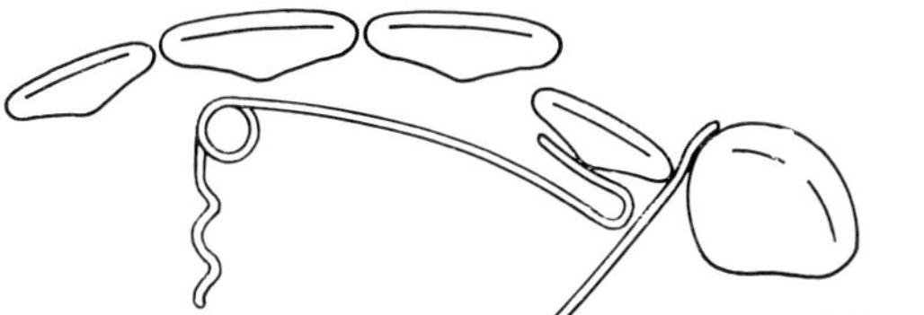

Fig. 141.—Recurved finger spring to push a tooth buccally or labially. The arm should be as long as possible and the recurved portion enables adjustment to be made in direction.

procedures are described for the alinement of instanding, outstanding, and rotated teeth.

Incisor Crowding.—Incisors may be crowded inside or outside the line of the arch. Where only one tooth is displaced in this way the centre line is towards that side. The single instanding upper incisor *associated with crowding* cannot be corrected with the use of the tongue spatula as described in Chapter VII. *Figs.* 140 and 141 show a case where the upper lateral incisor is trapped inside the bite, and also the appliance to effect alinement following premolar extraction and distal movement of the upper canine.

Incisors crowded *outside* the line of the arch are readily alined with a labial bow or fine wire springs from a high labial bow after sufficient space has been provided (*Figs.* 142 and 143).

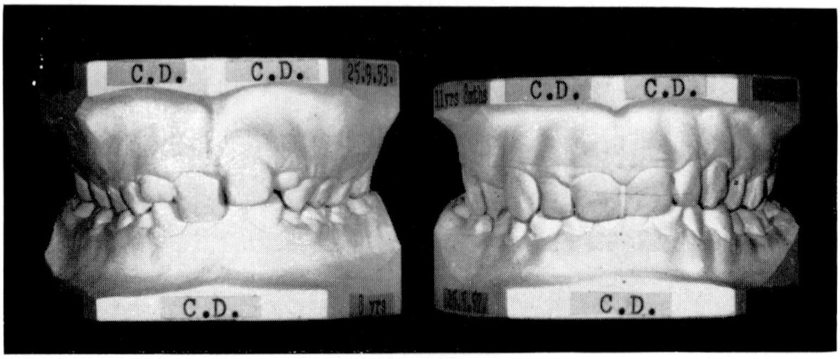

Fig. 142.—|1 outside line of arch, retracted by apron spring after space had been created.

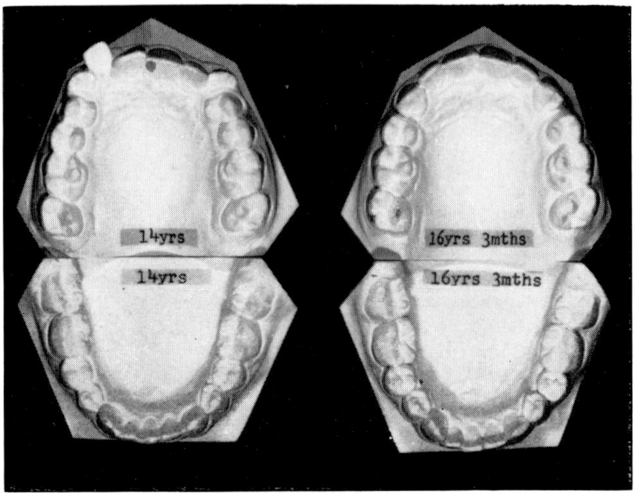

Fig. 143.—Outlocked 2| retracted after extraction of 4|4 and retraction of 3|3.

Rotations.—Many forms of apparatus are available to correct incisor rotations once sufficient space has been provided for their alinement. The simplest consists of a removable appliance with a labial bow and a spring on the palatal aspect, if necessary, to apply pressure to instanding corners of the crown. The application of these forces can be varied, depending upon the relationship of the crown of the incisor to the line of arch.

Thus, as in *Fig.* 144 A, B, if the axis of the incisor is in the line of arch, pressure can be applied both from a labial bow and from the

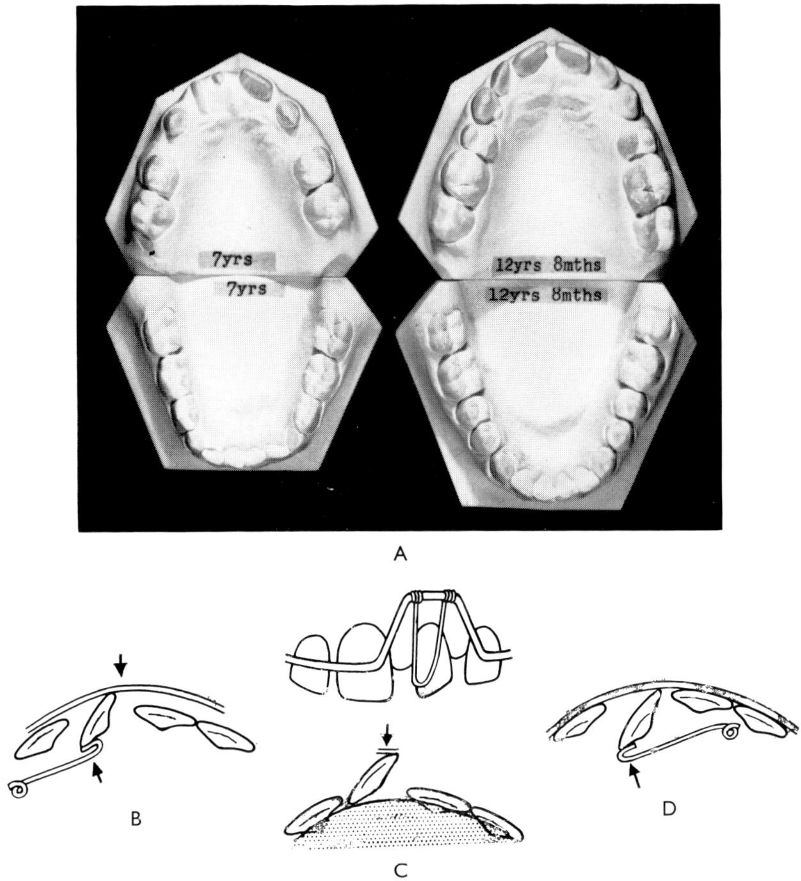

Fig. 144.—A, Models showing rotation of $\underline{1|}$ with removable appliance after removal of supernumerary tooth. B, Case where the axis of the incisor is in the line of the arch. C, Case where the axis of the incisor is outside the line of the arch. D, Case where the axis of the incisor is inside the line of the arch.

palatal spring. If the tooth is situated outside the line of the arch (*Fig.* 144 C), the instanding corner can be controlled by the appliance and pressure applied to the outstanding corner by the labial bow, or apron spring from a high labial bow. If it is related to the line of the arch, as in *Fig.* 144 D, the outstanding corner can be controlled by the bow without active pressure, and the spring is the active element.

Upper lateral incisors may be rotated by similar apparatus, but the mesiodistal flattening of the root in cross-section makes the rotation more difficult to correct, and *Fig.* 145 illustrates a more efficient

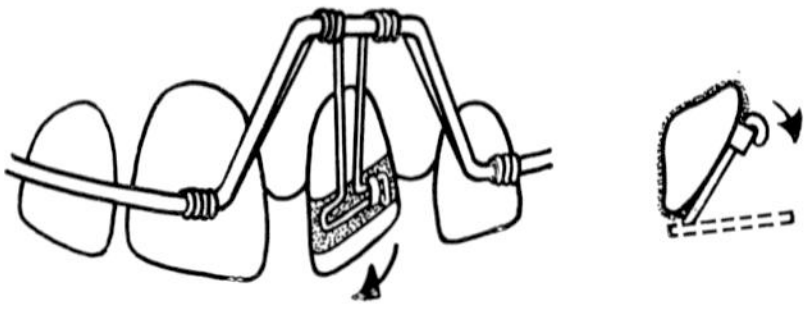

Fig. 145.—'T' spring from high labial bow in a 0·3-mm. wire. The incisor tooth is banded and has a hook soldered or welded on to the instanding corner. Torque is applied to fix arm of 'T' under hook.

mechanism which can be used with a removable appliance. A band carrying a hook is placed on the incisor.

Where all four incisors in the upper arch are rotated, the use of a labial bow to contact the outstanding corners and an 'S' spring on the palatal side to contact the instanding corners can provide a

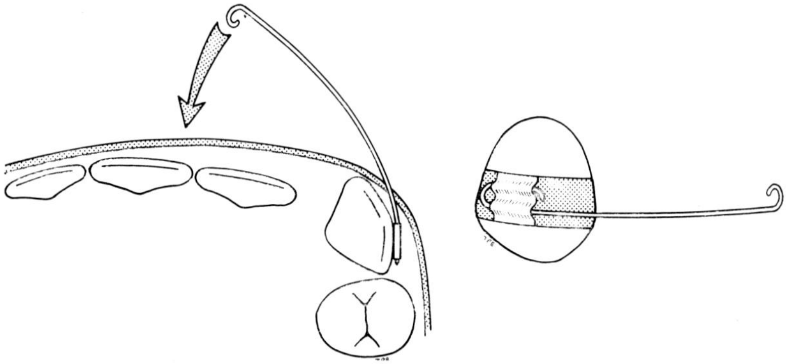

Fig. 146.—The 'whip' appliance incorporating a band on the canine in 0·35-mm. wire which is hooked under the labial bow of the removable appliance. As the wire attempts to straighten, the desired rotational movements occur.

satisfactory result. Another method of using a combined fixed and removable appliance to carry out rotation has been described in Chapter IX using a 'whip' (*Fig.* 146).

Rotation of lower incisors is not uncommon. They are not easily corrected with simple apparatus owing to lack of crown width which makes the application of torque difficult. Once space is made available for alinement the same principles of treatment apply as for upper incisors, although the placing of small lingual springs to apply counter pressures is more difficult. Multiple incisor rotations are more readily effected with fixed apparatus.

It is advisable to overcorrect all rotations, and to follow active treatment immediately with a retaining plate. This should have a bow to contact the labial surfaces, and the acrylic accurately fitting the lingual or palatal surfaces. This appliance must be worn continuously for a period of months whilst the supporting tissues adapt. Reitan has shown that residual torsion exists in the marginal free fibres of the periodontal tissues for many months. There is a great tendency to relapse, particularly where it has been difficult to obtain sufficient space for the alinement. *Fig.* 147 shows how a band can be fitted to the rotated tooth with soldered spurs mesially and distally to retain the tooth in its overcorrected position.

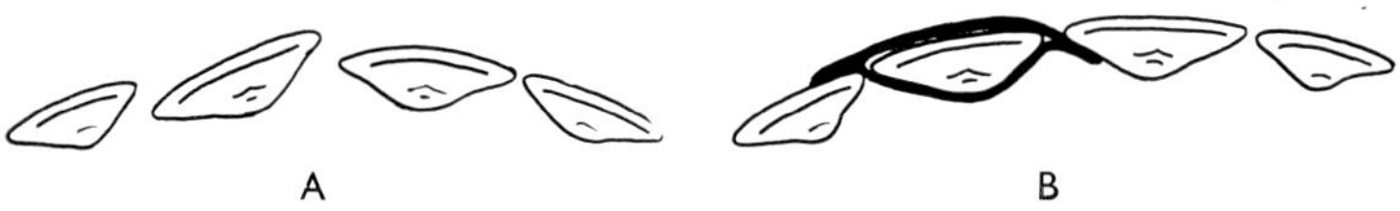

Fig. 147.—A, Rotation of $\underline{1}|$. B, After rotation a band with two soldered attachments mesially and distally is the best way of maintaining the tooth in a slightly overcorrected position.

Crowding in the Premolar and Canine Regions.—In both arches the canines are usually displaced buccally and the second premolars lingually or palatally. In the lower arch the first premolar may occasionally be displaced buccally. The lower second premolar may be found vertically impacted between the first premolar and the first permanent molar.

A palatally placed unerupted upper canine tooth can be associated with crowding but, as discussed in the APPENDIX, other factors must also be considered in this particular instance.

Canines Buccally Displaced.—*Fig.* 148 illustrates a case where the upper first premolar was extracted and an appliance inserted to retain the space and allow the natural alinement of the canine. In other cases the canine may have to be actively retracted. In an extreme case, as in *Fig.* 149, where the first premolar and the upper lateral incisor are in contact and the canine apex well forward, the canine itself may be extracted. The result is not aesthetically acceptable if the palatal cusp of the first premolar is visible.

In the lower arch there may be a buccal displacement of the canine or the first premolar, but the canine frequently erupts before the first premolar. Where the crowding is severe the first premolar may be

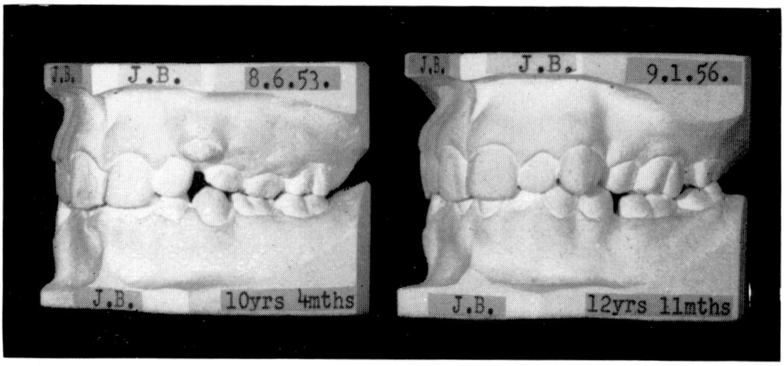

Fig. 148.—Model to show natural alinement of $|\underline{3}$ after extraction of $|\underline{4}$.

removed (*Fig.* 150) and an appliance is usually required to maintain the space and retract the canine. Occasionally where the canine already has a distal inclination and its apex is well forward, it is preferable to extract it and aline the first premolar.

Fig. 151 illustrates appliances which may be employed using buccal springs to retract the canines.

Premolar Crowding.—If apparatus is used to accommodate premolars in the lower arch, without extractions, the space is often obtained at the expense of lower incisor alinement or crowding in the molar region. Where the second premolar is displaced lingually or palatally it may be extracted, provided that the first permanent molar is of reasonable quality. Instanding premolars may move into the arch if the first permanent molars have to be extracted early. Where this movement is not complete, they can be assisted with recurved springs.

Where the second premolar is vertically impacted, the second molar may be extracted rather than resort to surgical removal of the premolar. It may not be necessary to use apparatus to move the first molar distally as a considerable thrust is exerted by the erupting premolar (*Fig.* 152 A).

The procedure is best carried out as soon after the eruption of the second molar as possible and the third molar must be present and not tilted too far mesially. The difficulties and pitfalls in the extraction of lower second molars have been described by Cryer (*see* Chapter VIII). The extraction of second molars may have been carried out to treat crowding in the upper arch, but if not, the upper second molars may over-erupt, if they are unopposed. This can be prevented by an occlusal rest extended back from an upper appliance.

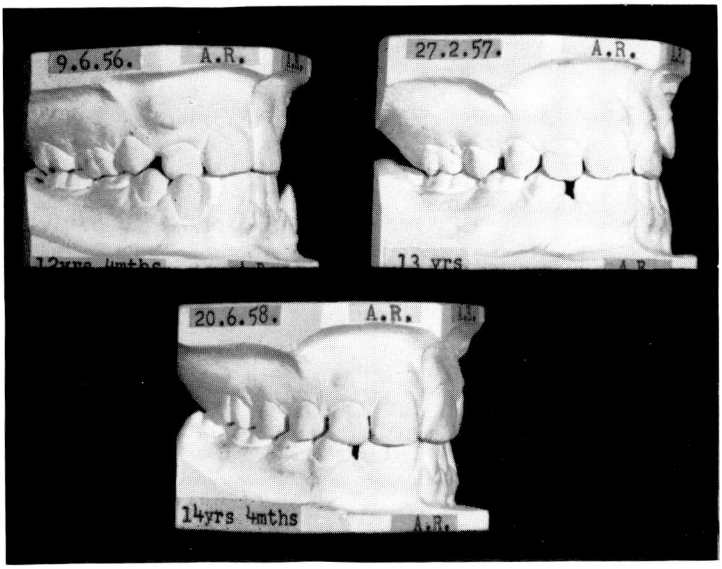

Fig. 149.—Extraction of $\frac{3}{3}|$ where they are grossly displaced.

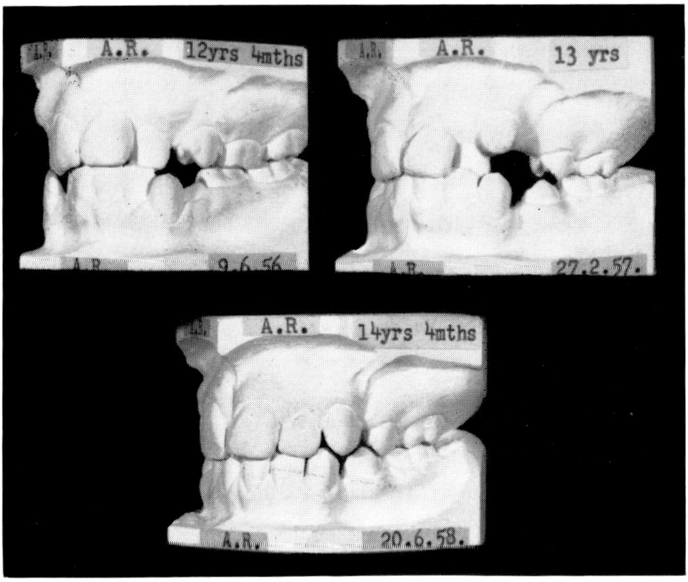

Fig. 150.—Retraction of $|\frac{3}{3}$ after extraction of $|\frac{4}{4}$.

General Arch Crowding.—The extraction of the first permanent molars in crowded arches has been discussed in Chapter VIII, p. 101. It has been shown that some spontaneous improvement in incisor and

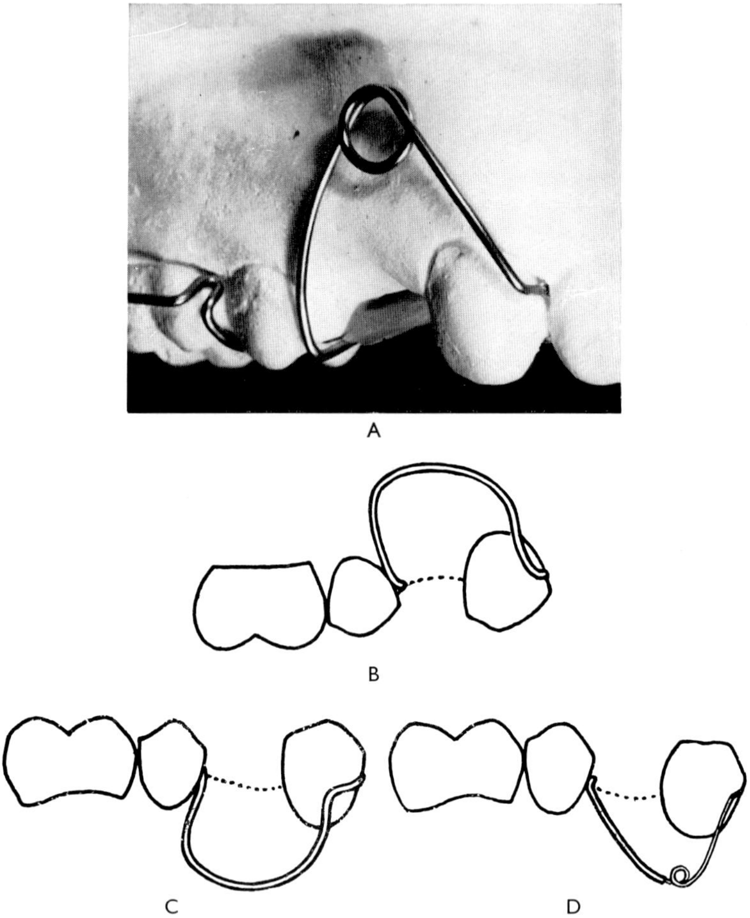

Fig. 151.—Buccal canine retractors: A, Buccal retractor with coil in 0·7-mm. wire. B, 'Fly-over' type of buccal retractor in 0·7-mm. wire. Note that the end is flattened to fit interdentally and some palatal movement can be obtained by allowing the spring to contact the buccal surfaces of the tooth. C, 'Fly-over' retractor used in lower arch. D, Buccal retractor with active portions in 0·5-mm. wire supported by tube into sulcus.

premolar alinement may be obtained provided these teeth are extracted between $8\frac{1}{2}$ and $9\frac{1}{2}$ years of age (*Fig.* 153).

In cases with severe crowding, apparatus is necessary if much of the space made available for the alinement of teeth is not to be lost by

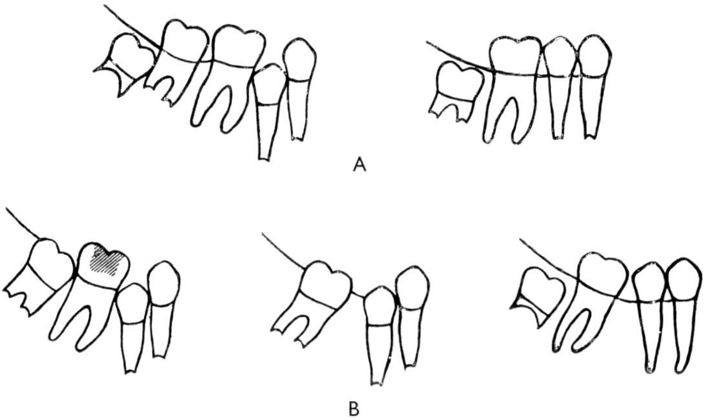

Fig. 152.—A, Tracing from X-ray showing $\overline{5}|$ reaching occlusion without appliance after extraction of $\overline{7}|$ at 13 years of age. B, Enforced extraction of $\overline{6}|$ at 11 years of age, allowing vertically impacted $\overline{5}|$ to erupt. Note that there is a tilt of the $\overline{7}|$ which occurs when the $\overline{6}|$ is extracted late, but this may improve with continued eruption.

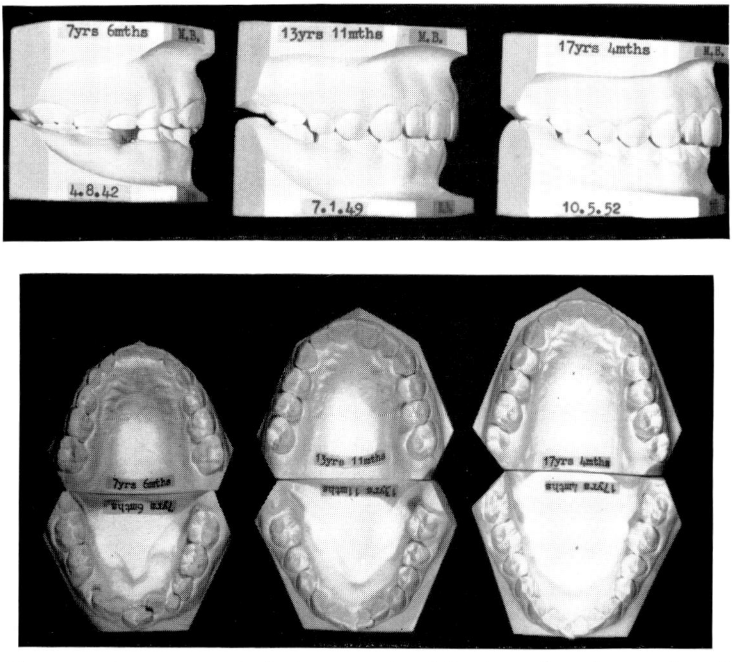

Fig. 153.—Improvement in incisor crowding following enforced extraction of $\frac{6|6}{6|6}$ at 9 years of age. No appliance.

mesial movement of the second permanent molars (*Fig.* 154). Where carious upper first molars have not been extracted and the case is seen after the age of 11 years, it is preferable to await the eruption of

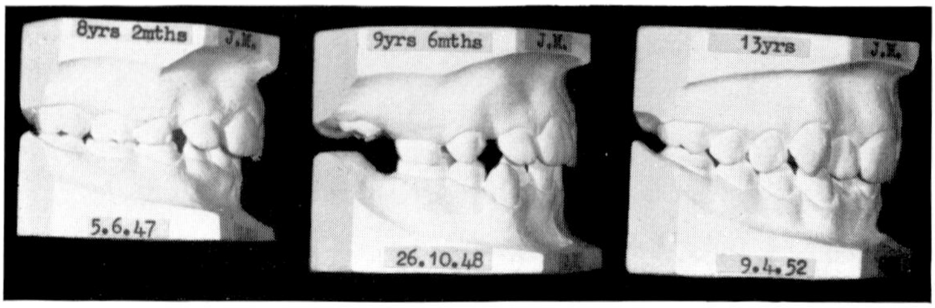

Fig. 154.—$\frac{6|6}{6|6}$ extracted at 9 years of age. Distal movement of upper premolars using screw appliance.

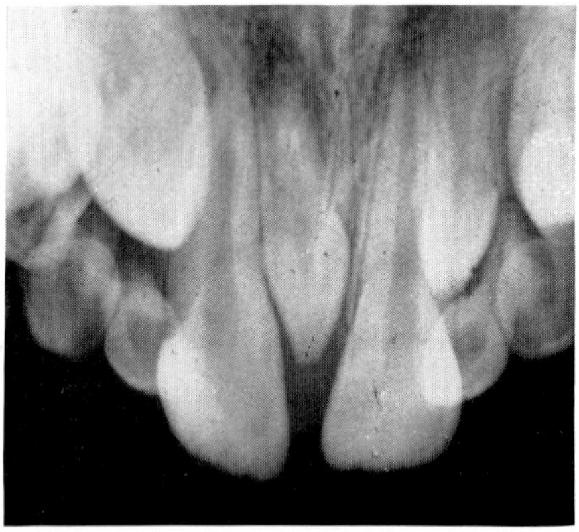

A

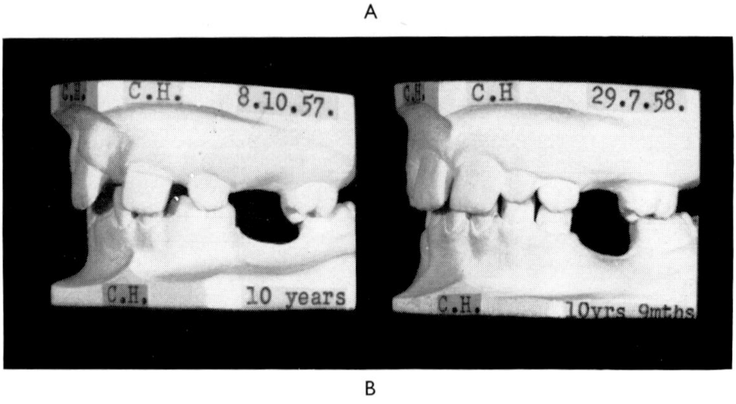

B

Fig. 155.—Cases illustrating some local causes of spacing: A, Missing $\underline{2|}$, rudimentary $\underline{|2}$ and midline supernumerary. B, Proclination of $\underline{1|1}$, with space closing when $\underline{2|2}$ erupt and incisors retracted.

second molars in order that they may be held while premolars and canines are moved distally and alined.

2. SPACING

The local factors producing spacing have been considered in Chapter V (*Fig.* 155). General spacing occurs where the basal bone is large in relation to the size of the teeth or where the tongue, lips, or thumb splay out the teeth.

Where spacing is very marked it is desirable from the aesthetic point of view to close the spaces in the upper incisor region with the object of placing one or two pontics where the space has thus been

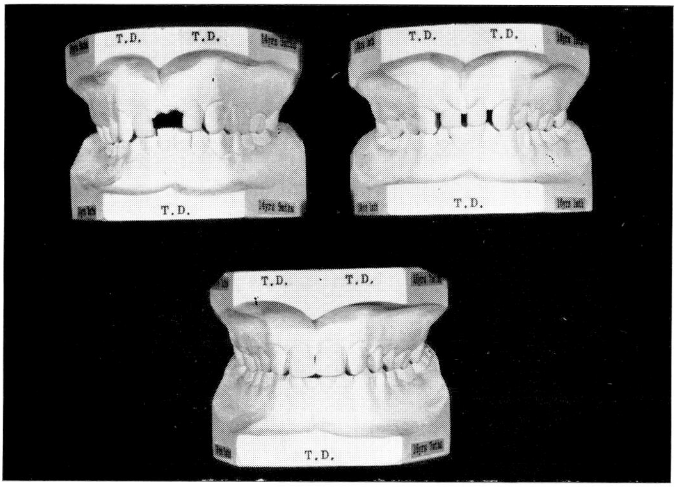

A

Fig. 156.—A, Traumatic loss of 1|1. Approximation of 2|2 which have been crowned to simulate 1|1. Treatment carried out by a modified 'pin and tube' apparatus. (*Continued on p.* 174.)

concentrated. *Fig.* 156 A illustrates a case where the lateral incisors were approximated and crowned to simulate central incisors. *Fig.* 156 B shows an appliance used to approximate incisors.

Spacing may be associated with splaying out of upper and lower incisors which is termed 'bimaxillary proclination' (*Fig.* 157 A, B). The posterior teeth are in Class I relationship and both the upper and lower incisors are inclined labially. This form of occlusion may be seen as a normal feature amongst the Negro races, where it is often associated with a true bimaxillary prognathism. It is also found amongst other ethnic groups as a racial characteristic. Amongst Western Europeans with this form of malocclusion the lips are often bulky and

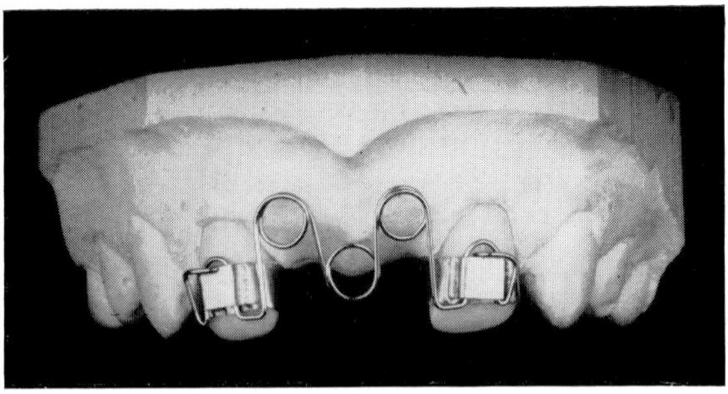

B

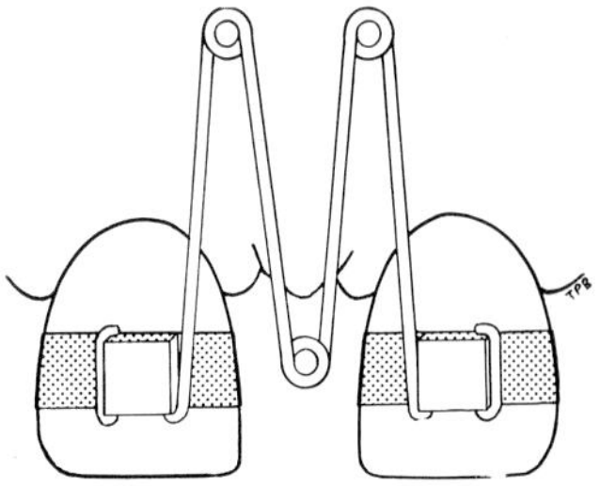

C

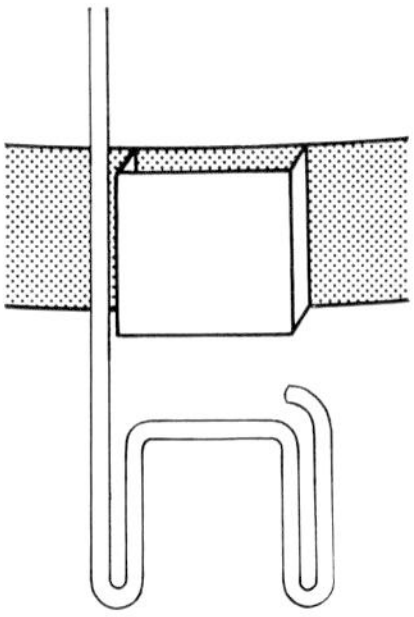

D

Fig. 156 *continued.*—B, Modification of a 'pin and tube' appliance used to approximate incisors. Lock of 2| not fully in place. C, A modified 'pin and tube' appliance to approximate upper central incisors. Spring in 0·5-mm. wire. D, Enlarged view of 'box' welded to incisor band.

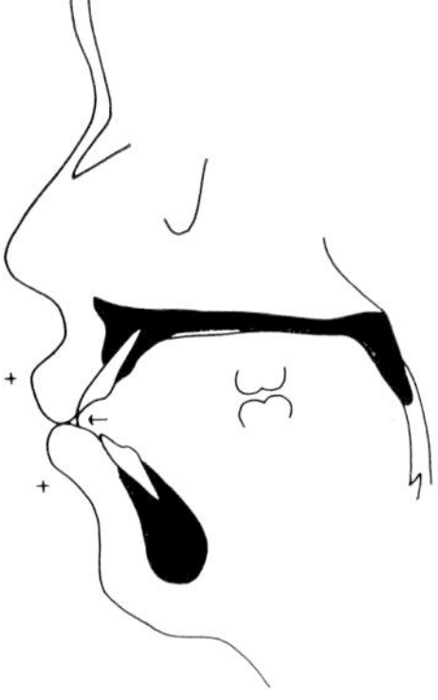

A

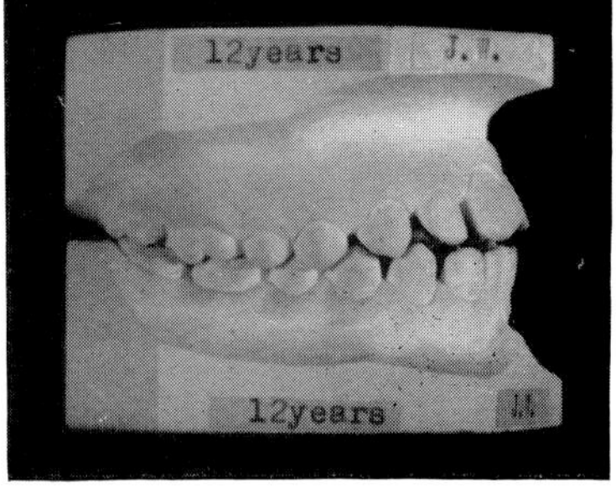

B

Fig. 157.—A, Tongue size and activity fostering bimaxillary proclination. B, Incisor spacing associated with bimaxillary proclination.

everted and take little part in expressive behaviour and the tongue is large and may be lolling (*Fig.* 157).

Such racial characteristics are strong and it is doubtful if any basic change can be made in the oromuscular behaviour. This, together with tongue size, suggests that the conditions producing the malocclusion will exist after treatment and will cause relapse.

Incisor teeth tend to become more upright with growth (*see* Chapter I). This may produce some aesthetic improvement with the passage of time and there may be some degree of space closure. Where the incisor teeth protrude between the lips, conscious effort on the part of the patient to effect a lip seal may play a part in effecting some improvement in the appearance at a later date without treatment.

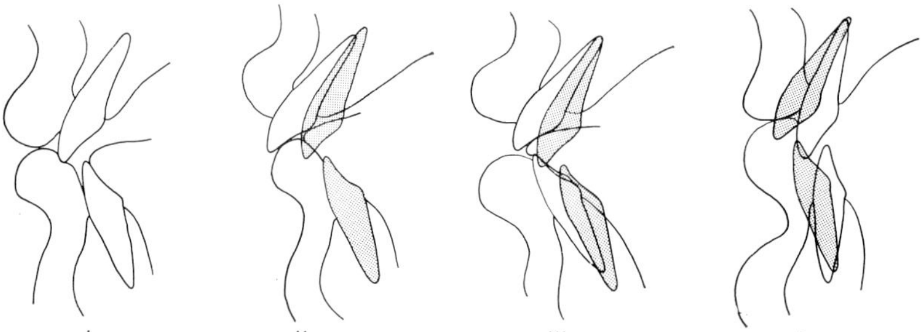

Fig. 158.—i, Incisor relationship showing normal axial inclination of incisors. Skeletal 1 base. ii, Due to habit, lower lip trapped under upper incisors maintaining an increased overjet. iii, Bimaxillary proclination of incisors with associated soft-tissue morphology. iv, Retroclination of upper and lower incisors showing associated lip morphology. Shaded teeth show position before soft-tissue influence.

There is a type of bimaxillary proclination without spacing. Such cases are sometimes treated with the extraction of four premolars and uprighting of the incisors. In some of the cases, if no treatment has been carried out, the natural uprighting of the incisors will result in incisor crowding in the late teens.

3. DERANGEMENTS OF OCCLUSION IN A RADIAL DIRECTION

Radial derangements are those in which there is a deviation from the normal buccolingual or labiolingual relationship of the upper and lower teeth. *Fig.* 158 illustrates the normal and extreme variations in occlusion of the anterior teeth in a Class I case. *Fig.* 160 illustrates the normal buccolingual relationship of the posterior teeth together with examples of deviations from normal.

Radial Derangements of Occlusion of the Anterior Teeth.—

Linguo-version of Upper Incisors.—The commonest derangement of this type, the upper incisor trapped inside the lower incisors, has

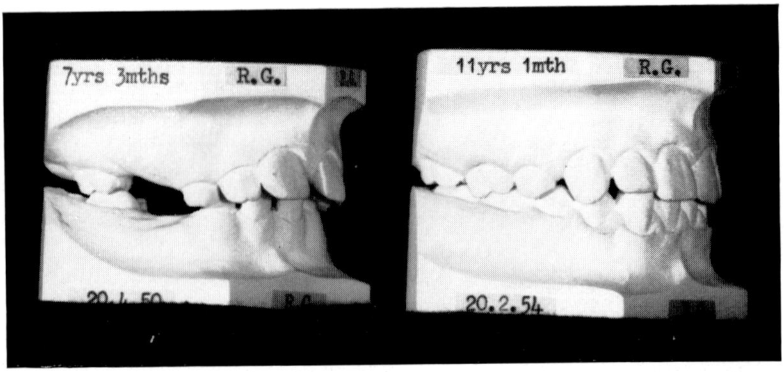

Fig. 159.—Upper incisors proclinated, early loss of deciduous molars. Treated by extraction of $\underline{4|4}$ and retraction of $\underline{3|3}$ and alinement of incisors. $\overline{2|2}$ missing.

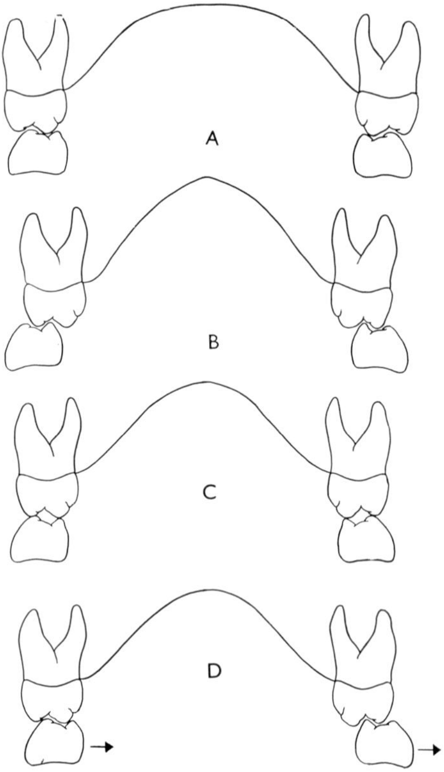

Fig. 160.—Disturbances in buccolingual relationship of posterior teeth. A, Shows normal buccolingual relationships where there is a broad upper arch. B, Bilateral cross-bite where the upper arch is narrow. C, A slightly narrow upper arch showing that there is a cusp-to-cusp relationship which encourages lateral deviation in the path of closure of the mandible so that it presents as a unilateral cross-bite (D).

been described in relation to local factors. This may result, as suggested in Chapter IV, from the retention of a deciduous tooth beyond its normal time of shedding so that it has deflected the permanent incisor from its normal path of eruption. It may also arise as an expression of crowding in the upper arch.

Proclination of Upper Incisors.—*Fig.* 159 illustrates a case in which there is a normal anteroposterior relationship of the cheek teeth but

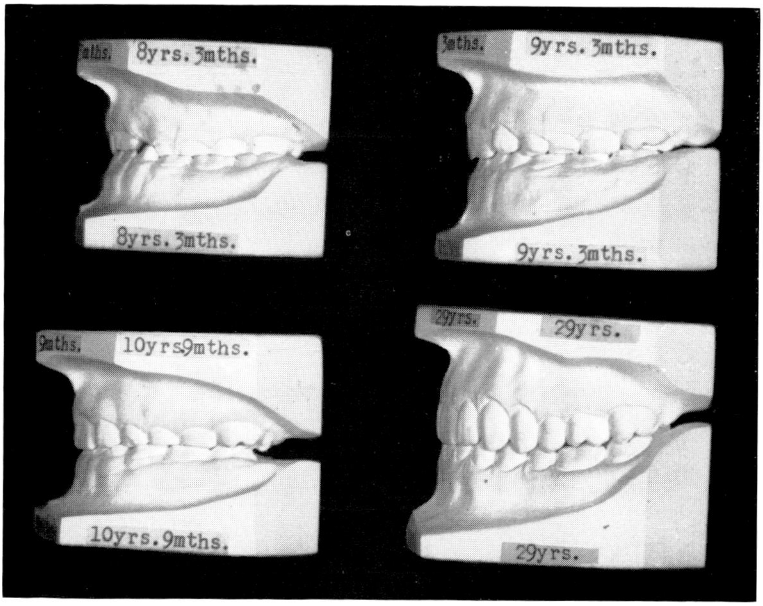

Fig. 161.—Case showing bilateral linguo-occlusion of cheek teeth. Treated by simple expansion with removable appliance showing stability of end-result at 29 years of age. (*By kind permission of Mr. K. E. Pringle.*)

there is a marked overjet with spacing of the upper incisors. The lower lip may become interposed between the erupting incisors following a thumb-sucking habit. Even when the sucking habit ceases and there is a fundamentally normal soft-tissue activity, the lower lip may still be trapped and maintain the overjet. In such cases mechanical reduction of the overjet will give a stable result.

If, however, the behaviour of the soft tissues is adverse, mechanical reduction of the overjet may be followed by relapse to some extent. It is certainly not advisable to reduce the overjet by attempting any degree of labial movement of the lower incisors where the lower lip is actively contracting to effect a lip seal, as they will relapse later.

Radial Derangements of Occlusion of the Posterior Teeth.—

Cross-bite.—In a cross-bite the buccal cusps of the upper teeth occlude between the buccal and lingual cusps of the lowers. It may be unilateral or bilateral. Where there is a slightly narrow arch, a normal path of mandibular closure could produce a cusp-to-cusp occlusion of the cheek teeth (*Fig.* 160 C). A lateral mandibular deviation may be induced in the last phase of closure so that a cross-bite is produced on one side with a normal cheek-tooth relationship on the other side (*Fig.* 160 D).

Where the narrowness of the upper arch is greater in degree centric occlusion is attained without any mandibular deviation, but there is a bilateral cross-bite (*Fig.* 160 B). The function of mastication is not impaired in such cases and the malocclusion is frequently accepted. *Fig.* 161 illustrates a treated case with a stable end-result.

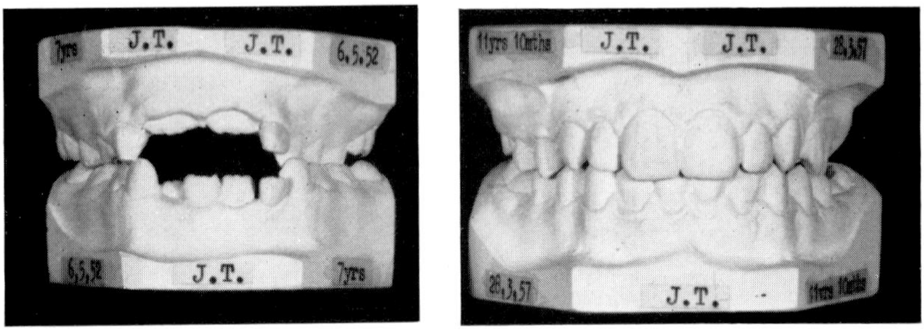

A B

Fig. 162.—A, Patient with unilateral cross-bite with mandibular deviation to the left; B, After expansion of the upper arch. Models 2 years out of retention.

Treatment of the bilateral cross-bite with lateral expansion of the upper arch where there is a narrow dental base will tilt the teeth buccally. They will not receive tongue support and will relapse. Cuspal locks between upper and lower posterior teeth cannot be relied upon to maintain any significant amount of lateral expansion.

Treatment of the unilateral cross-bite as shown in *Figs.* 160 D and 162, where there is a lateral deviation on closure, can be undertaken by simple lateral expansion of the upper arch. The upper buccal segments are already slightly tilted palatally and can be supported in an expanded position. These cases have symmetrical arches and should not be confused with true asymmetry of the jaws which is quite rare.

The simplest form of apparatus for producing lateral expansion of the upper arch is a well-stabilized removable appliance incorporating a screw in the centre of the palate. The screw can be turned by the patient. One quarter-turn is made once or twice a week. The plate must be thrust well home after each adjustment. *Fig.* 163 illustrates the type of appliance used where there is a symmetrical contraction of the upper arch.

Where the cross-bite is limited to the first permanent molars, simple reciprocal elastic traction with fixed bands may be used as illustrated in *Fig.* 164.

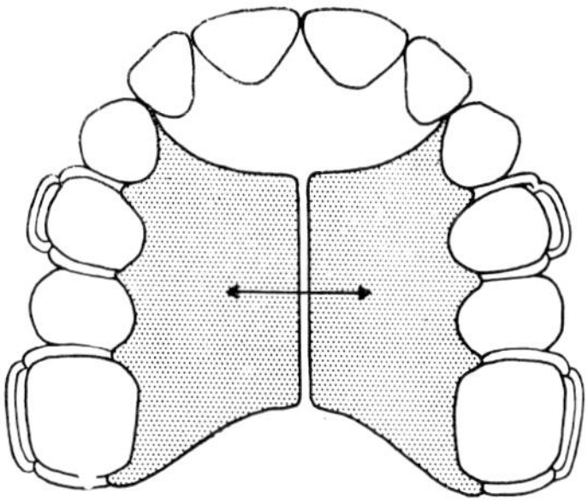

Fig. 163.—Simple expansion plate for symmetrical expansion of the upper arch. Note adequate clasping and siting of expansion screw in plate.

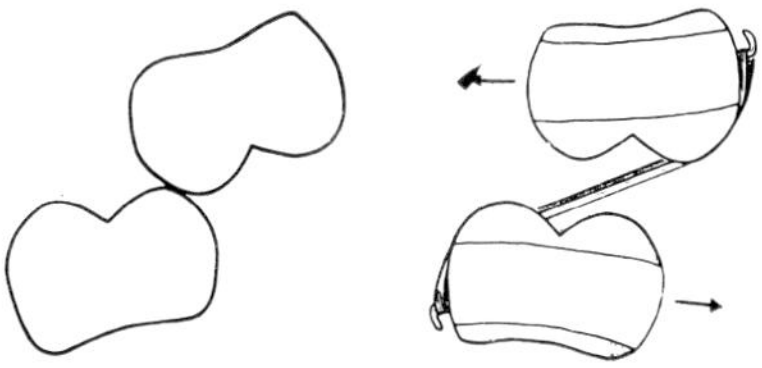

Fig. 164.—Reciprocal traction where upper and lower molars are in cross-bite. Molars are fitted with an elastic band stretched between them.

In the case with bilateral cross-bite there will be some reduction in the circumference of the upper dental arch and there may be crowding in the incisor region or in the canine and premolar regions. Because cuspal locks cannot always be relied upon to maintain expansion, the crowding may have to be relieved by extractions and a bilateral cross-bite accepted.

Linguo-version of Lower Posterior Teeth.—This is fortunately a rather rare condition which may be unilateral or bilateral (*Fig.* 165). It would appear to be an accident of eruption with adverse cuspal locks, but occasionally there is an obvious discrepancy in the width of the basal bones of maxilla and mandible. Where there is this obvious discrepancy in the width of the upper and lower dental bases, treatment is virtually impossible. If, however, the maxillary buccal segments are tilted buccally and the mandibular buccal segments are tilted lingually, treatment may be carried out with a removable or fixed appliance designed to reduce the maxillary arch width and to increase the mandibular arch width to establish a normal cuspal lock.

Removable apparatus in the upper arch may consist of a divided plate incorporating an open screw which can be used to contract the

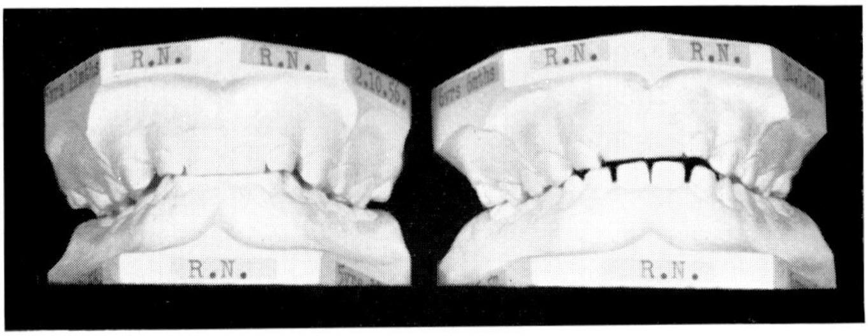

Fig. 165.—Case showing lower arch in complete linguo-occlusion to upper arch. Treated by expansion of lower arch and contraction of upper arch. (*By kind permission of R. D. W. Stileman.*)

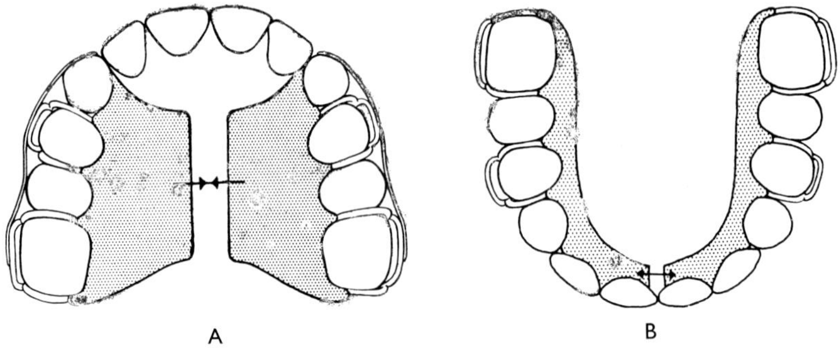

A B

Fig. 166.—A, Upper plate to contract upper arch by commencing with screw open and turning it to close. Note that adequate clasping and contact with the cheek teeth must be obtained. B, Lower expansion plate to expand lower arch. *N.B.*—Such an appliance is used only in cases where the lower cheek teeth have been tilted lingually by adverse lock with the upper cheek teeth.

upper arch laterally. It is important that clasping should embrace all the upper cheek teeth. *Fig.* 166 A illustrates an appliance having Adams cribs with extensions.

Removable apparatus may be used in the lower arch having a centrally placed screw with good clasping (*Fig.* 166 B). It would appear that most of the effect of the screw should be in the intercanine regions, but there is also a marked increase in arch width in the molar region.

4. DERANGEMENTS OF OCCLUSION IN A VERTICAL DIRECTION

Deep Overbite.—The term 'close bite' is now falling out of general use, and 'deep overbite' is substituted, because 'close bite' suggests that the condition is caused by overclosure. Deepening of the

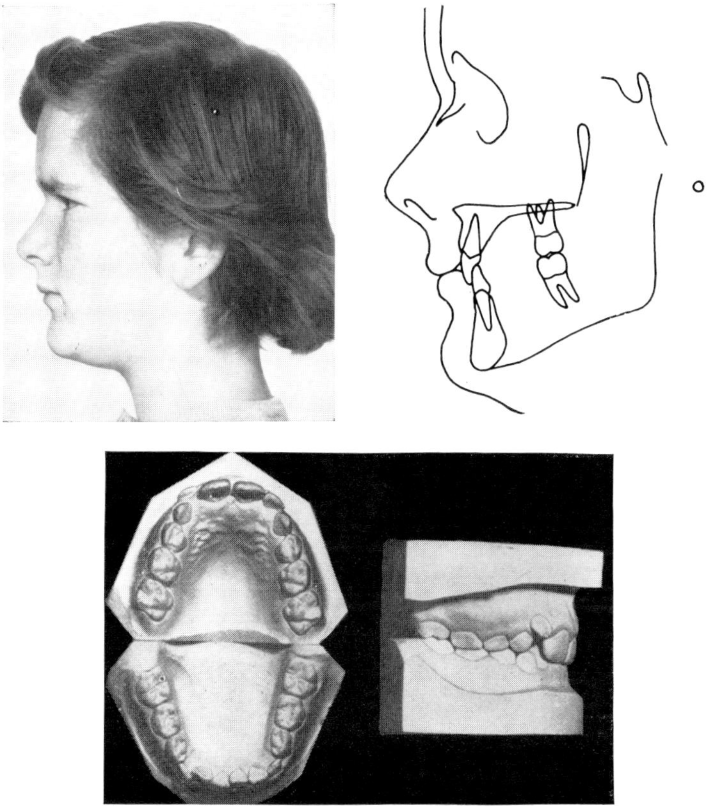

Fig. 167.—Patient with a Class I malocclusion showing deep overbite with crowding in both arches. The crowding in the lower arch is extremely difficult to improve without increasing the overbite further.

overbite can follow overclosure, but it is more commonly due to over-eruption of the anterior teeth, following a disturbance of the axial inclinations of the upper and lower incisors.

Fig. 167 illustrates a case of 'bimaxillary retroclination' of the incisor teeth with a Class I relationship of posterior teeth. The upper and lower arches are crowded in the incisor region and there is a deep overbite. Such a case often presents many of the features of a Class II, division 2 case—the facial form and the square-angled mandible—but the dental base relationship is usually Skeletal 1 or tending towards Skeletal 3. The soft tissues at rest and in activity also resemble Class II, division 2 with the lip line high up the labial surfaces of the upper incisors.

Fig. 168 illustrates the typical axial inclinations of the incisor teeth superimposed on a Skeletal 1 dental base. It will be seen that the lower incisors do not occlude with the cingulae of the upper teeth. These axial inclinations represent a position of stability between the muscle

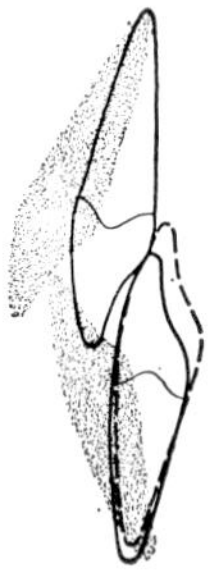

Fig. 168.—Diagram illustrating normal incisor relationship in the dark outline, and how a deep overbite can develop where upper and lower incisors are retroclined and the lower incisors are no longer held by cingulum contact so that they can over-erupt.

forces which are acting on them from the lingual and labial sides. Correction of these inclinations by labial tilting of the crowns will move them out of a position of muscular balance and will therefore invite relapse at a later date.

The only way in which this type of deep overbite can be reduced and maintained is by establishing a contact between the tips of the lower incisors and the cingulae of the upper incisors. As the crowns cannot be moved labially because of the lip morphology this must entail lingual movement of the apices of the incisors. This can only be achieved to any significant extent by means of multiband fixed appliances. The long-term results of such procedures are disappointing.

Treatment should aim principally at alinement of the upper incisor segment and is described in Chapter XII, dealing with Class II, division 2 cases. This type of case is difficult to treat and removable appliances are unlikely to achieve any permanent reduction in the overbite.

Open Bite.—This term is used when opposing segments of the upper and lower arches fail to meet each other in the vertical plane. When there is a degree of incisor overbite without contact of the lower teeth either with the upper incisors or the palate, this is referred to as an *incomplete overbite.*

Open bite may be partial, or true (skeletal) open bite.

The common type of partial open bite is one which is confined to the anterior segment of the arches and is labelled 'anterior open bite'. In certain instances there may be a failure of vertical contact of the buccal segments with the incisors in contact. This is referred to as 'lateral open bite'.

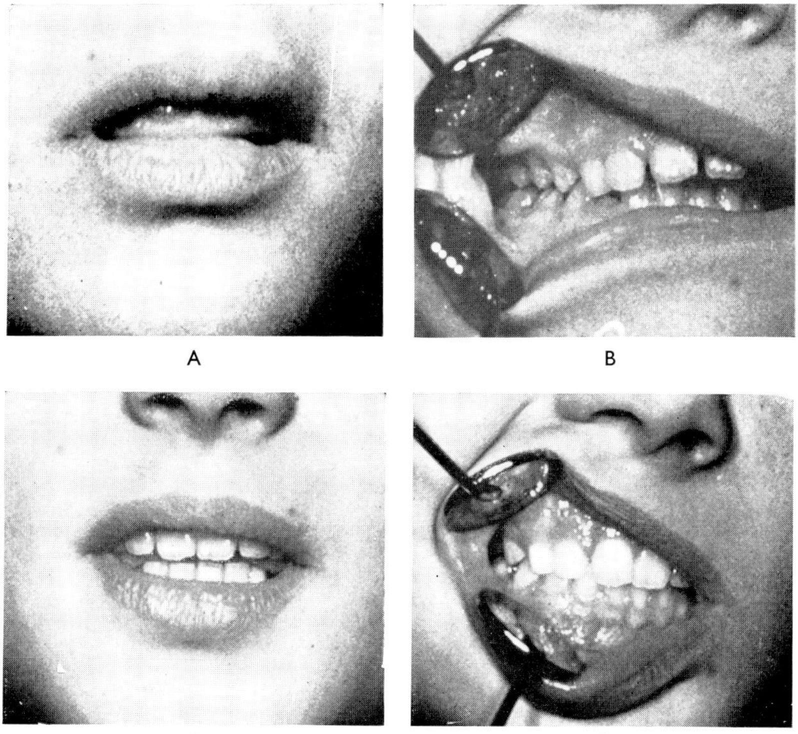

Fig. 169.—Extracted cine frames showing: A, Patient with forward tongue thrust in speech. B, Increased overjet and slight open bite due to thumb sucking. C, After 3 months' simple treatment to retract the incisors, no tongue thrust in speech. D, Resulting occlusion stable.

Anterior Open Bite.—A common cause of anterior open bite is the habit of sucking the thumb or fingers, or, less commonly, the tongue (*see* Chapter V, p. 70). In this chapter we are concerned with open bite as it occurs in Class I malocclusions. Sucking habits usually cause an asymmetrical condition reflecting the way in which the digit is inserted. There may be no discrepancy in the anteroposterior relationship of the incisors. In such cases, the open bite will often improve spontaneously when the habit is given up. Following the long-term observation of many cases without treatment, the authors are quite emphatic that no drastic deterrent methods should be used—*see* Chapter VII. Where there is a definite overjet and the lower lip falls under the proclined upper incisors, a simple plate to retract the spaced incisors will, in itself, tend to discourage the action of the thumb and will also deter a tongue thrust when this is merely a simple habit or adaptive modification (*Fig.* 169).

Persistence of the open bite, after a habit has been given up, indicates an underlying abnormal activity of the tongue which thrusts between the teeth to contact the lower lip, both at rest, in swallowing and during the sibilant sounds of speech. As described in Chapter V this is quite a rare cause of perpetual open bite and is more commonly found where there is a jaw discrepancy of the Skeletal 2 or 3 type.

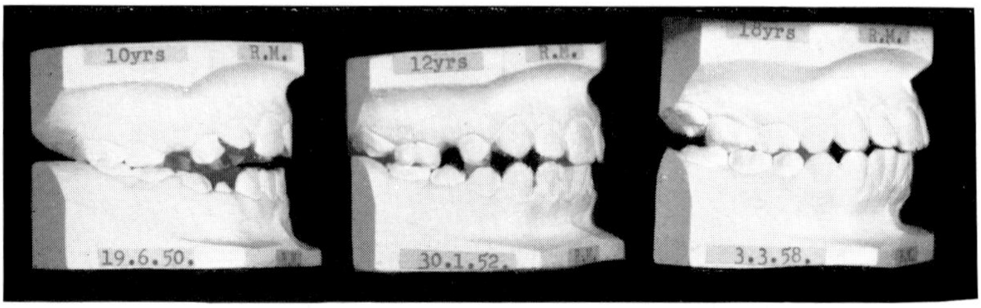

Fig. 170.—Anterior open bite associated with tongue to lower lip contact. There was also a finger-sucking habit initially. Note that by 18 years there is still a slight overjet with incomplete overbite.

Fig. 170 shows a case where the open bite became an incomplete overbite following the cessation of a sucking habit but incisor contact was prevented by the tongue.

There are many transitory cases between those which can be described as anterior open bite and those which come in the category of true or skeletal open bite where only the last molar teeth are in contact.

Ballard has shown that the posture of the tongue and the shape of the mandible appear to be related. In those cases where cessation of habit allows only a minor improvement in the incisor relationship, there is usually an increased anterior face height. The clinical picture may be dominated by the skeletal form with its secondary effect on tongue function. (*See Fig.* 180, p. 192.)

In some cases of open bite, the tongue size would seem to be significant. The sheer bulk of the tongue may contribute towards anterior thrust. Fortunately, such cases are rare and tend to improve with age as the tongue is more readily accommodated within the growing oral cavity.

Lateral Open Bite.—A number of teeth in either or both opposing buccal segments may fail to reach occlusion although there is incisor contact. This is known as 'lateral open bite' (*Fig.* 171).

The reasons may be:—

a. A local failure of eruption which may be seen in the deciduous dentition and may be followed by failure of the premolars to reach occlusion. (Relative submergence of one or two deciduous molars may be due to a definite ankylosis and is not followed by any disturbance in the occlusal level of the premolars.)

b. The tongue may spread over the occlusal surfaces of the cheek teeth at rest and in activity. This has been suggested as a causative factor, but it may be merely secondary.

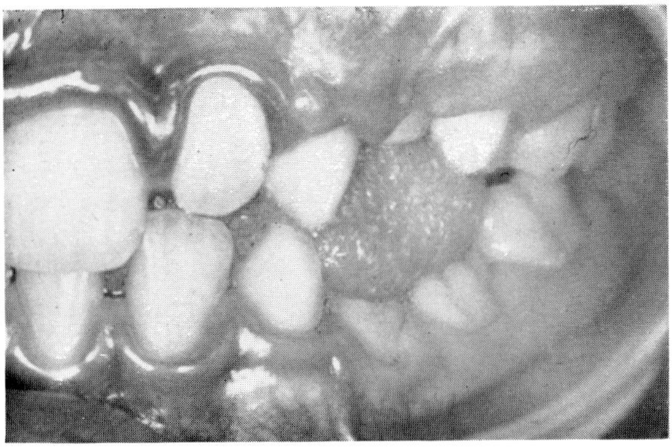

Fig. 171.—Lateral open bite. This patient showed a failure of occlusal rise of cheek teeth both in the deciduous and permanent dentition.

c. Faulty orthodontic treatment with use of overlays may produce a temporary lateral open bite which is rarely maintained unless there is some other abnormal factor operating. However, in some Class III cases with incisor contact which has been achieved by intermaxillary traction a lateral open bite may persist. Ballard and others have shown rare cases where the posterior teeth have failed to erupt across the intermaxillary space for no obvious reason.

Skeletal Open Bite.—This is specifically dealt with in the Appendix because apart from the intermediate cases already described, it usually occurs where there is a Skeletal 2 or Skeletal 3 relationship with gross morphological discrepancies outside the scope of this chapter.

CHAPTER XI

TREATMENT OF ANGLE'S CLASS II, DIVISION 1 MALOCCLUSIONS

The Occlusal Abnormality.—*Fig.* 172 illustrates the occlusal abnormality described as Class II, division 1. Although there may be a post-normal position of the lower arch to a normally placed upper, there may equally well be a prenormal relationship of the upper arch to a normally placed lower. It is, therefore, misleading to use the

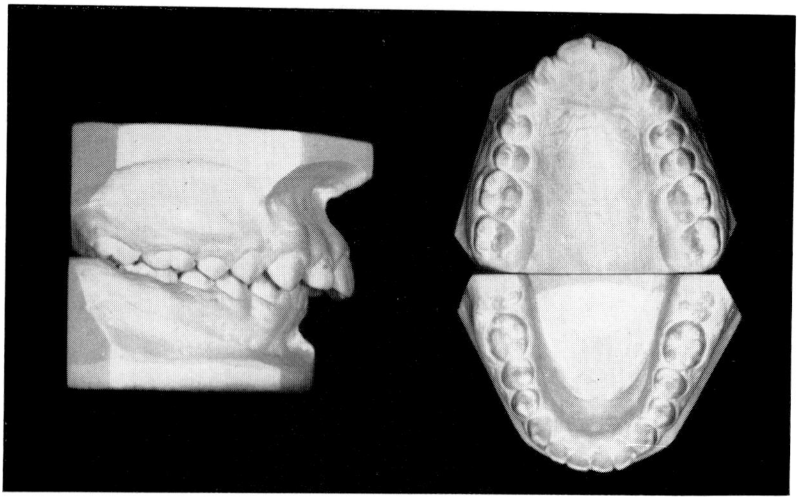

Fig. 172.—Models of Class II, division 1 malocclusion in permanent dentition. Good arches.

term 'post-normal occlusion' or 'disto-occlusion' and preferable to designate the occlusal relationship of the cheek teeth merely as 'Class II'.

In the particular case illustrated in *Fig.* 172 the arches are large and intact, but in the British Isles they are frequently crowded and this could be exaggerated by early loss of deciduous teeth (*Fig.* 173). There is usually a deep incisor overbite and marked overjet, but an anterior open bite is found in a number of cases. Unilateral or bilateral cross-bites are also present on occasions.

This type of dental irregularity is relatively common. In a recent survey of 1500 11-year-old schoolchildren, 329 (22 per cent) were classified as having a Class II, division 1 malocclusion. This condition does not always require treatment and a mild overjet is aesthetically quite pleasing in a girl. Only 141 of the 329 children were deemed to be in need of orthodontic treatment.

The Skeletal Relationship and Facial Form.—A Class II, division 1 malocclusion is most frequently associated with a Skeletal 2 facial pattern. The term 'Skeletal 2' does not differentiate between a

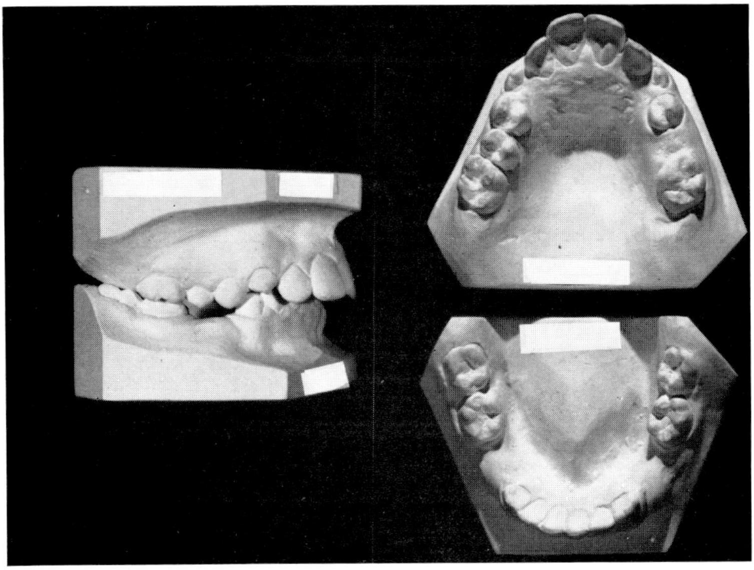

Fig. 173.—Models showing Class II, division 1 malocclusion with crowding in both arches. The lower arch is complicated by early loss of $\overline{\text{ED|DE}}$.

mandibular retrusion, a maxillary protrusion, or a combination of the two. In most cases there is a mild mandibular retrusion, but there are cases with no skeletal discrepancy with the upper dental arch forward of the maxillary dental base. *Fig.* 174 illustrates two common types of facial pattern. Only rarely is there a major discrepancy in jaw relationship as shown in *Fig.* 175. It is also rare, but possible, to find a Class II, division 1 malocclusion where the skeletal relationship is tending towards Skeletal 3 (*Fig.* 176).

The dental bases are usually rather short anteroposteriorly with consequent crowding in both arches, as in *Fig.* 173. The type of facial pattern where both jaws are large is rare in the British Isles.

It is usually confined to other ethnic groups, e.g., those originating from Eastern European countries.

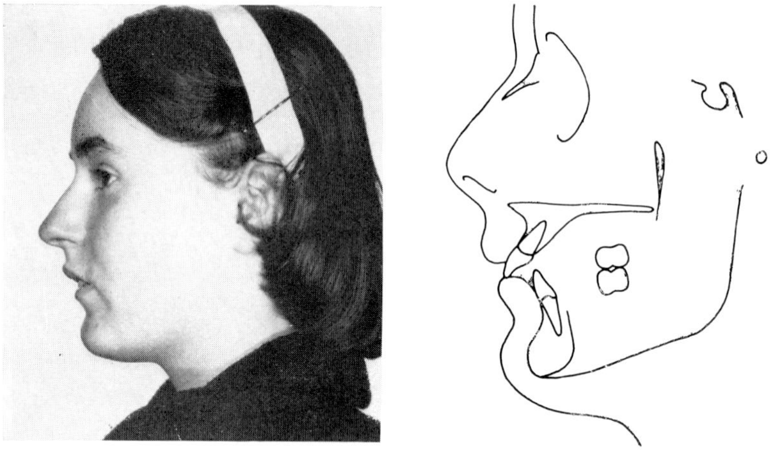

A

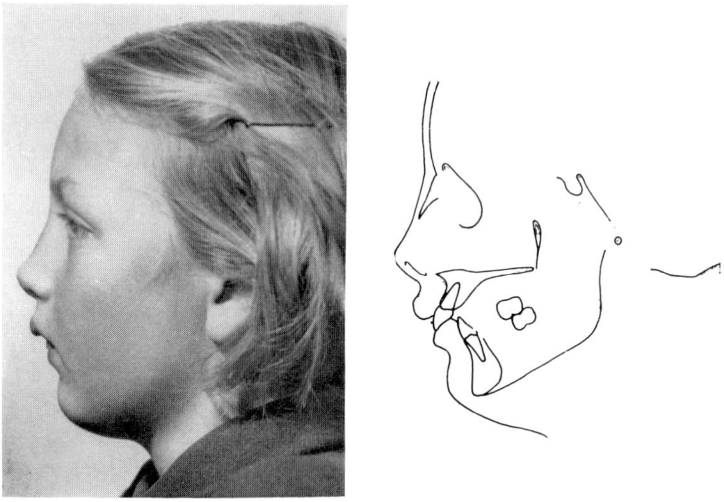

B

Fig. 174.—A, A patient with a typical Class II, division I malocclusion with minimal skeletal discrepancy. The upper dental arch is forward on the maxillary dental base. B, A patient with Class II, division I malocclusion with obvious skeletal discrepancy.

The mandible may vary considerably in its form particularly in relation to the condylar angle. *Fig.* 177 A shows an example of a case where the maxillary-mandibular-plane angle is low compared with the opposite type where the condylar angle is very obtuse so that the mandibular plane forms an angle of more than 30° with the Frankfort or the maxillary planes. These cases may be associated with anterior open bite. *See Fig.* 177 B.

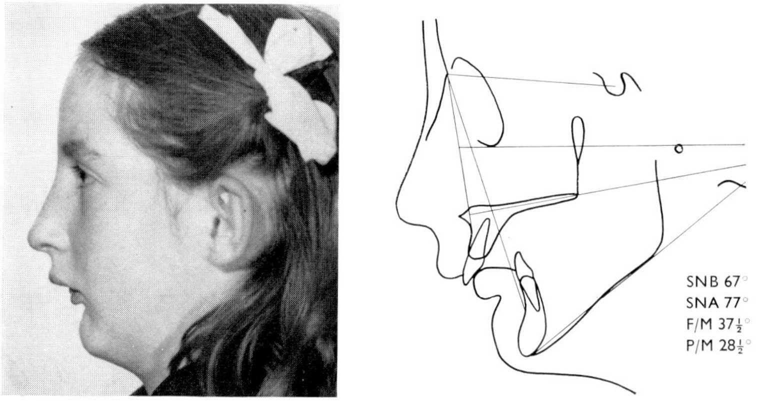

Fig. 175.—A patient with a Class II, division I malocclusion with very severe skeletal discrepancy and high maxillary-mandibular-plane angle.

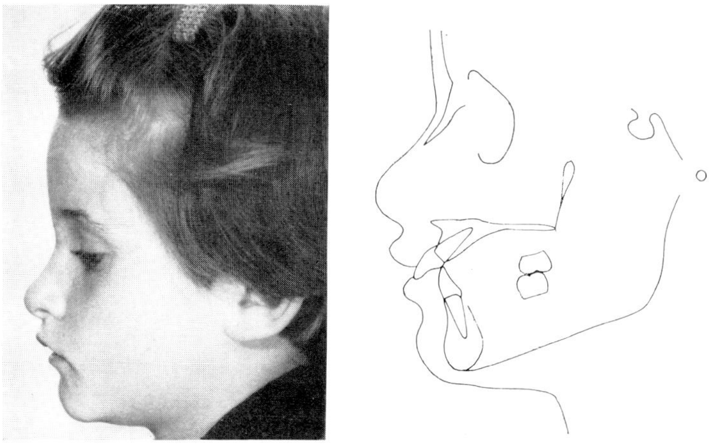

Fig. 176.—A patient with a Class II, division I malocclusion where the dental base relationship is mildly Skeletal 3. This is an unusual type.

In order to complete the assessment of the case it is necessary to study the position and behaviour of the soft tissues of the lips and tongue.

The Lips and Tongue.—In most Class II, division I cases the upper incisors are only partly covered by the upper lip and protrude over the lower lip at rest (*Fig.* 174). The lips may or may not be able to effect an anterior oral seal without conscious effort when the upper incisors have been retracted. If they are judged capable of effecting a seal they are referred to as 'potentially competent' (*Fig.* 178).

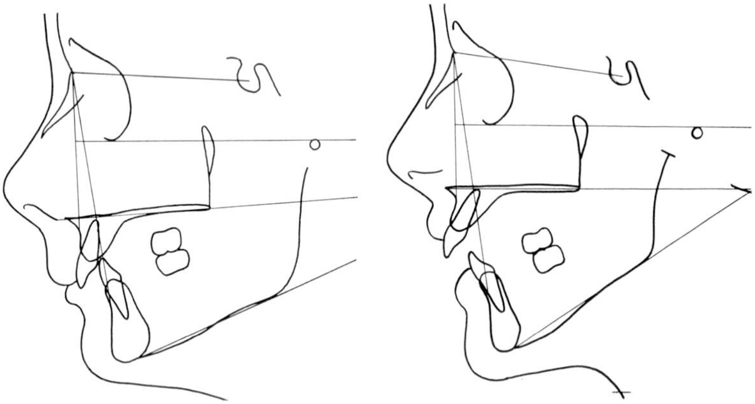

A B

Fig. 177.—A, Example of Class II, division 1 malocclusion with a Skeletal 2 dental base relationship. The maxillary-mandibular-plane angle is 20° and the Frankfurt-mandibular-plane angle is $23\frac{1}{2}$°. *Compare this with* B, Example of Class II, division 1 malocclusion on a Skeletal 2 dental base with poor facial pattern. The Frankfurt-mandibular-plane angle is 33° and the maxillary-mandibular-plane angle is 32°; anterior open bite associated with adverse tongue posture. (*See also Fig.* 180.)

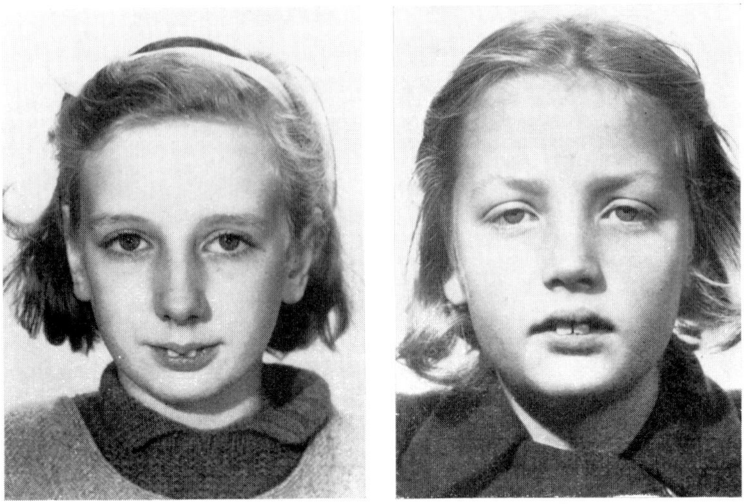

A B

Fig. 178.—A, Lips parted by upper incisors but capable of effecting a seal when upper incisors retracted. B, Short upper lip. Flaccid lower lip. Lips will fail to seal without conscious effort when the incisors are retracted.

In many instances, the lips are 'incompetent', the upper lip is too short, and the patient has to purse up the lower lip deliberately in order to effect a seal even after treatment. There are, however, some cases where the lips are of sufficient length to effect an anterior oral seal despite the increased overjet (*Fig.* 179).

Where there is a major discrepancy in the dental base relationship, a habitual forward positioning of the mandible may be adopted to facilitate an active lip seal.

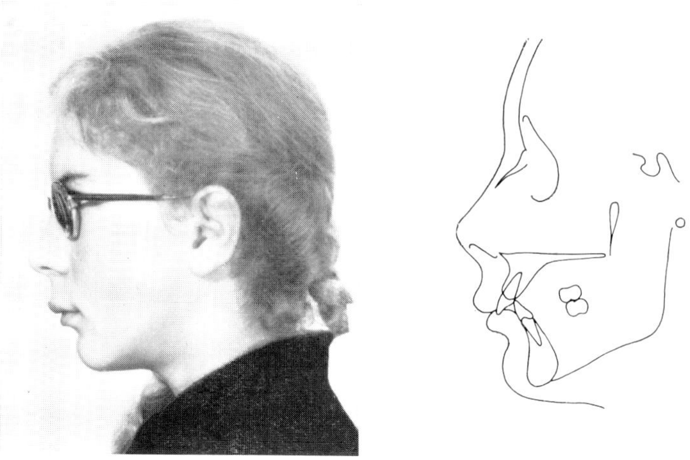

Fig. 179.—A patient with a Class II, division 1 malocclusion where upper and lower incisors are proclined and there is a Skeletal 2 dental base relationship, but the lips are of sufficient length to form an anterior oral seal without revealing the upper incisors. This type of case, if treated, frequently requires a multibanded technique.

In most Class II, division 1 malocclusions not only may the lower lip rest under the upper incisors, but it may also contract strongly under the upper incisors during various functional movements, particularly those of swallowing and in certain speech sounds. It may meet a forward thrusting tongue. *Fig.* 180 shows the type of activity described by Rix as a 'dispersing' activity where the upper and lower incisors fail to make normal contact, the upper incisors being splayed forward and, in some instances, the lower incisors are tilted lingually.

In many cases the overjet is primarily due to the malrelationship of the mandible to the maxilla, but where there is a normal skeletal relationship this activity of the lips and tongue has been considered of significance. Rix's explanation was that this might be akin to an infantile type of behaviour, reminiscent of the behaviour of the lower lip and tongue in the suckling infant. There is evidence to show that this is primarily an adaptive behaviour where the lips are incompetent and in making an anterior oral seal the lower lip scoops in to meet the

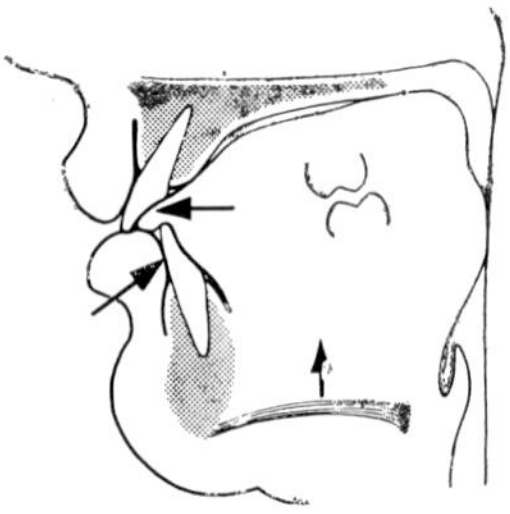

Fig. 180.—Diagram showing lower lip contracting to meet the tongue to effect an anterior oral seal. This type of activity may be changed by re-positioning the upper incisors to allow a lower lip to upper lip seal to be substituted, except in those cases where there is continuous forward tongue posture.

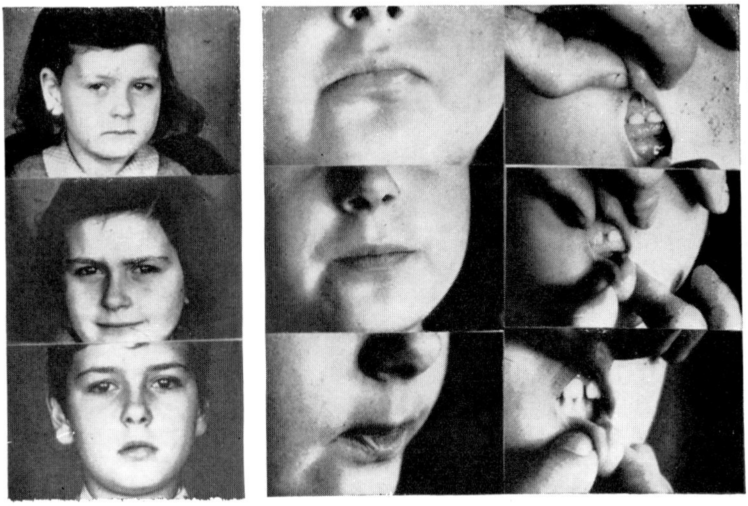

Fig. 181.—*E.S.* Extracted cine frames showing facial changes between 5½ and 10 years. Very strong lip-sucking habit at 5½ with secondary tongue-thrust and lower lip contraction under the upper incisors still present at 7½; still strong contraction of lower lip at 10, but labial to upper incisors, and tongue-thrust has disappeared.

tongue. Where there is any skeletal discrepancy the mandible may come forward so that the teeth are out of occlusion in swallowing activity. In other words, this is a secondary rather than a primary factor.

Whatever may be the reason for this activity, the important fact to establish is whether it is likely to exercise an adverse effect on the incisor relationship when treatment has reduced the overjet.

Fortunately these soft-tissue factors are not always adverse. *Fig.* 181 shows a case where there was considerable thrust of the tongue in swallowing and in speech to meet the contracting lower lip, but as soon as the incisor relationship was corrected the lower lip was brought up

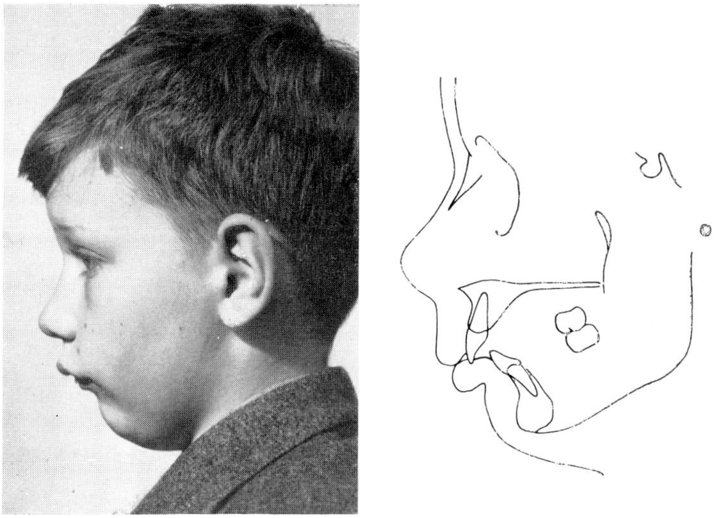

Fig. 182.—A patient with a Class II, division 1 malocclusion where there is a Skeletal 2 relationship and a particular type of lip morphology referred to by Ballard as an 'expressive' lower lip. The upper incisors cannot be moved into a position of stability without appliance therapy to move them bodily.

on to the labial surface of the upper incisors and the tongue-thrust disappeared. There was no anterior open bite.

From a recent survey of Class II, division 1 malocclusions, only 4 per cent showed adverse soft-tissue features which were likely to prevent permanent improvement in the incisor relationship.

At this stage it is convenient to describe two grossly adverse soft-tissue features which must be recognized in treatment planning. First, where the lower lip forms a taut sling spreading from the zygomaticus group of cheek muscles. This will make correction of the overjet extremely difficult, particularly when there is a severe skeletal discrepancy. *Fig.* 182 shows a typical example. Ballard has described this as an adverse 'expressive' behaviour because it is particularly noticeable during various expressive movements of the facial musculature.

Considerable importance must be attached to the 'lip line' in relation to the occlusal plane. If the upper labial segment cannot be placed into a position where the inner contour of the lower lip can control the labial surfaces, relapse will occur, and this will be referred to in detail on p. 196.

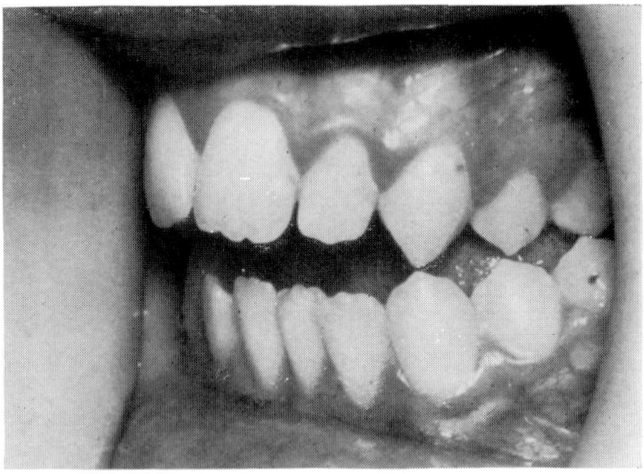

A

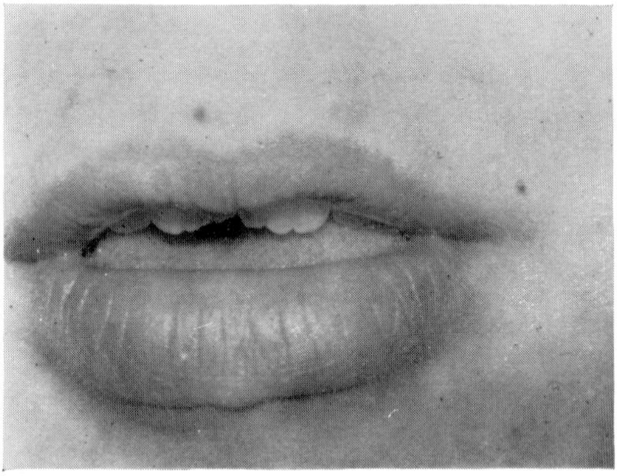

B

Fig. 183.—A, Shows patient with anterior open bite, Class II arch relationship. B, Tongue to lower lip contact at rest, in speech, and in swallowing.

Secondly, *Fig.* 183 shows a difficult case where there is a continuous forward resting position of the tongue in contact with the lower lip, a forward thrust of the tongue to meet the lower lip in swallowing and in the sibilant sounds of speech. There is also a Skeletal 2 relationship of the mandible to the maxilla, and a high angle between the mandibular and the maxillary planes. There is a discrepancy between the anterior and posterior face heights with a severe open bite, only partially due to a persistent thumb-sucking habit (*see Fig.* 177 B, p. 190).

It must be emphasized that the tongue-thrust in swallowing and a marked lisp in speech are not significant unless they are associated with the morphological features described above (*see* Chapter V).

Fig. 184 illustrates some of the possible variations in incisor position where there is a Skeletal 2 dental base relationship. It shows how the already existing overjet may be influenced by the soft tissues of the lips and tongue.

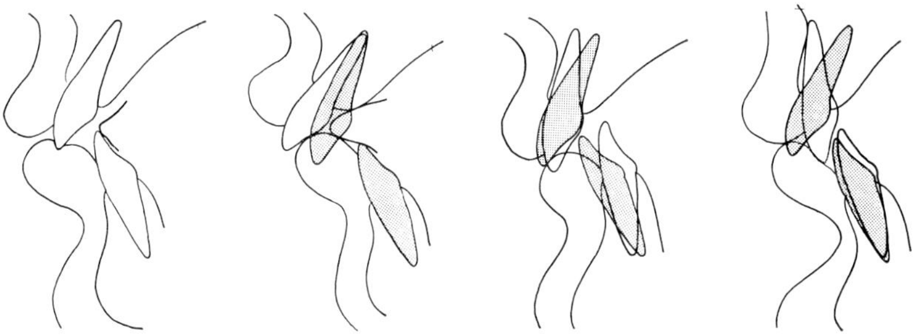

i ii iii iv

Fig. 184.—i, Skeletal 2. Incisors with normal inclination showing increased overjet. ii, Increased proclination of upper incisors through lip action. Tongue posture preventing lower incisors from erupting. iii, Unusual type of Class II, division 1 with strong lower lip action causing retroclination of lower incisors. Upper incisors upright. iv, Class II, division 2 type of lip morphology causing retroclination of both upper and lower incisors. Shaded teeth show position before soft-tissue influence.

Path of Mandibular Closure.—In most cases there is a simple hinge movement at the condyle from rest to occlusion, but it has been pointed out that some patients with a marked Skeletal 2 abnormality adopt a forward posture to mask their retrusive appearance and effect a lip seal. Brodie refers to this descriptively as 'the Sunday face'. In these cases the mandible shows a relative distal movement on closure from the forward habitual position. This is not a true posterior displacement and distal displacement from a normal rest position is thought to be rare.

Local Complicating Factors.—

Habits.—Sucking of fingers, thumb, or lips may be an additional factor contributing to the abnormal incisor relationship. Despite the views of some writers this is not commonly the only aetiological factor, but one to be considered when planning treatment, for it tends not only to add to an abnormal incisor relationship but also adds to conditions favouring a Class II relationship of the cheek teeth. With few exceptions the habit is given up when an appliance is fitted, and difficulties are principally encountered where the underlying behaviour of tongue and lips is abnormal.

Early Loss of Deciduous Cheek Teeth.—As in all other cases, premature loss of deciduous cheek teeth will allow forward movement of the teeth posterior to the site of extraction and movement of anterior teeth around the arch. Where there is crowding in the upper arch and the upper incisors have been proclined, loss of deciduous cheek teeth will allow the first permanent molars to move forward into a Class II relationship even when the facial pattern is Skeletal 1. The previous contention that premature loss in the lower dental arch tends to allow the lower incisors to fall lingually and over-erupt can no longer be substantiated. They are already in a position of linguofacial balance.

TREATMENT

General Principles.—In planning treatment of a Class II, division 1 malocclusion the main objective is retraction of the upper labial segment to an acceptable aesthetic position where they will be stable. Stability is only possible if the lower lip can act on the labial surfaces of the incisors and does not contract under the incisal edges (*Fig.* 185). Where there is a Skeletal 2 relationship, the upper incisors may have to be retroclined to achieve this. In these cases a satisfactory

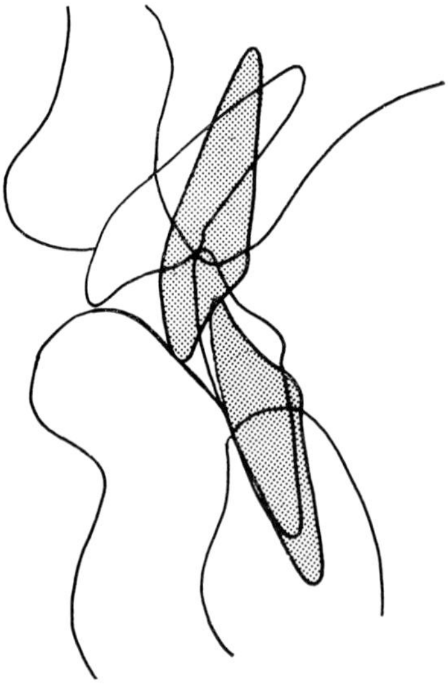

Fig. 185.—Outline shows Class II, division 1 incisor relationship and position of lower lip. Shaded outline shows positions which must be achieved if the upper labial segment is to remain in a stable position. This type of tooth movement can usually be carried out with removable appliances. In some forms of malocclusion this position can only be achieved with the use of appliances which can move the teeth bodily.

end-result is not judged by achieving upper and lower incisor contact, but by a position of the upper incisors which is stable in their new soft-tissue environment. Thus it is really the soft tissues which determine the prognosis for aesthetic improvement in the incisor region. A case with a Skeletal 1 relationship of the dental bases with tongue-thrust and strong lip contraction may be extremely difficult to treat and maintain. However, the case with some degree of Skeletal 2 relationship but lips and tongue which favour incisor retention after retraction gives a much more favourable prognosis. *Fig.* 182 (p. 193) illustrates the type of case described by Ballard where the upper incisors cannot be brought into the correct relationship with the inner surface of the lower lip without bodily movement. This type of movement can only be produced by multibanded appliances.

Naturally a case with any major discrepancy in dental base relationship has a poor prognosis for facial aesthetics, but it may still be possible to improve the incisor position if the soft tissues allow.

Where there is no significant skeletal discrepancy and there is no crowding, the change in axial inclination of incisors may be achieved together with a change in relationship of the whole upper to the lower arch, producing a Class I molar relationship. However, where there is a skeletal discrepancy there is no functional or aesthetic reason why the molars should not be left in Class II relationship and extractions in the upper arch allow the upper incisor segment to be retracted.

There are no grounds for the belief that the mandible can be encouraged to grow beyond its inherent potential size. Using the appliances described in this book, changes are confined to the dental arches, and if this is considered as a basic, if rather dogmatic, principle, treatment planning will be better appreciated.

Extractions in the upper arch are undesirable where there is considerable spacing of the teeth and no marked skeletal discrepancy.

The Mechanics of Treatment.—There are three basic mechanisms which can be employed to improve the incisor relationship:—

1. *Extra-oral Traction with Fixed or Removable Apparatus*: Distal traction on part or whole of the upper arch with or without a reduction in the number of teeth, obtaining anchorage from a head cap or cervical strap.

2. *Intermaxillary Traction by Fixed or Removable Apparatus*: Distal traction on the whole or just the anterior segment of the upper dental arch using the lower arch as anchorage.

3. *Intramaxillary Traction*: This involves the extraction of a tooth on either side of the upper dental arch and the retraction of the incisor segments against the anchorage of the posterior teeth and palate.

1. Extra-oral Traction.—Some clinicians, particularly in the U.S.A., use this as a 'guiding' treatment in the mixed dentition with a labial bow attached to molar bands. A removable bite plate may also be worn if necessary. The principle is to restrain the forward development of the maxillary dentition during part of the growth period.

It may also be used to retract segments of the upper dental arch, or to reinforce anchorage where active apparatus is being used to achieve these movements (*see* Chapter IX). Mechanically the principle is excellent and this form of anchorage cannot cause undesirable forward movement of teeth in either arch. The main disadvantage is that patients may be reluctant to wear a conspicuous appliance of this type.

2. Intermaxillary Traction.—If the lower dental arch is used as anchorage to retract the upper dental arch, there are many disadvantages which can only be overcome by multibanded techniques. The simple 'labiolingual' type of apparatus, where only the first molars are banded and traction applied from a simple lower lingual arch to an upper labial arch, is no longer acceptable. This method produces a forward movement of the lower buccal segments and the lower incisors are proclined and placed in an unstable position.

Even with a multiband technique where the teeth are connected in compound anchorage, there is still the possibility of the lower teeth being moved forward. (In certain types of multiband techniques, e.g., the edgewise arch, the anchorage is prepared by first tipping back the lower buccal segments.)

Tweed, finding this difficulty with the lower arch, developed the technique of extracting both upper and lower first premolars, allowing forward movement of the lower buccal segments to close the space and thus preventing the lower incisors from receiving any forward component of force. In fact they are uprighted if necessary. Details of this type of treatment can be obtained from texts devoted to the edgewise technique.

The only form of intermaxillary traction which will be described in this book is that produced by the monobloc, also known as the Andresen appliance or the Activator, to be described on page 210. When used to treat a Class II, division 1 malocclusion it is usually reserved for those cases where the arches are of good size and where there is no major skeletal discrepancy.

It must be emphasized by stating again that intermaxillary traction in whatever form it is used does not 'bring the mandible forward' to establish a new position of occlusion which is permanent.

3. Intramaxillary Traction.—Most patients in the British Isles have a very short upper dental base with a tendency to crowding as well as an increased incisor overjet. The cheek tooth relationship is usually a full premolar unit Class II. The teeth most favoured for extraction are the upper first premolars as this allows space to be made available as near the labial segment as possible and the canine can then be tilted distally into the first premolar space followed by retraction of the upper labial segment.

However, it is most important to establish that the first permanent molars are sound teeth with good prognosis, that the upper second premolars are present, and that the upper canines are not displaced.

The first appliance which is used is designed to retract the upper canines and to reduce the overbite (*Fig.* 186). There are a variety of designs but the one described here has been shown to be the most

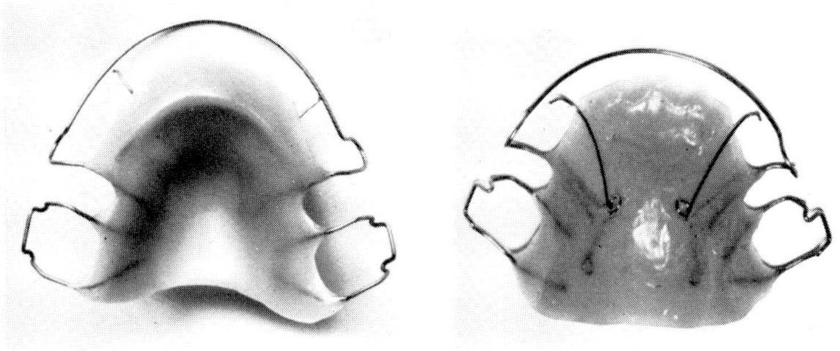

A B

Fig. 186.—A type of appliance used to retract 3|3 and reduce the overbite with a bite plane after 4|4 have been extracted. Bow constructed in 0·7-mm. wire and palatal finger springs in 0·5–0·6-mm. wire. A, Surface view of appliance; B, Fit surface view of appliance.

satisfactory in the authors' hands. The plate must be adequately stabilized, using Adams cribs on the first molars, and have a well-fitting base plate. The anterior portion is thickened to form a biting surface which is slightly inclined.

The low labial bow constructed in 0·7-mm. wire is desirable and should be positioned as shown in *Fig.* 187 so that it is low on the labial surface of the upper incisors and therefore the incisors are held by the arch and low down on the palatal aspect by the appliance. This reinforces the anchorage and tends to minimize any forward tilting of the incisors as a reciprocal effect of the distal movement of 3|3. There are many different forms of labial arch and *Fig.* 186 shows one which is brought out of the acrylic, mesial to the upper second premolars. If the placing of this is carefully considered it will not prevent the full retraction of 3|3. Some authorities prefer to use a short labial bow brought out of the plate distal to 2|2 which acts like an anterior clasp. There is no doubt that this may hold up the anterior portion of the plate in a more satisfactory way than the more flexible longer bow but does not allow any improvement in the position of 2|2, if they are in a slightly crowded position. *Fig.* 188 shows a better appliance with good anterior retention but 2|2 are still free to drift distally around the arch.

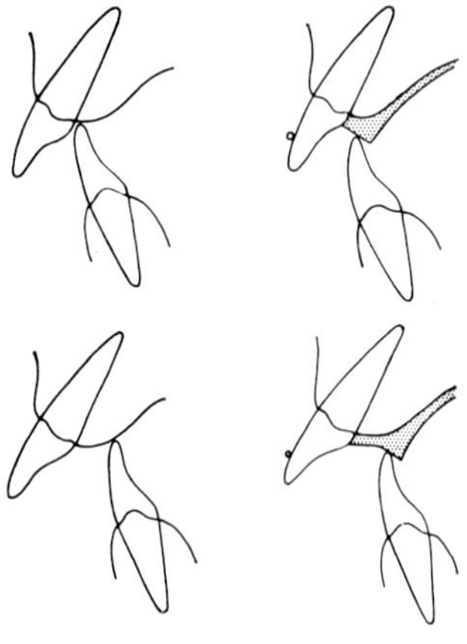

Fig. 187.—Two types of anterior bite plane used to reduce the overbite during retraction of 3|3. Note that the labial bow should be nearer the incisal edge.

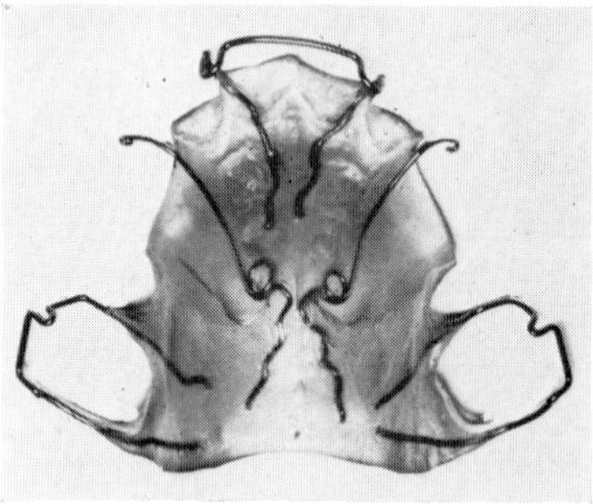

Fig. 188.—Alternative appliance to *Fig.* 186 with anterior clasp to 1|1 or a simple fitting short bow. This is preferred by some authorities as it gives better anterior retention to the appliance than the rather long and flexible bow shown in *Fig.* 186. It still allows 2|2 to drift distally around the arch. Finger springs in 0·5-mm. wire, clasps in 0·7-mm. wire.

If the canines are in the general line of the arch they are most effectively retracted by simple finger springs as described in Chapter IX. These springs are constructed in 0·5-mm. wire and are boxed in under the appliance. They should not be too short and should have a clear path of action.

Where the canines are buccally displaced the use of the forms of buccal retractor constructed in 0·7-mm. wire should be used (*Fig.* 189).

Anterior biting surfaces should allow the cheek teeth to be separated little more than the normal interocclusal clearance. It is doubtful whether there is any active depression of the lower labial segment, but this discourages their continued eruption and permits over-eruption of posterior teeth and has the general effect of temporarily separating the upper and lower incisors (*Fig.* 188).

When the upper canines have been fully retracted into a normal relationship with their lower counterparts and the overbite has been reduced, it is preferable to fit an appliance specifically designed to retract the incisors. The canines can be included with the anchorage teeth and held by mesial spurs. The acrylic should be cut well back from the incisors where possible, and there should not be a sharp leading edge to the acrylic which tends to cause the gingival tissues to be pinched between the cingulum of the upper incisors and the appliance producing the type of situation shown in *Fig.* 190.

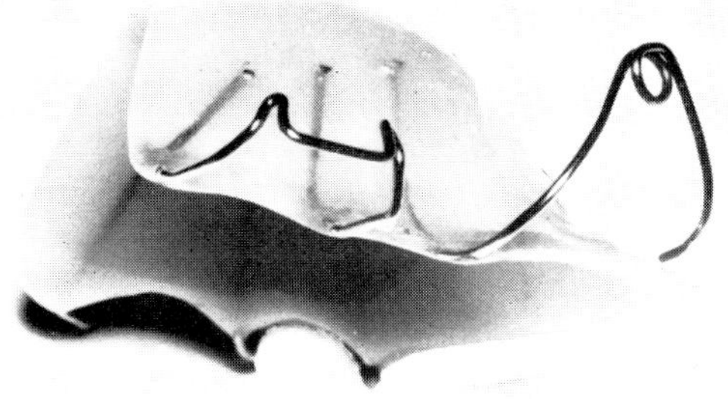

Fig. 189.—Type of retractor used for a buccally placed canine constructed in 0·7-mm. wire.

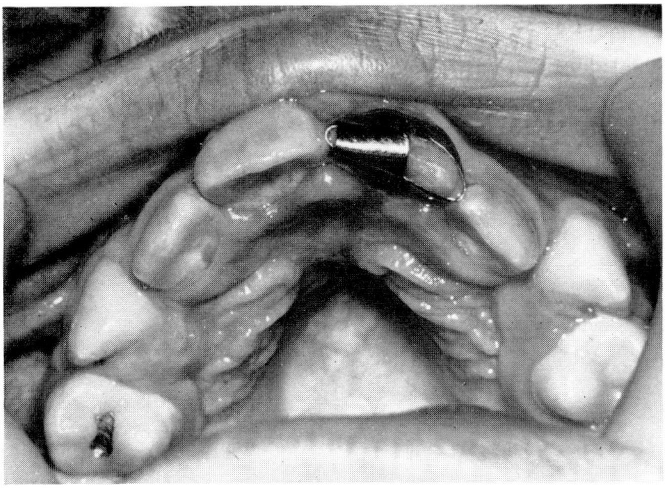

Fig. 190.—Gingival hyperplasia palatal to the upper incisors where the plate has been incorrectly trimmed back to a full saddle.

There are many methods which can be used to retract the incisors. The important consideration is the anchorage to prevent undue forward movement of posterior teeth. This can be achieved by an accurately fitting plate contacting all the teeth and the palatal vault. Inclined facets which receive the bite of the lower canines may be a helpful adjunct.

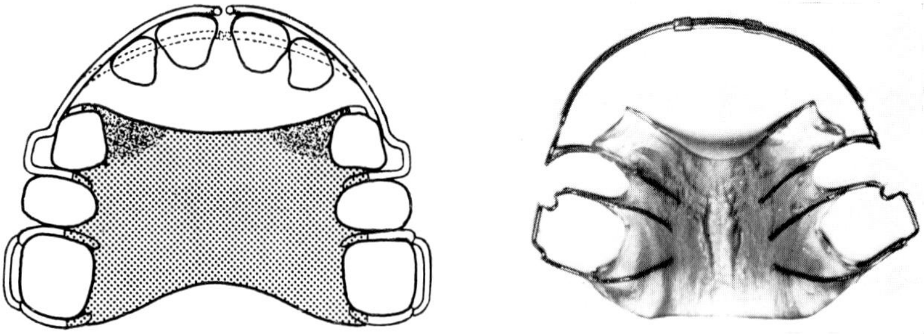

A B

Fig. 191.—Divided labial bow used to retract $\underline{21|12}$. A, Diagram showing free ending arms used as long flexible springs. B, Actual appliance showing how tape sleeves can prevent instability of the arms.

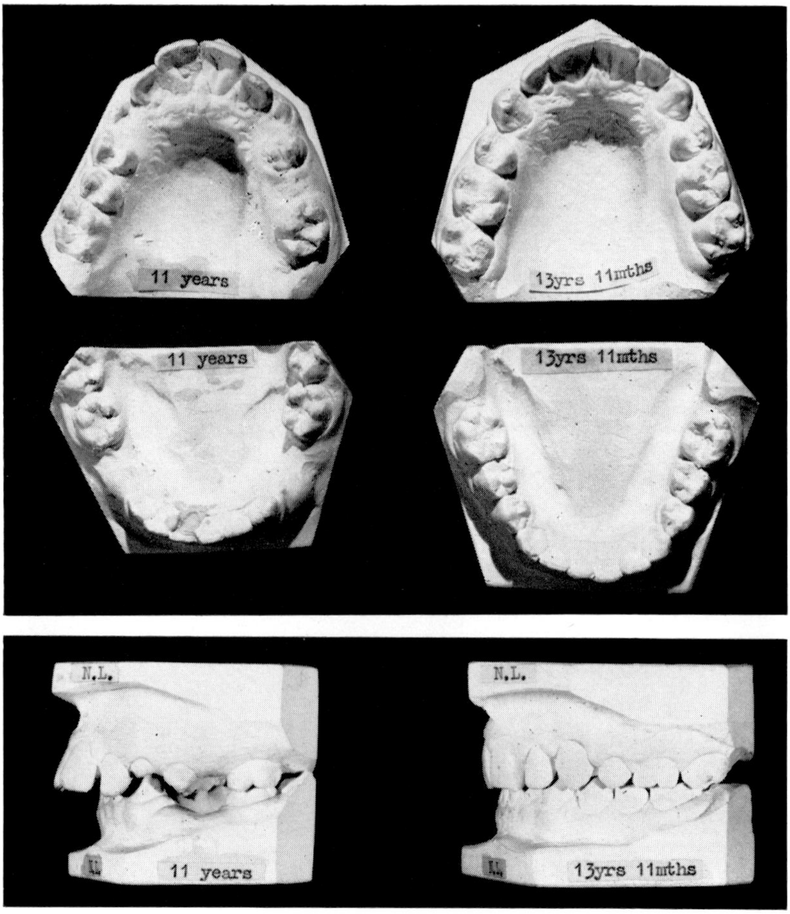

Fig. 192.—Class II, division 1 malocclusion treated by the extraction of $\underline{4|4}$. Two appliances used: (*a*) To retract $\underline{3|3}$ and reduce overbite, (*b*) To retract $\underline{21|12}$. No lower appliance. (*See also Fig.* 193.)

The simple labial arch with take-up loops is not very efficient if it is used to retract the incisors. Tension applied by tightening the take-up loops will only move the teeth for a very short period of time and frequent adjustments are necessary. There is also a great tendency to

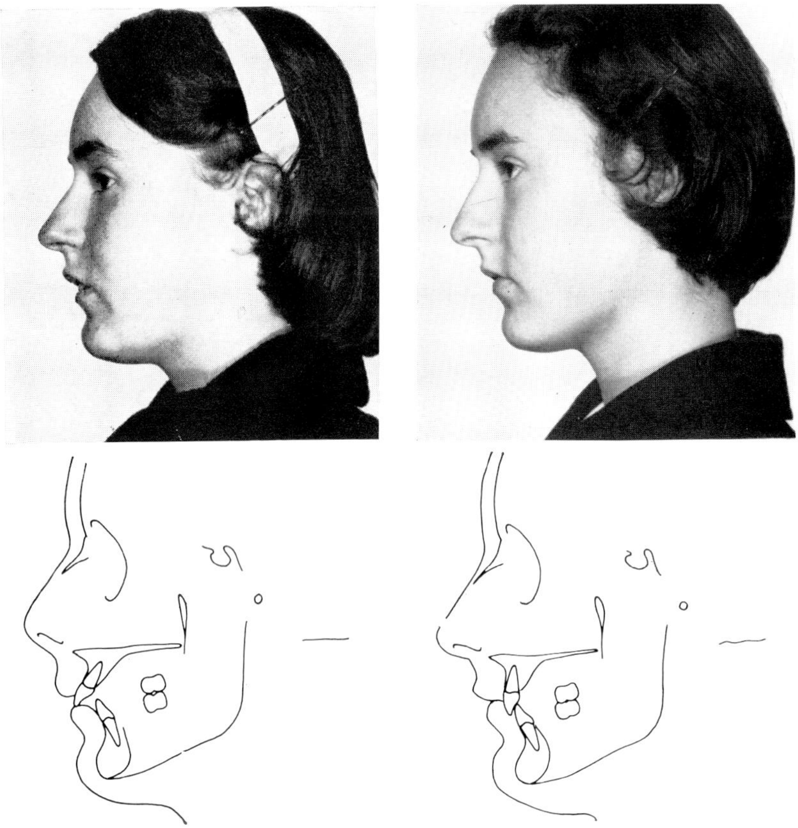

Fig. 193.—Class II, division I malocclusion. Skeletal I dental base relationship. Treated by extraction of $\underline{4|4}$ and retraction of $\underline{3|3}$, followed by retraction of incisors. There was no excessive contraction of lower lip or thrust of tongue prior to treatment, and upper incisors are well controlled by lower lip after treatment.

bring about reciprocal forward movement of the posterior teeth. There are many other ways of retracting the upper labial segment and in Chapter IX examples have been shown, including the type of labial arch described by Mills. (*See Fig.* 119, p. 143.)

'Self-straightening' wires, as described in Chapter IX, can be used to apply a light continuous force, but these wires do require careful adjustments and if they are displaced they may cause gingival damage. The authors favour the use of the high labial bow with apron springs wound in 0·4-mm. wire (*Fig.* 194). This is less obtrusive and gives a gentle force over a period of time. A small apron can be wound initially to retract the upper central incisors if they are not in line with the laterals.

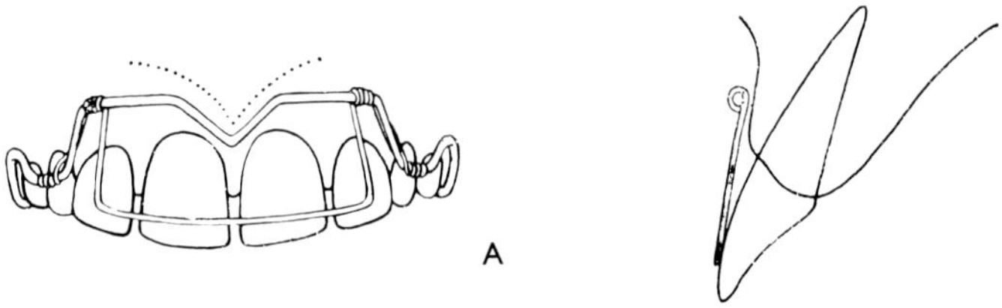

A

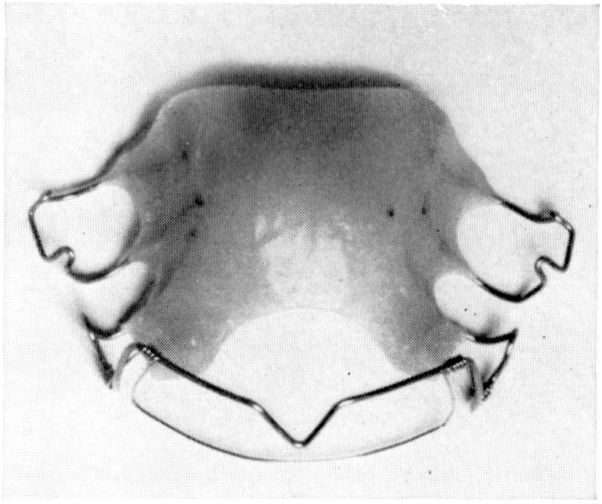

B

Fig. 194.—Apron spring from high labial bow. Alternative method of retracting upper incisors. Bow in 0·8-mm. wire, apron spring in 0·3-mm. or 0·4-mm. wire.

Walther has described the use of elastic bands made from sections cut from Paul's tubing which is a fine latex surgical drain. This can be obtained in three sizes and stretched from two buccal hooks in the canine region (*Fig.* 194). It has the advantage of being almost invisible and is therefore welcomed by the older patient. The main disadvantage to this is that in the initial retraction of very proclined incisors it may tend to ride up gingivally.

In Chapter IX the use of extra-oral anchorage has been discussed to reinforce intramaxillary anchorage. In the authors' opinion this is only needed in a few cases where the extraction of upper first premolars does not give sufficient space or where the space is critical and no forward movement of buccal segments can be tolerated.

In these circumstances a tube can be soldered to the bridge of the Adams crib or bands can be placed on the first molars and an extra-oral appliance used at night time to hold back the buccal segment.

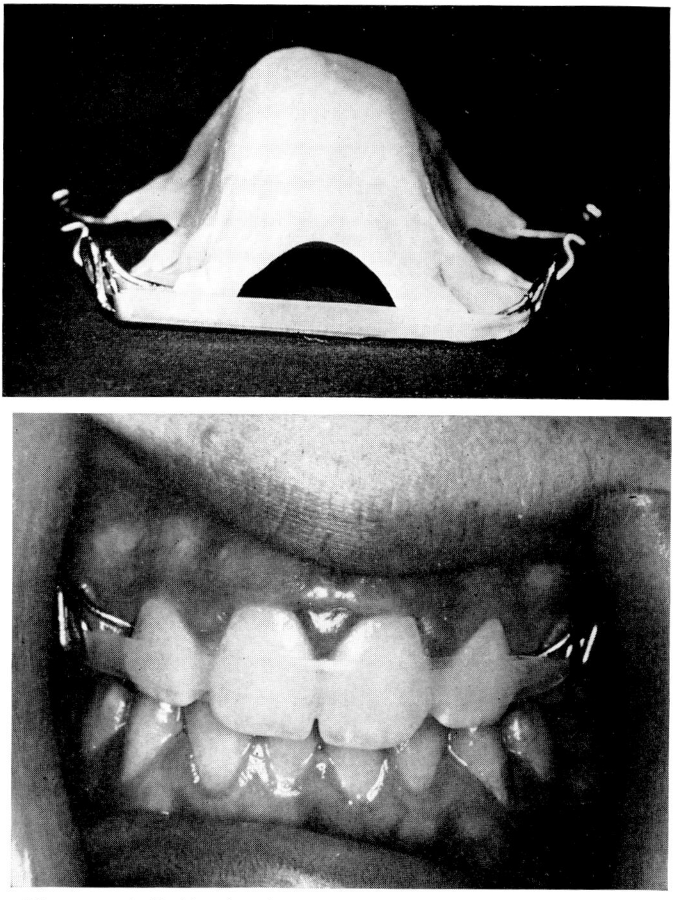

A

B

Fig. 195.—A, Rubber band cut from Paul's tubing attached to adjustable buccal hooks as described by Walther. B, Note trauma to interdental papilla where the elastic has slipped up. It should be adjusted to lie about 2 mm. from the incisal edge.

Choice of Upper Extractions in Association with Intramaxillary Traction: Although the main emphasis is placed on the extraction of first premolars, the upper second premolars may sometimes be missing and in such cases the upper second deciduous molar is extracted and an appliance used to retract 43|34. The second premolar is not usually the tooth of choice for extraction. Even if considerable care is taken the upper first molars tend to tilt mesially and the upper first premolars distally, producing an unsatisfactory contact (*Fig.* 196).

If the upper first molars are carious in a Class II, division 1 case and are unsavable, they should, where possible, be retained until the second molars erupt (*Fig.* 197). If this is not done, the second molars may move forward before they can be clasped or banded, and take up all the space made available by the extraction of first molars. Moving upper second molars distally is a complication which adds to the treatment.

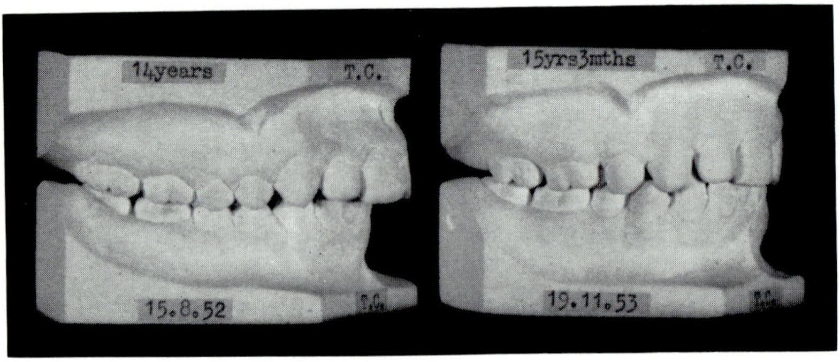

Fig. 196.—Class II, division 1 malocclusion treated by extraction of 5|5, retraction of 43|34 followed by retraction of incisors. Note poor contact between 6| and 4| and mesial tilt of 6|.

There are cases where one or more upper incisors have been traumatized or knocked out. Each of these cases has to be judged on its merits, but there are definite indications for extracting an incisor tooth on one side and a premolar on the other. It is really a question of when endodontic treatment and crowning is justified, and also whether the supporting tissues of the teeth are healthy and there is sufficient tooth substance on which the orthodontic appliance may act. *Fig.* 198 shows one of these problems.

Unilateral Class II, Division 1.—The so-called unilateral Class II, division 1 is fundamentally a Class II malocclusion with asymmetrical arches so that the Class II cheek tooth relationship is seen on one side only. It must be distinguished from a case where there has been early loss of deciduous teeth on one side with local drift of first molars and those cases where there is a deviation in the path of closure.

The treatment of these asymmetrical cases is difficult. A unilateral extraction on the side of the upper arch where the cheek tooth relationship is abnormal is rarely sufficient to reduce the overjet and to correct the upper centre line. Bilateral extractions in the upper arch disturb the normal cuspal relationship on one side, but this has to be accepted

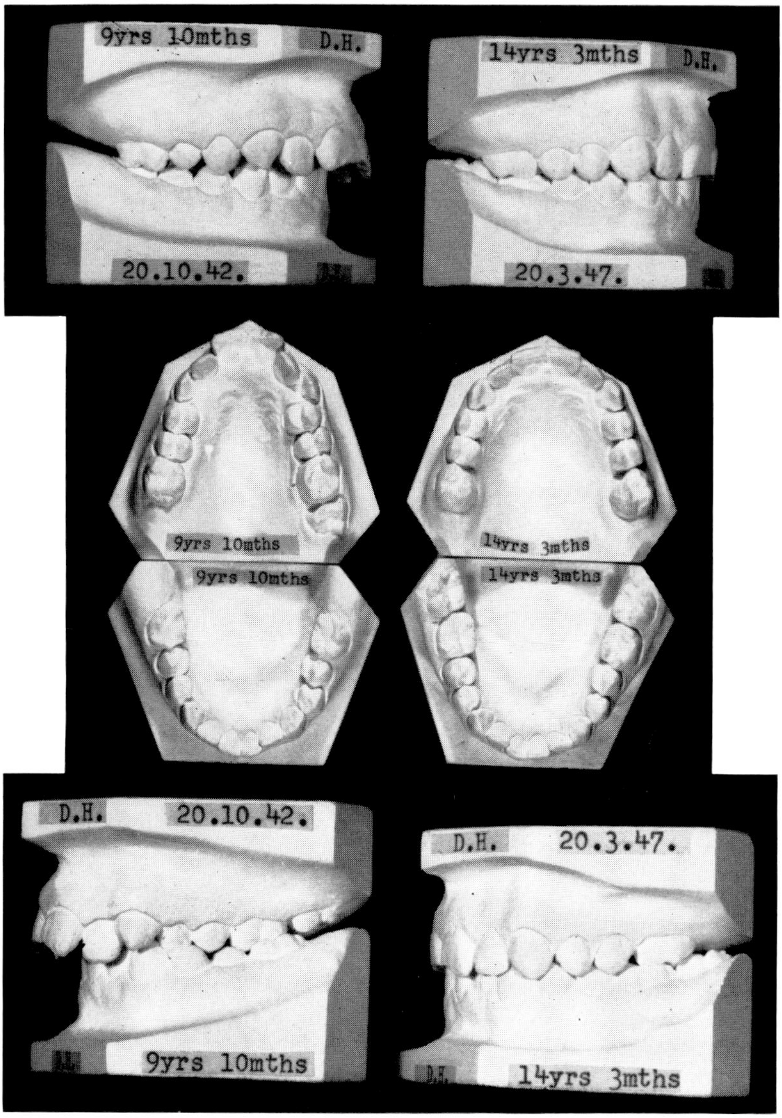

Fig. 197.—Case treated by removable appliance following extraction of $\underline{6|6}$ after eruption of $\underline{7|7}$. $\underline{543|345}$ moved distally prior to retraction of incisors.

and the upper arch adapted as well as possible to the asymmetrical lower unless elaborate fixed-appliance therapy is instituted.

The Complications of Crowded Arches.—Crowding in one or both arches may complicate the treatment of a Class II, division 1 malocclusion.

The Crowded Upper Arch.—Where, for example, the upper second deciduous molars have been extracted at an early age, the upper first permanent molars will have moved forward so that the second premolars may erupt palatally. The extraction of these instanding teeth will not make any space available for retraction of the incisors. Ideally, the first molars should be moved back to their original position, a movement

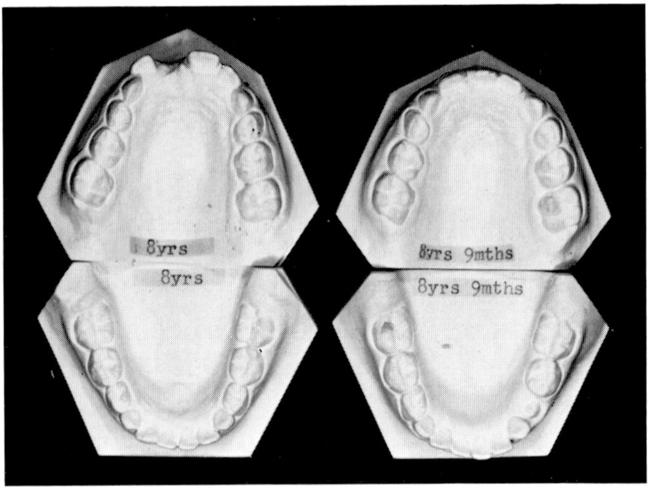

Fig. 198.—Traumatic loss of $\underline{1|}$. The three remaining incisors were collapsed palatally. Such a patient may require the removal of a premolar on one side to correct the centre line and $\underline{|2}$ may be positioned for a jacket crown later.

which does require careful anchorage and may require the assistance of extra-oral traction. Where upper second molars have erupted and can be held back, the extraction of the first molars may allow sufficient space for alinement of an instanding premolar and incisor retraction if the overjet is not marked.

If the upper first molars have had to be extracted early owing to caries, instanding second premolars may move into the arch and the upper second molars move forwards and occupy the space without benefit to the front of the arch. In *rare* cases with *very severe crowding* exaggerated by early loss, two premolars may have to be extracted from each side, one to relieve the crowding and the other to allow space for the retraction of the incisors.

The Crowded Lower Arch.—Early loss of deciduous cheek teeth will exaggerate any crowding that may be present in the lower arch. The crowding may be concentrated so that the second premolar is

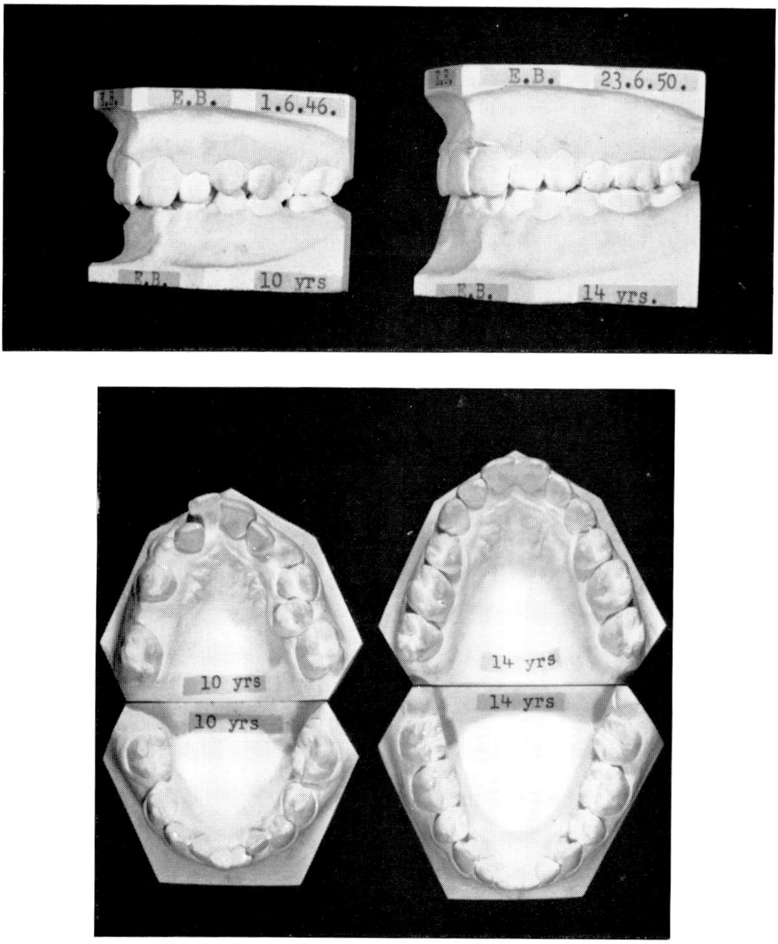

Fig. 199.—Class II, division I malocclusion treated by the extraction of $\frac{4|4}{4|4}$ owing to gross crowding in the lower arch. No lower appliance. Upper arch treated by two upper appliances: (*a*) To retract $\underline{3|3}$ and reduce overbite, (*b*) To retract $\underline{21|12}$.

displaced lingually. If impacted vertically it may attempt to erupt into the arch at the expense of lower incisor alinement.

Where the second premolar is markedly displaced lingually it is better to extract this tooth. However, sometimes the lower first premolar is displaced buccally following the premature loss of the first deciduous molar. *In the past attempts have been made to avoid extractions near the front of the lower arch, but there is no doubt that it is better to extract the lower first premolar on each side than to face severe incisor crowding. These extractions do not have the adverse effect on the incisor overbite which was, at one time, thought to be inevitable.* (*Fig.* 199.)

It is not possible to recreate space to overcome crowding in the buccal segments without employing extractions somewhere in the lower arch.

If lower incisors are ever actively proclinated to obtain space for premolars they will relapse in the face of lip pressure. Slight crowding with slipping contacts in the incisor region of the lower arch at the age of 12 years heralds a worsening of this condition at the time of eruption of the third molars. One form of treatment advocated to prevent deterioration of lower incisor alinement was the extraction of the lower second molars which gave an opportunity for lower third molars to erupt in those cases described as favourable by Cryer (*see* p. 124). It is the authors' opinion that this form of treatment should no longer be practised except in a limited number of cases. Extensive appliance therapy is required to relieve crowding anteriorly, and usually the labial segment of the lower arch does not benefit to the full extent and the path of eruption of the third molars cannot be guaranteed.

It is surprising how well the lower canines will move distally following extraction of lower first premolars and many of the incisor irregularities are self-correcting. There is less need for complex multibanded techniques to retract lower canines and aline the incisors, particularly as it is not necessary to move buccal segments forward to support the lower labial segment and a small space in the first premolar region is a useful 'safety valve'.

The first permanent molars are so frequently carious that the extraction of all four may be a practical necessity in a Class II, division 1 case. Where there is a crowded lower arch and the patient is seen by $8\frac{1}{2}$ years of age, the results are not as unfortunate as previously thought if the monobloc can be used to apply traction to the upper teeth to reduce the overjet and control the movement of lower teeth.

The Andresen Appliance.—This is a modification of the monobloc originally used by Pierre Robin in the early part of this century. He used it as a splint between upper and lower jaws, holding the mandible in a forward position to relieve the airway for those children who had difficulties in breathing. An active method of using this appliance was devised by Andresen in Norway and Haupl in Germany and there have since been many modifications. In certain European centres this type of appliance is used to treat many forms of malocclusion. It may have auxiliary devices for individual tooth movements. In this book the authors intend to limit its use to those cases suitable for inter-maxillary traction.

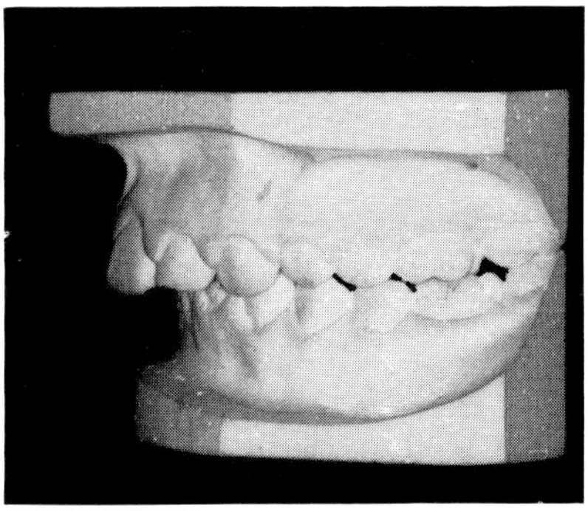

A

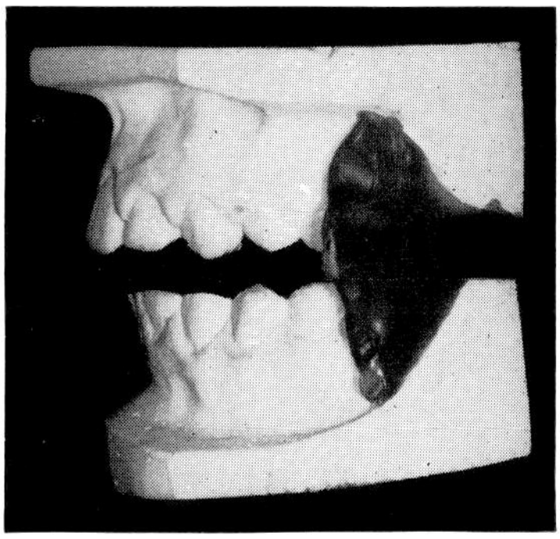

B

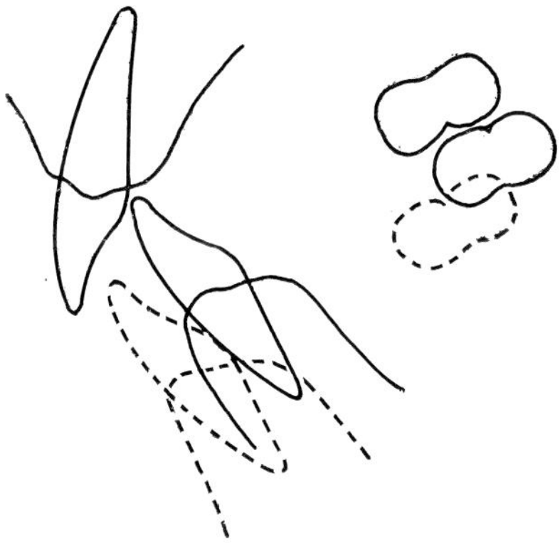

C

Fig. 200.—A, Class II, division I malocclusion with good arches. Suitable case for monobloc. B, Position of models in 'working' bite. C, Tracing to show incisor and molar relationship; solid line indicating occlusion position, dotted line indicating position of forward 'working' bite.

The general principles have been described in Chapter IX and some detail has been given concerning the methods of construction. It is a combined upper and lower appliance which fits loosely in the mouth. It is worn at night and as much as possible during the evening. In order to produce traction on the upper dental arch it is constructed to a forward 'working' bite as shown in *Fig.* 200 B, C. The cheek teeth are empirically separated by 3–4 mm. in order to exceed the freeway space or 'inter-occlusal clearance'. The amount of forward bite registered is usually sufficient to bring the cheek teeth into Class I relationship and the lower incisors should not be advanced beyond the upper incisors. The bite is taken with a firm horseshoe of wax about 6 mm. in thickness. This may be reinforced by inserting thin pieces of wooden spatula, but it is usually sufficient to have it thoroughly chilled. The mandible should be advanced symmetrically and no attempt should be made to correct any severe discrepancies in upper to lower centre lines. Any lingual undercuts on the lower models should be eliminated. The labial arch is constructed in 0·9-mm. wire.

When the appliance is in place the mandible is forced to adopt a forward position, even at rest. Because it encroaches beyond the freeway space, the mandibular elevators and retractor muscles exert a steady pull which has been demonstrated by the electromyograph. This pull is transmitted to the upper dental arch and the anchorage is derived from contact with the crowns of the lower teeth and contact in the lingual sulcus.

Apart from this general effect on the upper dental arch, the appliance acts as a complex bite plate, when it is forced into place during swallowing and idle movements. Certain trimming of the appliance will encourage movement of individual teeth. The methods of trimming are controversial and the authors will describe those modifications which have been found to be useful.

Usually there is a deep overbite in the cases suitable for treatment by this method. The lower incisors are therefore prevented from further eruption by keeping a lip of acrylic over their incisal edges. The upper incisors, which are to be tilted distally, have the acrylic freed from behind their crowns, far up on to the palate (*Fig.* 201 A). The upper labial arch should not be activated but merely rest in contact with the labial surface of the upper incisors, one-third of the distance from the incisal tip to the cervical margin. The acrylic is trimmed away from the occlusal surfaces of the upper cheek teeth so that they are free to erupt. This trimming takes the form of a gully which is directed slightly distobucally and a well-defined mesial contact is kept for each upper tooth (*Fig.* 201 C). Some authorities do not trim away acrylic over the lower cheek teeth. This would not appear to be a critical factor. If they are trimmed occlusally, the gully should not allow any mesial movement as it is essential for the teeth in the lower arch to be compounded together as firm anchorage. This will lessen the forward movement of the lower dental arch, which would place the incisors in an unstable position (*Figs.* 202, 203).

This appliance appears disarmingly simple, but unless the technique and case selection are fully appreciated the results are disappointing.

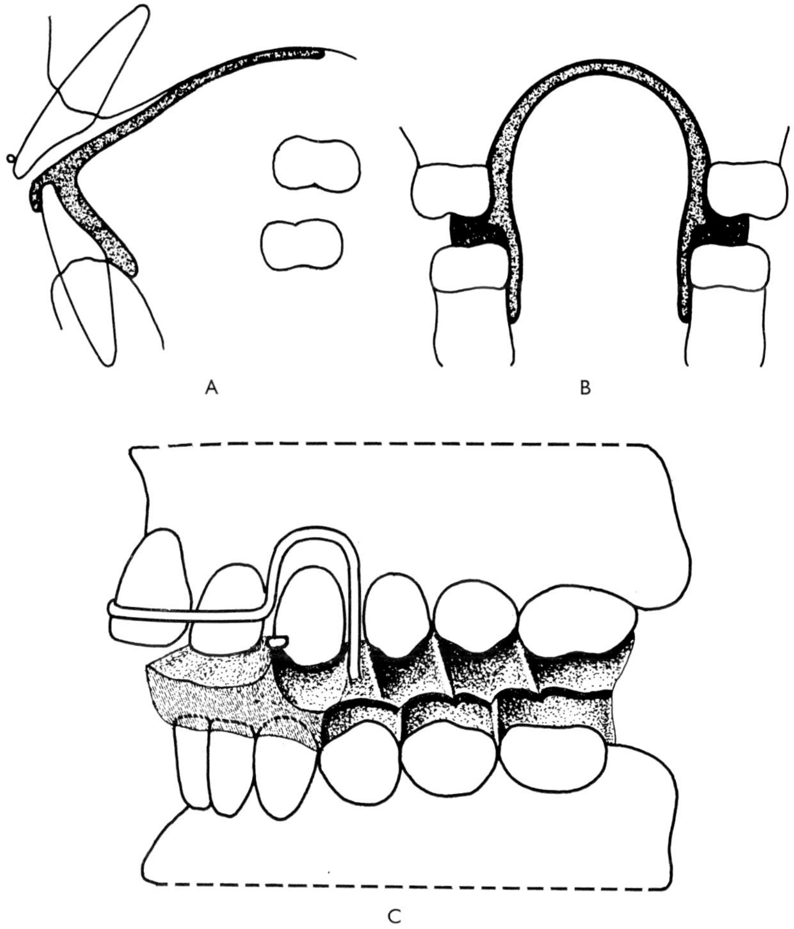

Fig. 201.—A, Sagittal section showing way in which plate is trimmed away beyond the upper incisors and lip kept over the lower incisors. B, Transverse section showing how the plate is trimmed over the occlusal surfaces of the cheek teeth allowing the upper molars to be on a buccal inclined slope and the lower molars to be free occlusally. C, Side view of monobloc on models to show trimming of facets allowing continued eruption of cheek teeth with buccal inclinations of upper facets. Mesial contacts with all upper cheek teeth allow them to be 'dragged' distally transmitting the pull of the mandibular elevator muscles. (*Continued on p.* 214.)

Fig. 204 shows an ideal case which has been followed up for a number of years to show the stability of the end-result. There is no doubt that this appliance in experienced hands has many advantages. Treatment can be carried out in the mixed dentition before the first molars

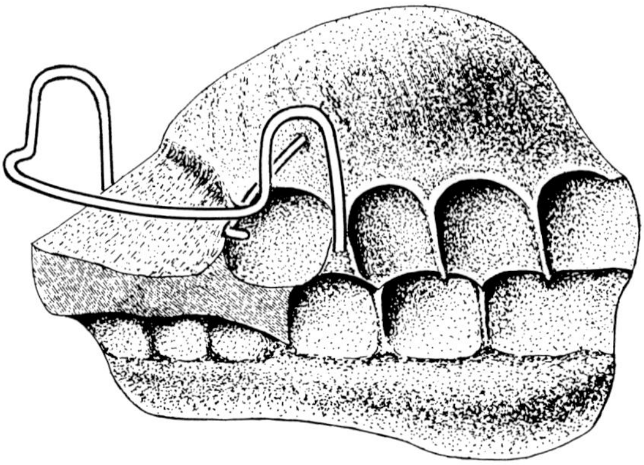

D

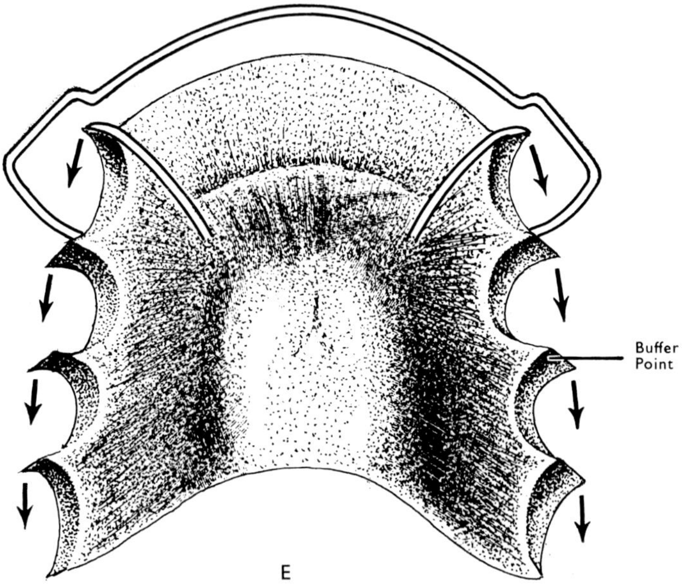

E

Fig. 201 (*continued*).—D, Lateral view of monobloc showing wire insert to provide good mesial contact for upper canines and acrylic removed palatal to upper incisors. E, View of monobloc from above showing buffer points for mesial contact with upper cheek teeth: dark shading indicates burnished facets where upper teeth contact the acrylic.

are well erupted and an abnormal incisor relationship can be intercepted.

Prognosis.—It has been explained that it is possible to predict whether the upper labial segment can be moved into a position where it can be stable in labiolingual balance, and when it is not possible to achieve a perfect incisor relationship. In a limited number of cases a multibanded technique is required to move the incisor segments bodily so that the upper labial segment can be contained by the inner surface

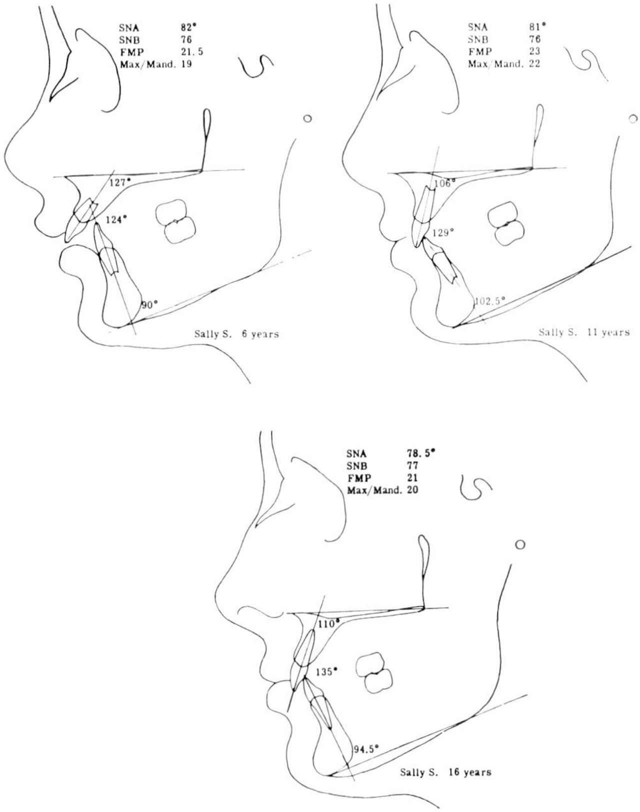

Fig. 202.—Tracings of a Class II, division 1 malocclusion treated by Andresen appliance. Note slight relapse of upper incisors to stable position; lower incisors were proclined by the appliance but did not relapse to original inclination; note that there was no tongue-thrust in this case. (*See also Fig.* 203.)

of the lower lip. It is not possible to predict skeletal growth but it can be said with certainty that a Skeletal 2 relationship will never turn into a Skeletal 1 with or without orthodontic treatment. Particular care has to be taken in those cases where there is a Class II, division 1 malocclusion with a Skeletal 3 pattern. Such a case is seen in *Fig.* 205, where

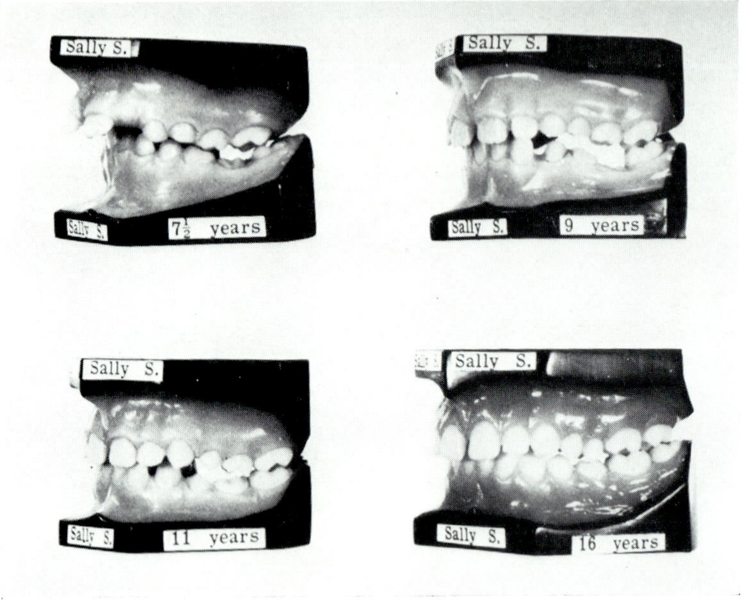

Fig. 203.—Serial models of Class II case treated by monobloc. Models of patient whose tracings are shown in *Fig.* 202. There was rapid improvement in the early stages of treatment. Last model four years out of retention shows slight relapse. $\overline{5|5}$ are missing and $\overline{E|E}$ are retained, hence the slight abnormality in cuspal relationship.

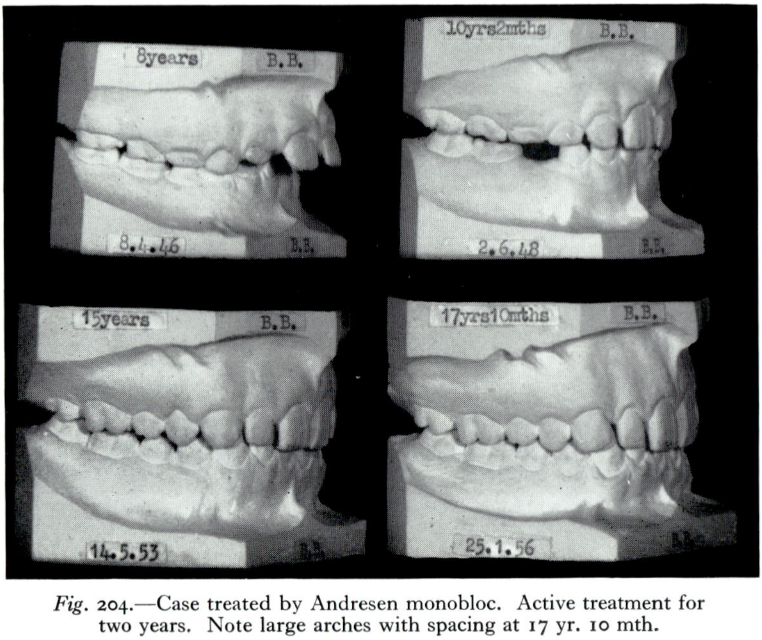

Fig. 204.—Case treated by Andresen monobloc. Active treatment for two years. Note large arches with spacing at 17 yr. 10 mth.

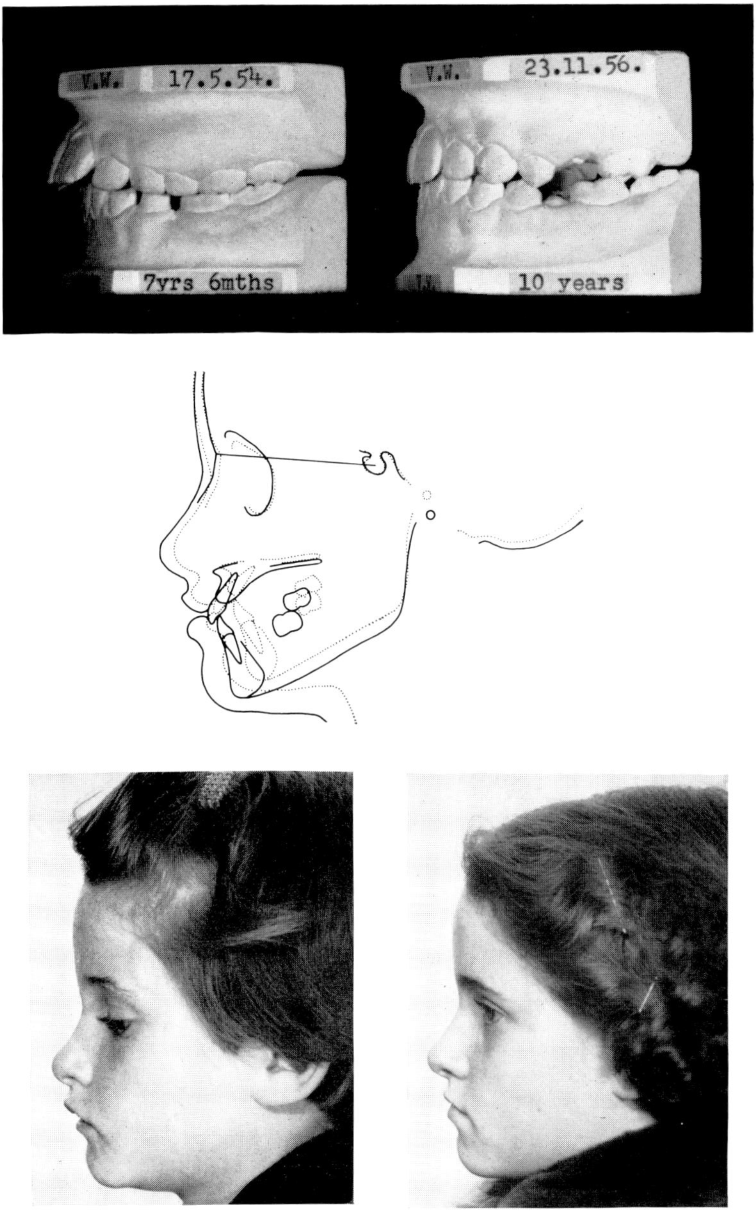

Fig. 205.—Class II, division 1 malocclusion, early loss of $\overline{D|D}$ showing Class I molar relationship with slight Skeletal 3 dental base relationship. Treated by monobloc. Note mandiblar growth with the Skeletal 3 pattern. *Not the result of wearing a monobloc.*

the arch relationship was changed with the Andresen appliance and the incisor relationship is nearly edge to edge after treatment.

The Timing of Treatment.—It is unwise to commence treatment in the complete deciduous dentition. Clinical experience indicates that this is a complete waste of time.

If the patient is attending for routine dental treatment there can be a strong case for intercepting a Class II, division 1 relationship when the incisors erupt, using a monobloc. It may not, however, prevent the need for further treatment in the permanent dentition. An alternative treatment in the mixed dentition is to extract upper deciduous canines and correct the incisor relationship. This will allay the parents' worries and diminish the likelihood of fracture of the upper incisors, but a further period of active treatment may be required following the extraction of upper first or second premolars to complete the alinement of the canines.

Apart from appeasing the parents and reducing the possibility of damage to the incisors it is much better to await eruption of the upper premolars and canines before commencing active treatment.

BIBLIOGRAPHY

BALLARD, C. F. (1957), 'A Symposium on Class II, division 1 Malocclusion—Morphology in Relation to Treatment Planning', *Dent. Practit.*, **7**, 269.

— — (1967), 'The Morphological Bases of Prognosis Determination and Treatment Planning', *Trans. Brit. Soc. Orthodont.*, **11**, 95.

BJØRK, A. (1951), 'The Principles of the Andresen Method of Orthodontic Treatment—A Discussion based on Cephalometric X-ray Analysis of Treated Cases', *Amer. J. Orthodont.*, **37**, 437.

PRINGLE, K. E. (1955), 'Long Term Results of Orthodontic Treatment', *Dent. Practit.*, **5**, 297.

RIX, R. E. (1953), 'Some Observations upon the Environment of the Incisors', *Dent. Rec.*, **73**, 427.

CHAPTER XII

TREATMENT OF ANGLE'S CLASS II, DIVISION 2 MALOCCLUSIONS

The Occlusal Abnormality.—*Fig.* 206 illustrates the occlusal abnormality described as Class II, division 2. The relationship of the

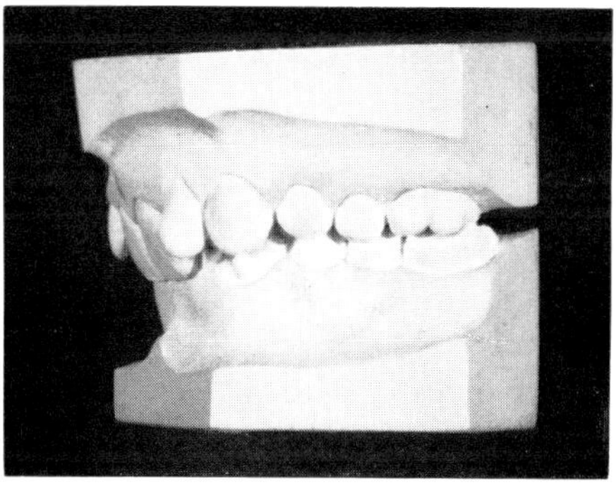

Fig. 206.—Model of a typical Class II, division 2 malocclusion.

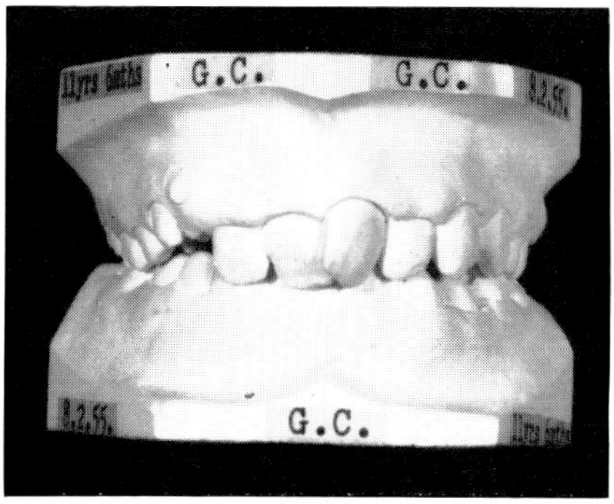

Fig. 207.—Model showing atypical incisor crowding in Class II, division 2 type of malocclusion.

cheek teeth being Class II, four instead of six lower teeth occlude with four upper incisors which are not supported on the lower lip as in Class II, division 1. In its classic form the upper central incisors are closely applied to the lowers and the upper laterals are proclinated and overlap the centrals. There are other atypical forms of incisor crowding in this group where all the upper incisors are retroclined, overlapping, and are closely applied to the lowers (*Fig.* 207).

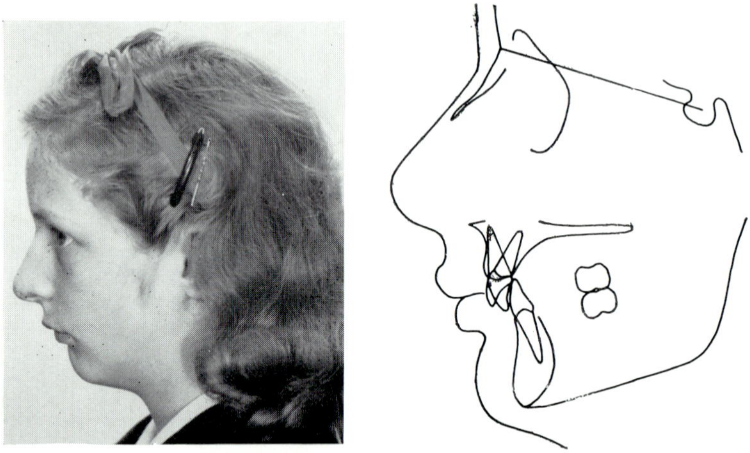

A

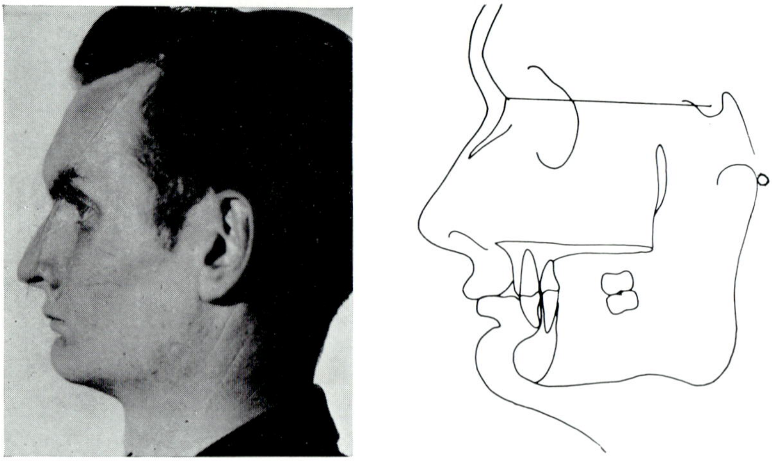

B

Fig. 208.—A, A typical profile and lateral skull tracing of a patient with Class II, division 2 malocclusion on a Skeletal 2 dental base. B, A very severe type of Class II, division 2 which is almost a caricature of the classic facial form with an excessively deep overbite.

The lower arch is flat anteriorly, and both arches are usually broad so that a cross-bite is uncommon. The upper central incisors are retroclined, but the lowers are not necessarily so. The overbite is almost invariably deep, but not usually traumatic to the palatal or lower labial gingivae. The upper central incisors often show a definite angulation between the crown and root. They also have an ill-defined cingulum which may account for the lower incisors being 'wedged' lingually and continuing to erupt under certain circumstances. (*See* p. 182.)

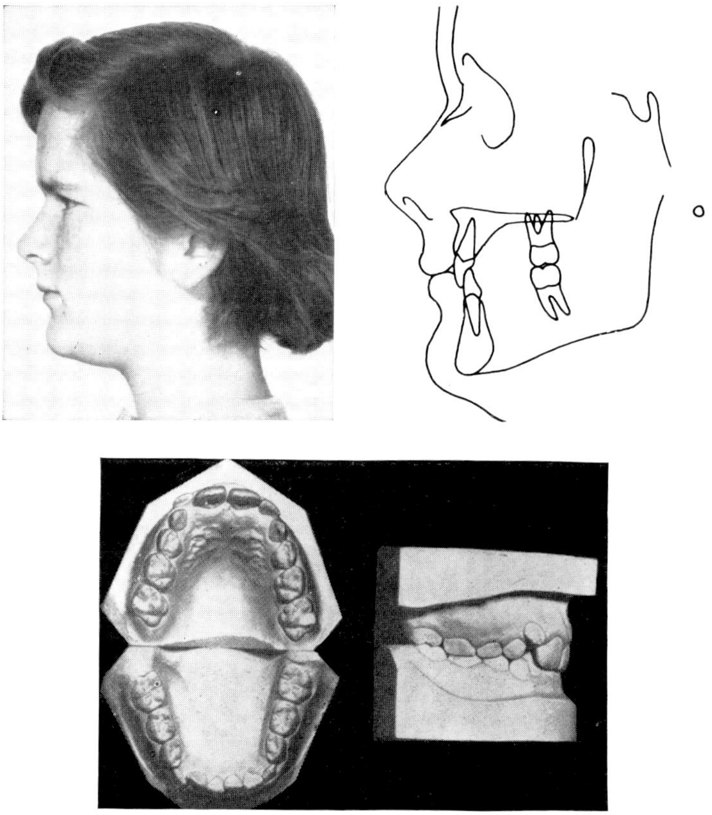

Fig. 209.—Patient with a Class I malocclusion showing deep overbite with crowding in both arches. The crowding in the lower arch is extremely difficult to improve without increasing the overbite further. Skeletal 1 dental base (*see Fig.* 218).

The Skeletal Relationship (Anteroposterior Relationship of the Dental Bases).—This type of malocclusion is most frequently associated with a Skeletal 2 dental base relationship (*Fig.* 208 A), but it may also occur on a Skeletal 1 or even a Skeletal 3 dental base, in which case the lower incisors are retroclined as in the Class I case shown in *Fig.* 209. This type of malocclusion has many strong familial features. *Fig.* 208 B shows an extreme example with a very low Frankfort-mandibular-plane angle, the condylar angle being almost 90°. The malar eminences are prominent, and the face is broad. There is usually a well-defined mental eminence.

The Lips and Tongue.—The lips are usually sealed at rest and the upper lip is rather long and flat. There is a marked depression beneath the lower lip, and the lip line at rest is high on the labial surface of the upper central incisors. *Fig.* 210 shows how little of the central incisors is visible when the upper lip is pulled away.

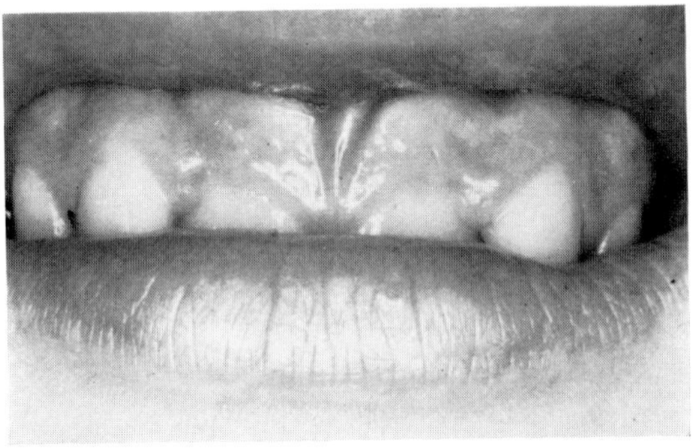

Fig. 210.—Upper lip retracted showing position of lower lip at rest in relation to upper incisors.

The soft tissues foster contact of upper and lower incisors rather than dispersing them as in Class II, division 1. In only a few cases is there any excessive contraction of the lips. There is no forward tongue-thrust but some cases show lateral tongue-thrust and lateral sigmatism in speech. The effects of the muscular environment on the incisors are illustrated in *Fig.* 211. The lips do not exert lingual pressure continuously, but they have certain morphological features which cause them to act like thick curtain drapes. This prevents any active proclination of the incisors from being maintained.

Path of Mandibular Closure.—At one time it was thought that most patients with a Class II, division 2 malocclusion and deep overbite showed a true posterior displacement of the mandible when closing from the rest position into occlusion. The initial contact of the lower incisors with the palatal surface of the upper incisors was thought to produce a reflex avoiding action. This might have a deleterious effect on the function of the temporomandibular joint and might produce painful symptoms. Ballard has shown that in most cases there is an habitual mandibular rest position which is downward and forward from the true 'endogenous' postural position.

Closing from this forward position into occlusion gives the false appearance of posterior displacement.

True posterior displacement is thought to be quite rare. When it does occur treatment to improve axial inclinations of the upper incisors

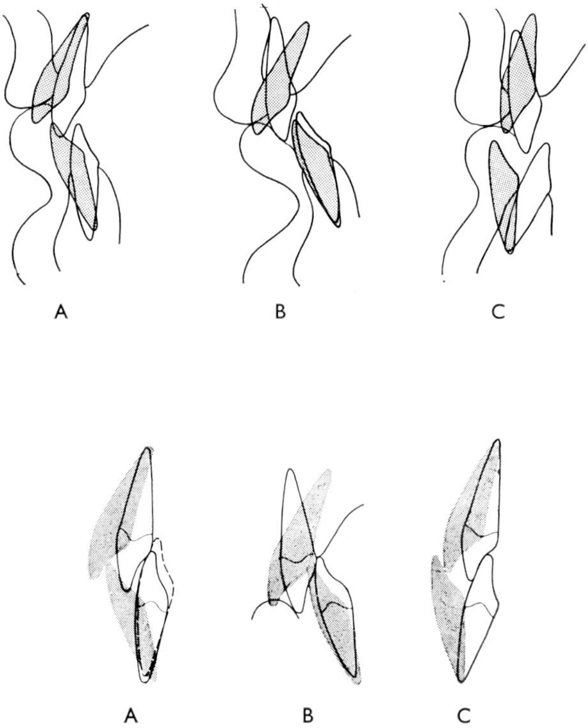

Fig. 211.—Diagram to show moulding effect of soft tissues. Note how axial inclinations of the incisors may be influenced on: **A**, Skeletal 1 base; **B**, Skeletal 2 base; **C**, Skeletal 3 base. The stippled teeth indicate the position the teeth would assume with normal soft-tissue influence. *N.B.*—Most Class II, division 2 malocclusions on a Skeletal 2 base will not show excessive lip contraction.

may allow some slight forward movement of the mandible and this probably accounts for the considerable improvement in the case illustrated in *Fig.* 212.

Local Complicating Factors.—

Sucking Habits.—Sucking habits are rarely encountered, and when they do occur are not usually persistent enough to mask the underlying malocclusion. Once the habit ceases there is rapid reversion to the typical incisor position, as the lips and tongue do not perpetuate the dispersal of the incisors. (*See Fig.* 68, p. 91.)

Premature Loss of Deciduous Cheek Teeth.—Early loss of deciduous cheek teeth in the *upper* dental arch may foster crowding in the premolar region but may allow some improvement in the position of the lateral

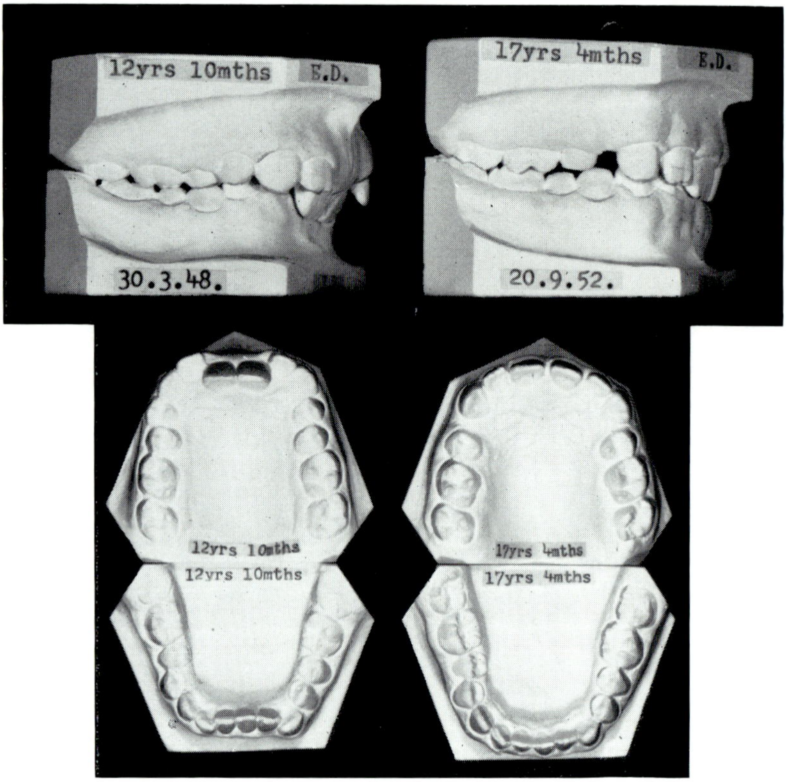

Fig. 212.—Rare case with true distal displacement on closure, treated by extraction of $\underline{4|4}$ and retraction of $\underline{32|23}$, with some labial movement of $\underline{1|1}$. Note residual spacing.

incisors in less severe cases. Early loss in the lower dental arch may localize crowding to the premolar region and could exaggerate the overbite to the extent that it becomes traumatic to the soft tissues of the palate. This is somewhat controversial, but there is clinical evidence to show this can happen when the overbite is complete and excessively deep. This may be encouraged because of the lack of well-formed cingulum palatal to the upper incisors.

As stated above, trauma to the soft tissues is rare, but *Fig.* 213 shows one very gross type of Class II, division 2 with severe gingival damage.

TREATMENT

General Principles.—The main aims of treatment are to aline the upper incisors and to make some reduction in the overbite where possible.

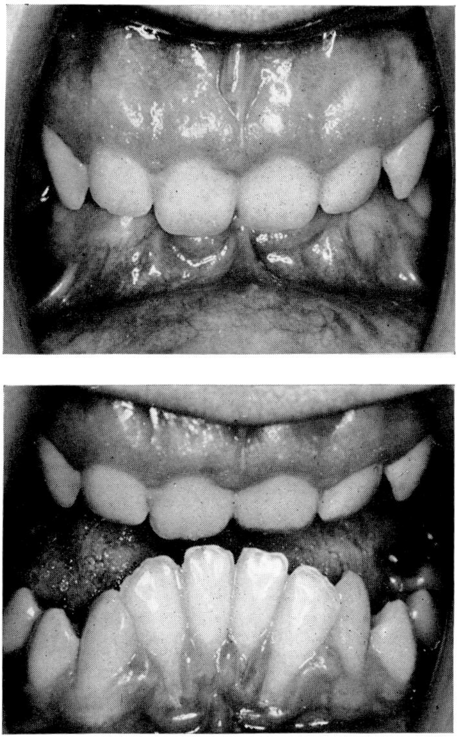

Fig. 213.—Very extreme case of Class II, division 2 showing trauma to the lower labial gingivae.

Forward movement of the upper central incisors will relapse owing to the influence of the lower lip. In general, the position of the upper centrals has to be accepted and bilateral extractions in the upper arch are required to obtain room for the alinement of the outstanding laterals. It is true to say that the inclination of the upper central incisors can sometimes be slightly improved, particularly in rare cases where there is a true distal displacement of the mandible on closure from rest to occlusion (*Fig.* 212). With complex multiband techniques, it is possible to move the central incisor apices palatally and maintain the position of their crowns in linguo-labial balance. Evidence for the permanence of such results is far from satisfactory except in those cases where there was a true posterior displacement of the mandible.

The Mechanics of Treatment.—Extra-oral and intermaxillary traction can be used to move the upper buccal segments distally, but only those methods which employ intramaxillary traction will be described here. There are two procedures, of which the first is the most direct and reliable:—

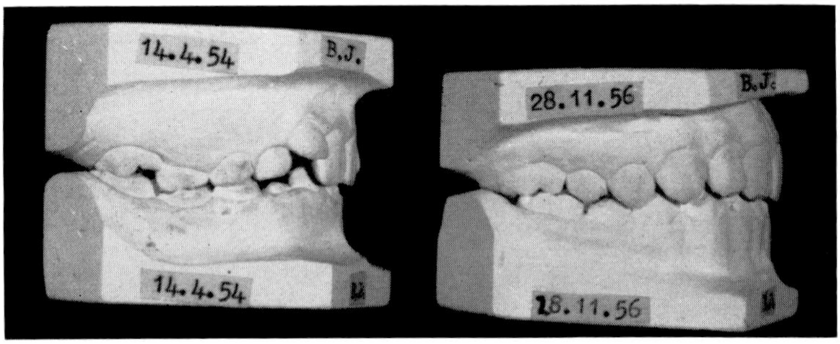

Fig. 214.—Case treated by serial extraction of $\underline{C|C}$ and $\underline{6|6}$. No appliances.

1. Upper first premolars may be extracted and the canines and lateral incisors retracted and alined.
2. The cheek tooth segments may be moved distally, coupled with the extraction of upper second molars, allowing room for alinement of the upper lateral incisors.

Premolar Extractions and Alinement of Anterior Teeth.—This form of treatment may be initiated in the mixed dentition by employing serial extractions in the upper arch. Upper deciduous canines are extracted and the upper lateral incisors alined, using an appliance with free-ending buccal arms, incorporating a short, steep, inclined plane. Later, upper first premolars are extracted and the upper canines alined. In rare circumstances, some cases can be resolved by serial extraction in the upper arch without recourse to appliances, but it would be wrong to highlight these mild cases. (*Fig.* 214.)

Fig. 215 shows the type of apparatus used. The basic appliance has palatal canine retractors boxed in under the plate. Short buccal arms in 0·7-mm. wire can retract the upper lateral incisors when the canines have been retracted. A short, steep, anterior bite plane makes a temporary reduction in overbite and sometimes does produce a slightly better position of the incisors.

Where the upper first permanent molars are very carious but can be conserved until the second molars erupt, the second molars can be clasped and included in the anchorage when the first permanent

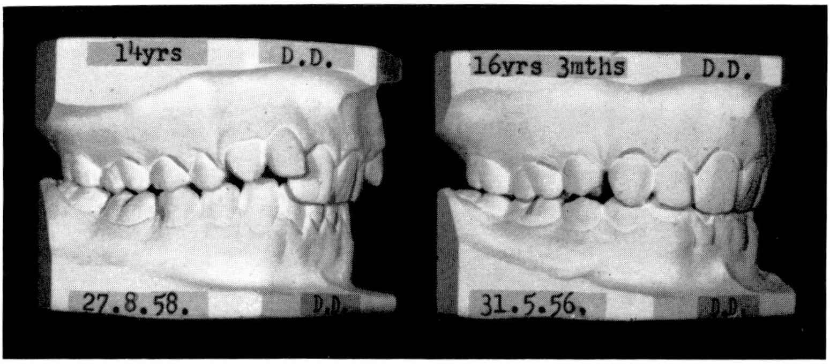

A

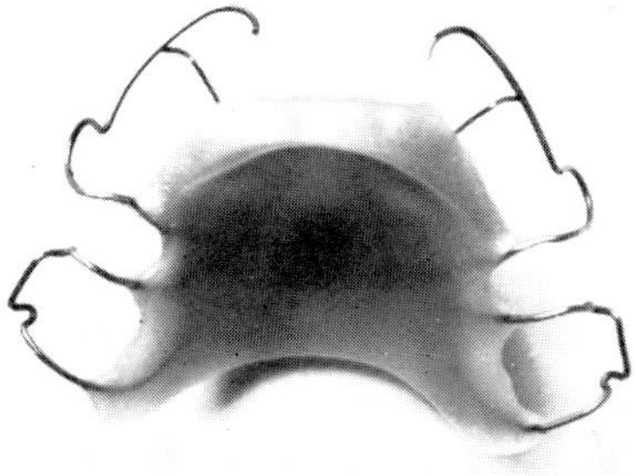

B

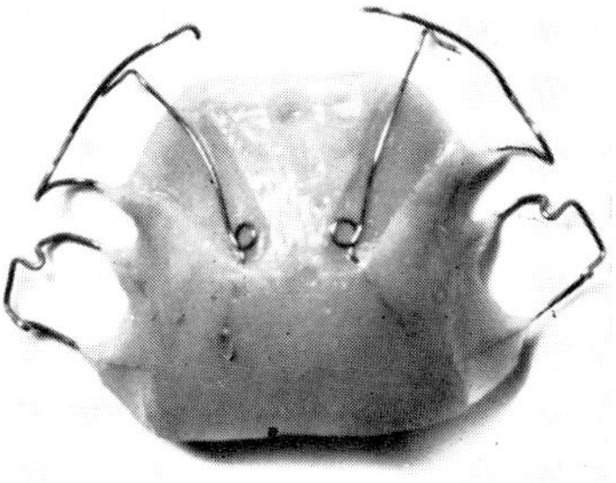

C

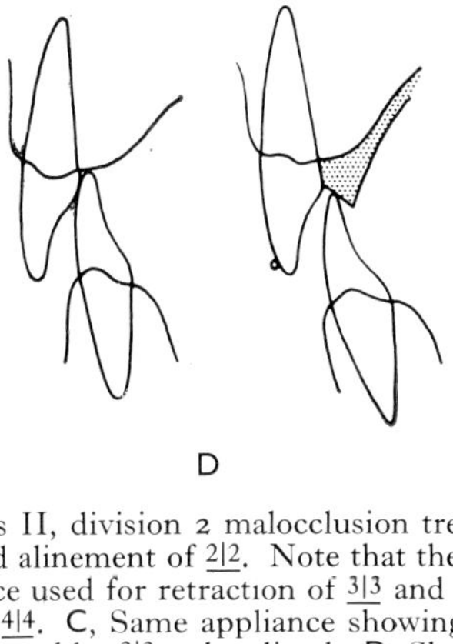

D

Fig. 215.—A, Class II, division 2 malocclusion treated by extraction of 4|4, retraction of 3|3, and alinement of 2|2. Note that there is a residual space distal to 3|. B, Appliance used for retraction of 3|3 and later alinement of 2|2 following extraction of 4|4. C, Same appliance showing fit surface. Careful use of free ending arms enables 2|2 to be alined. D, Short steep anterior bite plane used in this type of case.

molars are eventually extracted. The premolars can then be moved distally, followed by the retraction of upper canines and lateral incisors. *Fig.* 216 A illustrates a form of apparatus which can be used in these circumstances. This enforced extraction of upper first permanent molars must inevitably increase the treatment time. *Fig.* 216 B shows an example of a treated case.

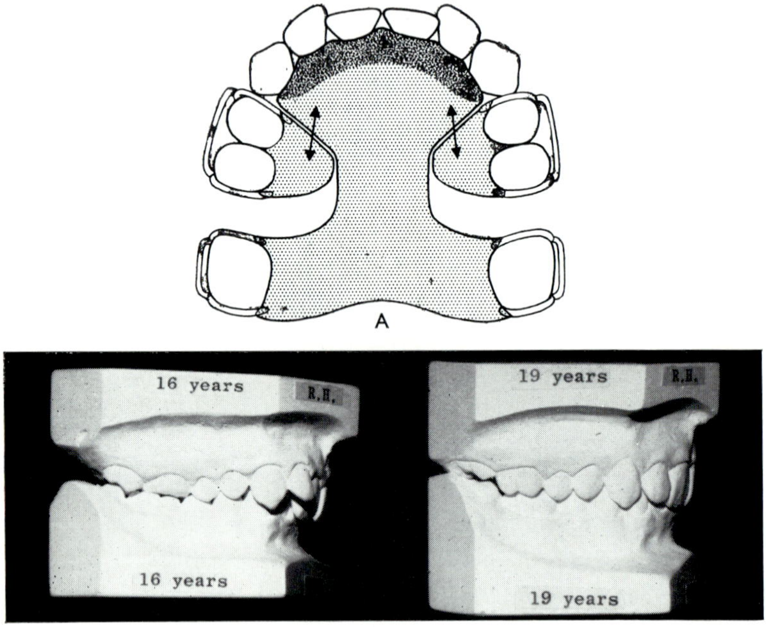

A

B

Fig. 216.—A, Upper appliance to move 54|45 distally after extraction of 6|6. Note that 7|7 are adequately clasped and a short steep inclined plane minimizes the forward component of thrust on the upper incisors and reinforces anchorage. B, Case treated after 16 years by extraction of 6|6 and 7|7. Active treatment for 14 months.

Distal Movement of Upper Buccal Segments with Extraction of Second Molars.—*Fig.* 217 B illustrates the type of appliance which can be used to move both buccal segments distally. This should only be used in association with extraction of upper second molars in cases *where the upper first molars are not already distally inclined.* Anchorage is reinforced by using a steep anterior inclined biting plane, and if only one buccal segment is moved at a time, there will be less likelihood of moving the upper incisors forward into an unstable position. *Fig.* 217 A shows this treatment in the mixed dentition, which requires extraction of the upper second molars on eruption.

Where there is actual trauma to the palatal or lower labial gingivae some stoning of the lower incisors and the use of a bite plane may help. There may be a temporary oedema of the mucosa aggravating the condition which will clear up with treatment.

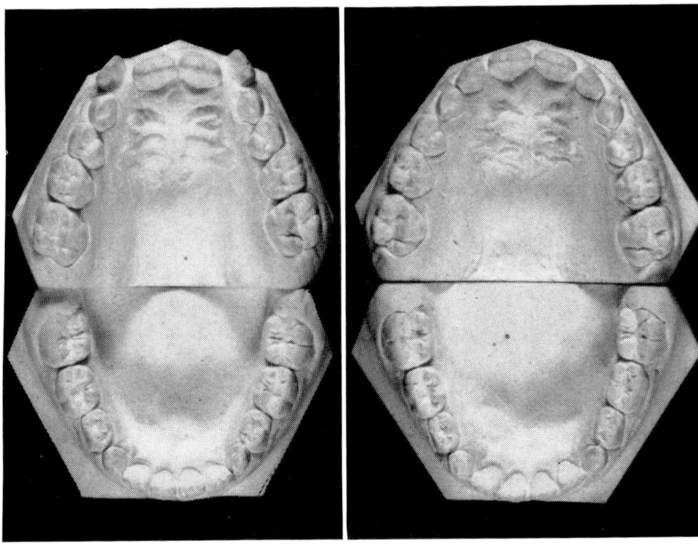

A

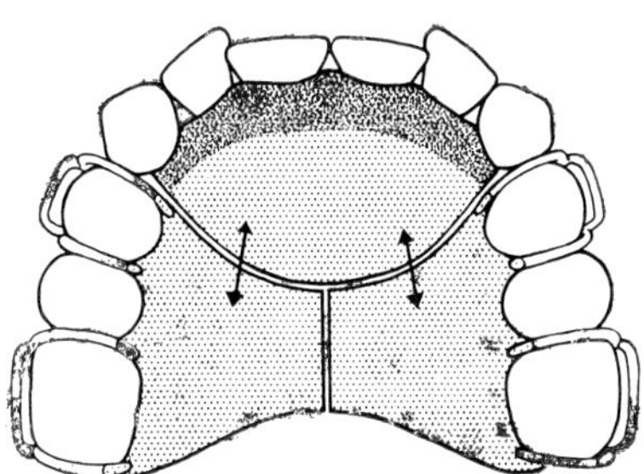

B

Fig. 217.—A, Case treated by distal movement of buccal segments; to have $\underline{7|7}$ extracted. B, Appliance to effect this movement.

Where there is severe trauma a permanent overlay may have to be fitted. (*See Fig.* 213.) These overlays are well tolerated, but it is advisable to construct one in acrylic first to test the bite opening and follow this with one constructed in chrome-cobalt.

The Complications of Crowded Arches.—As in the treatment of Class II, division 1 malocclusions, complications may arise where the arches are crowded. Fortunately, there is less tendency to crowding in the lower arch.

The Crowded Upper Arch.—The crowding in the upper arch is usually revealed by the outlocking of the upper lateral incisors. Although early loss in the buccal segments may have allowed some improvement in the position of the incisors, this does not occur in the gross cases. Any improvement of the lateral incisors is at the expense of

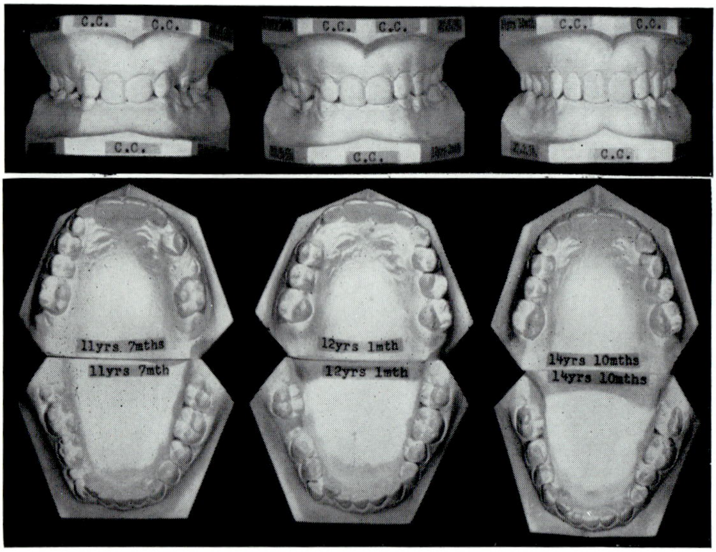

Fig. 218.—Model to show how lower canines crowded outside arch may complicate alinement of upper lateral incisors. This type with lower crowding is difficult to treat. Owing to the forward drift of the buccal segment, the molar relationship may be Class I. Extraction of $\frac{6|6}{6|}$ enabled the incisors to be alined. $\overline{543|}$ were retracted with a screw plate. The overbite has not increased.

space for a premolar or a canine. Where there has been no improvement in the position of the laterals and where the second premolar is displaced palatally, extraction of this tooth will not provide sufficient space for the complete alinement of upper laterals without mechanical distal movement of the upper molars.

The Crowded Lower Arch.—Early loss of deciduous cheek teeth in the lower arch may exaggerate crowding. The problems are similar to those described in the lower arch in Class II, division 1 malocclusions. The major problem is that extractions to relieve crowding may permit an increase in the overbite so that it becomes traumatic to the soft tissues and therefore some slight degree of crowding should be accepted. Extraction of lower second molars to allow third molars to erupt and prevent deterioration of the mildly crowded lower arch is very limited in its application. *See* contra-indications on p. 124.

The lower second premolar, which is displaced so far lingually that the first molar and first premolar are in contact, may be extracted when the mechanical treatment of the upper arch has been completed.

In most Class II, division 2 cases on a Skeletal 2 dental base the lower arch is well formed. Crowding in the lower arch is more likely to be seen where the malocclusion occurs on a Skeletal 1 tending to a Skeletal 3 base where the lower incisors are markedly retroclined and the lower buccal segments have drifted forward so that the malocclusion could be more correctly termed Class 1 (*see Fig.* 209). The outlocking of lower canines complicates the alinement of upper lateral incisors. These cases are very difficult to treat. Where all the first molars are carious, their early removal allows lower second molars to erupt without tilting and some space is available to allow the lower premolars and canines to be moved distally if a similar treatment is instituted in the upper arch. It is important to get the upper premolars moved distally to a normal relationship with the lower premolars (*Fig.* 218).

Hereditary Pattern and Relapse.—The clinical picture is dominated by the hereditary facial form and many cases show a measure of relapse even if retained for a prolonged period. The upper lateral incisors may move forward, although there is adequate space for them in the arch, and the overbite may increase. Many cases show a definite angulation between the crown and the root of the central incisors. This is probably an inherent morphological feature rather than a product of lip pressure as these teeth erupt.

Relapse will occur when the overbite has been reduced by proclining the upper and lower incisors, thus moving the crowns of the teeth out of balance with their soft-tissue environment.

There is no doubt that many mild cases are better left untreated unless they are very aesthetically displeasing. The deep overbite *per se* is not deleterious as trauma to the gingival tissues is extremely uncommon.

BIBLIOGRAPHY

BALLARD, C. F. (1956), 'Morphology and Treatment of Class II, division 2 Malocclusions', *Trans. europ. orthod. Soc.*, **32**, 44.

LEECH, H. L. (1957), 'The Treatment of Angle's Class II, division 1 and Class II, division 2 in Identical Twins', *Trans. Brit. Soc. Orthodont.*, 60.

RIDLEY, D. R. (1960), 'Some Factors concerned with the Reduction of Excessive Incisor Overbite in Angle's Class II, division 2 type of Malocclusion', *Ibid.*, 118.

CHAPTER XIII

TREATMENT OF ANGLE'S CLASS III MALOCCLUSIONS

The Occlusal Abnormality.—*Fig.* 219 illustrates the occlusal abnormality described as Class III where the labial segments may have a reduced overbite, an edge-to-edge bite or, more commonly, there may be an 'anterior cross-bite'. Like all other malocclusions there may be considerable variations with cross-bite in the buccal

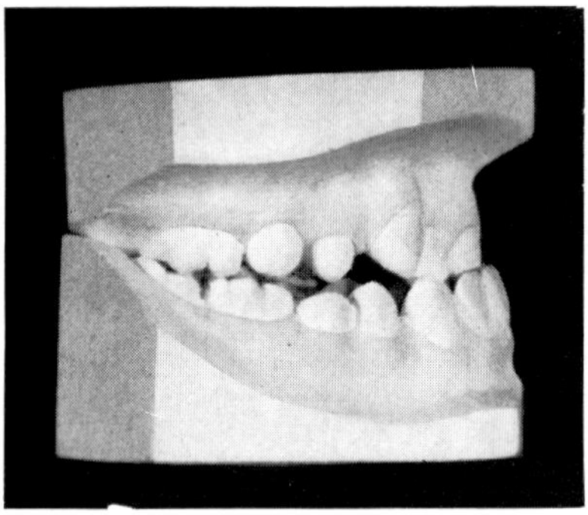

Fig. 219.—A Class III malocclusion associated with a true Skeletal 3 dental base relationship.

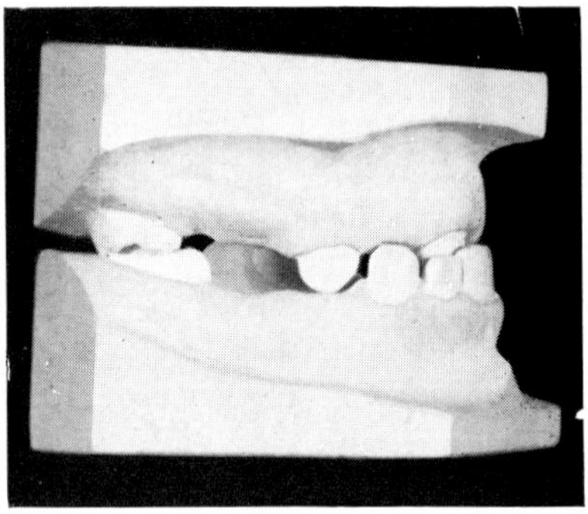

Fig. 220.—A pseudo-Class III malocclusion with excessive incisor overbite produced by overclosure.

segments and arches which may be large or small, crowded, or spaced. It has been customary to refer to the pseudo-Class III malocclusion (*Fig.* 220), where there is a deep reversed overbite exaggerated by a mandibular overclosure. There may also be some initial mandibular forward displacement and this will be discussed more fully in due course. It is important to emphasize that the term 'pseudo-Class III' or 'postural Class III' is merely a descriptive term.

The Skeletal Relationship.—Probably in Class III cases more than in any others the inherited jaw form is evident (*Fig.* 222). The Hapsburg family have always been quoted as the classic example. True Class III malocclusions occur with a Skeletal 3 relationship generally associated with a mandibular protrusion or in some cases a degree of maxillary retrusion. There is, however, considerable variation in skeletal form. For the purpose of classification, McCallin described three groups. Group 1 comprises those cases with small maxilla, excessive anterior face height, and a mandible which is long and presents a high Frankfort-mandibular-plane angle. There is usually a degree of anterior open bite (*see Fig.* 225).

Group 2 includes the opposite end of the scale where both maxilla and mandible are large. There is true mandibular prognathism and a normal to low Frankfort-mandibular plane (*see Fig.* 226).

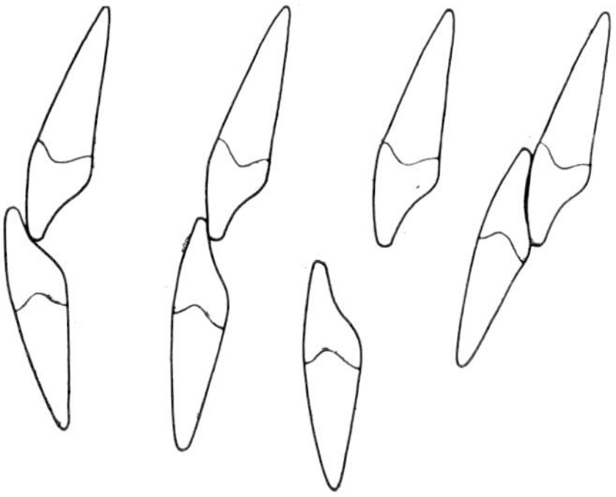

Fig. 221.—Variations in incisor overbite that may be found in Class III malocclusions. A, Mild Skeletal 3 abnormality with some degree of overclosure. B, Marked Skeletal 3 relationship with near edge-to-edge bite. C, Marked Skeletal 3 relationship with open bite. D, Marked Skeletal 3 relationship with overclosure showing excessive reverse overbite.

Group 3 comprises the pseudo-Class III cases with a mild Skeletal 3 pattern and mandibular form as seen in Group 2. In these cases there has usually been loss of deciduous teeth in the buccal segments at a critical stage in the development and an initial contact has fostered some slight forward movement and overclosure, with the upper central incisors erupting lingual to their lower counterparts. In these cases the patient can bite back into an edge-to-edge incisor position and there is a good prognosis for establishing an incisor overbite as the upper incisors are tilted lingually and the lower incisors labially.

It is true to say that all Class III malocclusions have some degree of Skeletal 3 pattern which may become more marked in the later stages of growth. This grouping is merely for the sake of classification and there are many intermediate examples (*Fig.* 221).

The Lips and Tongue.—In most cases the lips are sealed at rest but the upper lip may be short and the lower everted and rather flabby as in the classic Hapsburg profile (*Fig.* 222). The relative length of the

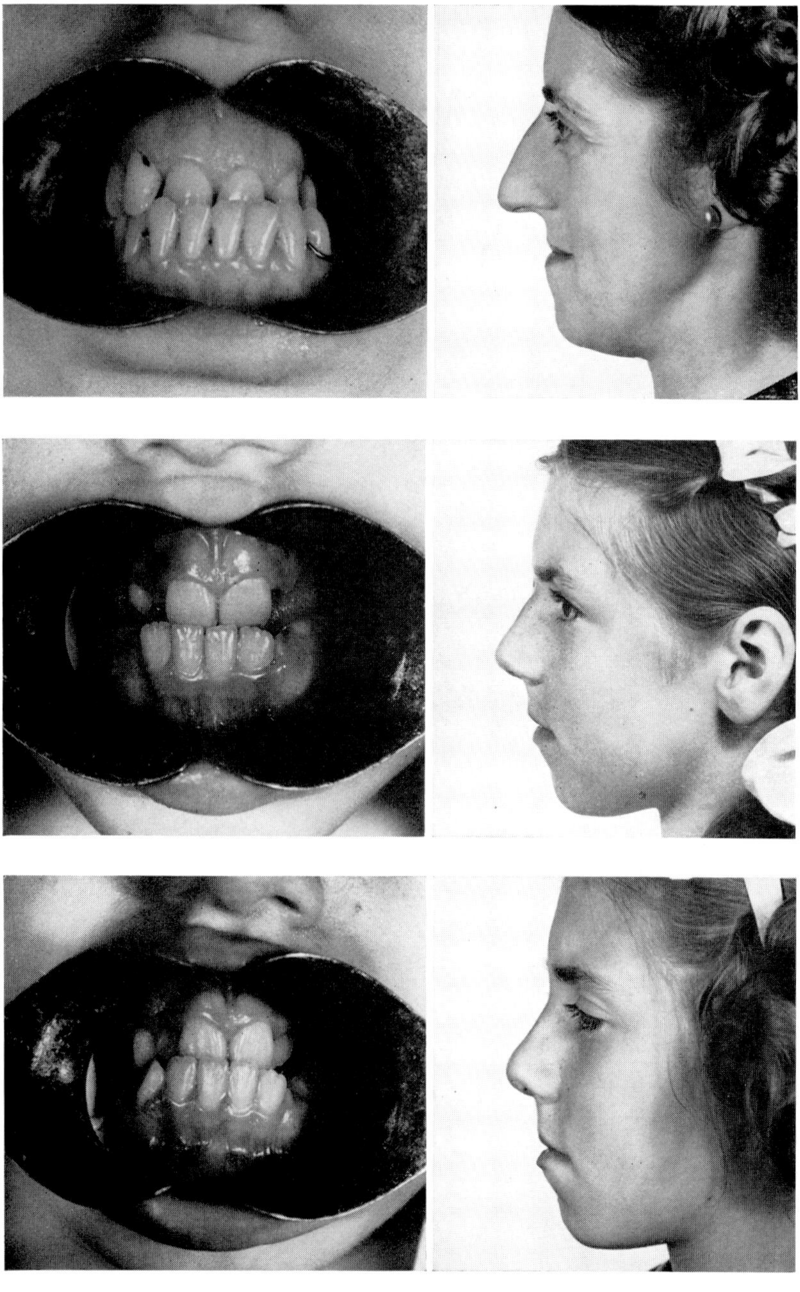

Fig. 222.—Mother and twin daughters showing familial pattern of Class III malocclusion. (Twins are not uni-ovular.)

lips tends to reflect the size of the underlying skeletal structures of either jaw. In *Fig.* 226, although both jaws are rather large there is adequate lip cover of the labial segments. In the patient with the long

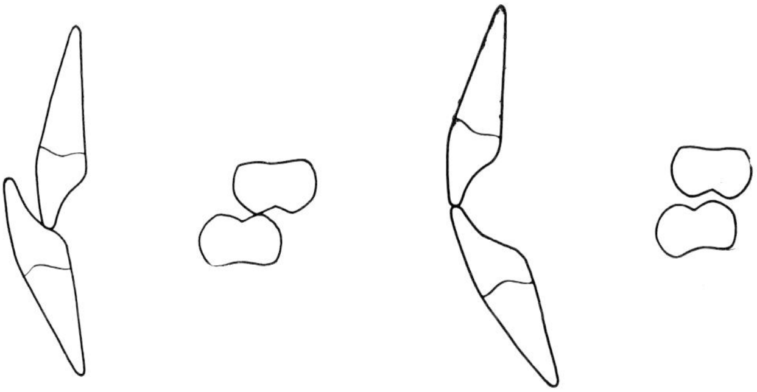

A B

Fig. 223.—A, Diagram showing pseudo-Class III relationship in occlusion where upper incisors are retroclined and lowers proclined. B, A better assessment can be made of the skeletal relationship when biting in an edge-to-edge position.

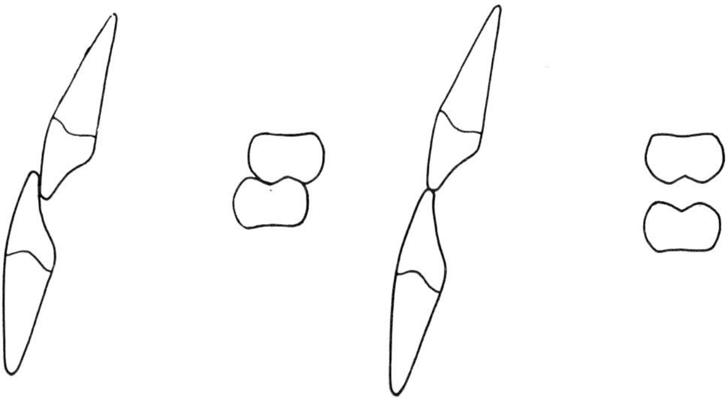

A B

Fig. 224.—A, Diagram showing overclosure complicating a Skeletal Class III malocclusion. B, When biting edge-to-edge upper incisors have normal inclination, lower incisors appear retroclined, demonstrating the Skeletal 3 relationship.

face (*Fig.* 225), there is frequently a deficiency in lip length compared with face height with consequent 'incompetence' of the lips.

Tongue size tends to reflect the size of the lower jaw and therefore many Class III cases may have a large tongue. It often adopts a low resting posture particularly in those cases of the Group 1 type and this posture may be a secondary adaptive pattern in forming an anterior oral seal both at rest and in deglutition. In speech there may not be any interdental sigmatism as the tip of the tongue will make contact with the lower surfaces of lower incisors adapting to the abnormal

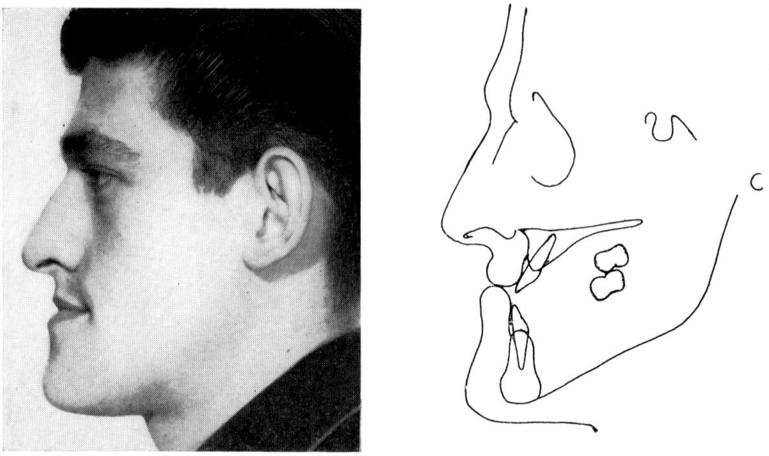

Fig. 225.—Example of patient with long face and small upper jaw and skeletal open bite. Compare with *Fig.* 226 where the face is squarer. (*By courtesy of Mr. D. M. Macdonald.*)

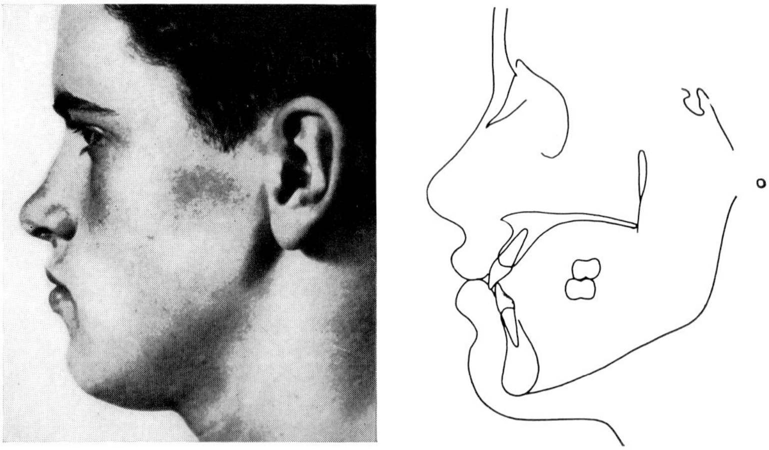

Fig. 226.—Patient with Skeletal 3 relationship with compensating proclination of upper incisors presenting a virtually 'normal' occlusion with reduced overbite. Patient sucked thumb for 16 years.

skeletal pattern. Others may have an interdental position of the tongue tip with some degree of sigmatism purely as a secondary factor.

The form and behaviour of the soft tissues are not a major problem in planning treatment except in those cases where a large tongue maintains the contour of the lower arch and there is spacing between the teeth. In such cases there is little chance of reducing the perimeter of this arch by any form of treatment.

Paths of Closure of the Mandible.—In the true Class III malocclusion the path of closure from rest position to occlusion is the result of a simple hinge movement at the condyle. However, a displacement of the mandible with overclosure may occur in some cases. Loss

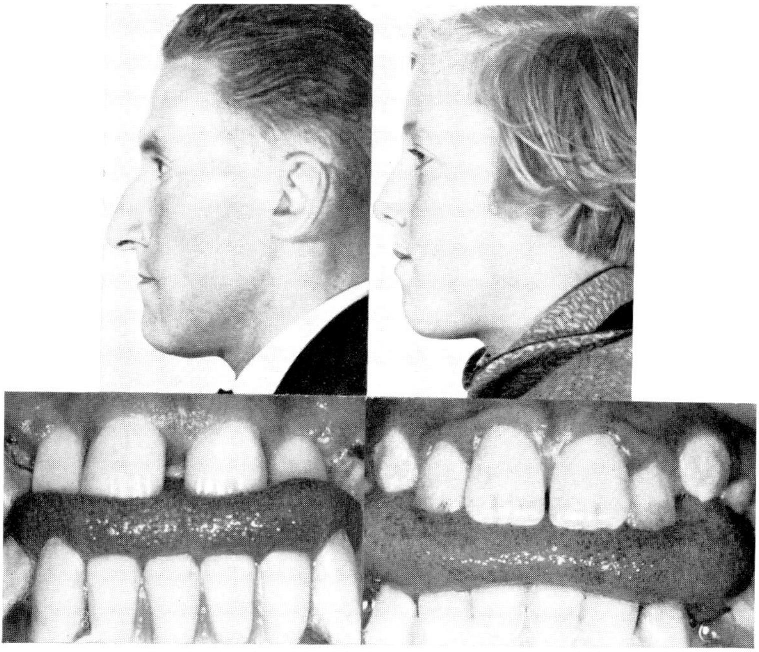

Fig. 227.—Father and daughter with Skeletal 3 relationship with persistent tongue-to-lower-lip contact at rest and in speech. (From the *American Journal of Orthodontics.*)

of posterior teeth and initial contact on the deciduous canines prior to the eruption of the permanent incisors may facilitate overclosure (*Fig.* 228).

Experimental evidence derived from radiographs of the temporomandibular joint is far from conclusive, owing to inaccuracies in the method. It would tend to show a pure hinge movement at the condyle, indicating that there is mainly overclosure with rotation of the condyle about an axis which maintains a normal fossa/condyle relationship.

Any permanent forward displacement of the mandible is eliminated by the mechanical action of the lower incisors sliding up the labial surfaces of the upper incisors as they erupt (*Figs.* 223, 228). The upper incisors become retroclined and the lowers proclined as they erupt.

Where there is a slight narrowing of the upper arch there may also be a lateral deviation as described for Class I cases, producing a unilateral cross-bite.

Local Complicating Factors.—

Finger- and Thumb-sucking.—Thumb-sucking in Class III malocclusions may be a helpful rather than a hindering factor. *Fig.* 226 shows a case where the thumb was sucked for 16 years, and it may have been responsible for maintaining the upper incisors over the lowers despite a Skeletal 3 relationship. The insertion of the thumb or finger

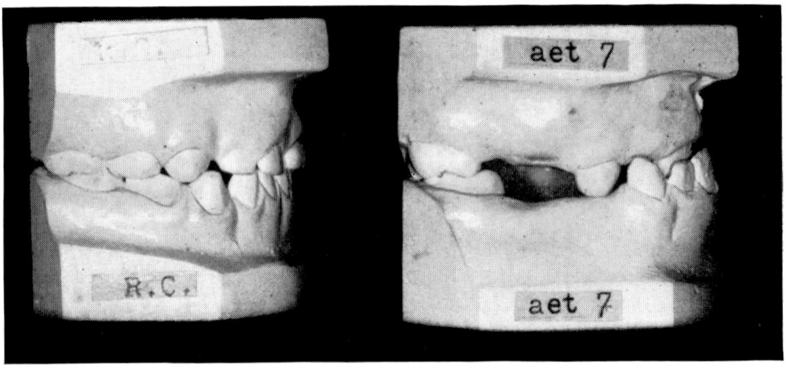

Fig. 228.—Models at 5 years and 7 years showing loss of deciduous molars prior to eruption of permanent incisors and first permanent molars. Subsequent overclosure with reverse overbite and production of pseudo-Class III malocclusion with exaggeration of the malocclusion on a mild Skeletal 3 base.

may buttress the upper incisors forward so that a pseudo-Class III malocclusion does not occur.

An open bite in a Class III case is generally associated with a major skeletal discrepancy and possibly with an abnormality in tongue size and behaviour. If there is also a sucking habit, any improvement which follows its cessation indicates the degree to which the habit was responsible for the open bite.

Premature Loss of Teeth.—Premature loss of *upper* deciduous cheek teeth will tend to exaggerate the crowding where the arch is already small. It may allow the upper incisors to fall inside the bite in a case which might have had a very reduced overbite or edge-to-edge bite. Premature loss of *lower* deciduous cheek teeth may have little effect on the lower arch if there is a large dental base and large tongue. However, if the upper arch is intact and of reasonable size and the lower arch is slightly crowded, early extractions may induce some slight lingual movement of the lower incisor crowns. This will depend on the soft-tissue environment of the incisors. If this movement occurs it may enable an edge-to-edge bite or a slight overbite to be maintained, providing it is followed by lower premolar extractions.

TREATMENT

General Principles.—In a true Class III case, as the relationship of the dental bases cannot be changed, the main objective is to move the

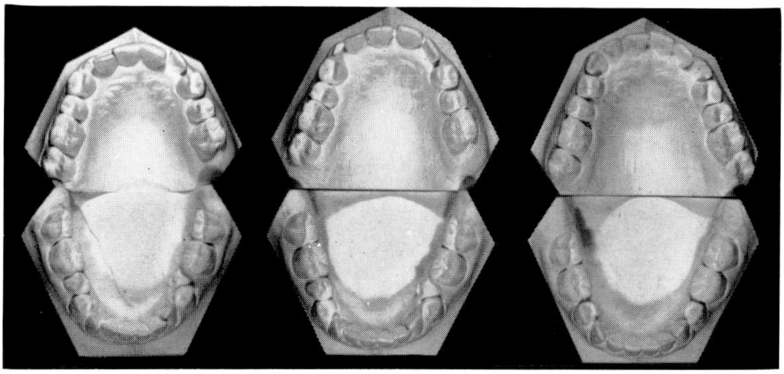

Fig. 229.—Class III malocclusion showing upper incisors moved forwards and $\underline{3|3}$ accommodated within the arch without extractions. $\overline{5|5}$ were extracted and slight shortening of the lower dental arch was possible in this case.

upper incisors forwards over the bite and increase the anteroposterior dimensions of the upper dental arch. As a general principle upper extractions should be avoided if at all possible, but where there is marked crowding extractions will be inevitable.

In some cases the anteroposterior length of the lower arch can be reduced by extractions (*Fig.* 229). Where there is a major discrepancy in the size and relationship of the dental bases and a large tongue, lower extractions do not permit any retraction of the incisor segment.

Although the bony profile cannot be changed, where there is a Skeletal 3 relationship the flattened contour of the upper lip does improve when the upper incisors move forward and does to some extent mask the prominent chin (*Fig.* 230). Lateral expansion of a small upper arch, where there is a bilateral cross-bite, is undesirable as it cannot compensate for the lack of width of the maxillary base. Some authorities advocate rapid expansion techniques which split the inter-maxillary suture and claim satisfactory results. This form of treatment, however, is certainly not generally advocated. Where there is a unilateral cross-bite with only slight narrowness of the upper arch and a deviation in the path of closure, lateral upper expansion may allow this to be corrected.

Where there is overclosure of the mandible and a very mild Skeletal 3 dental base relationship, moving the upper incisors over the

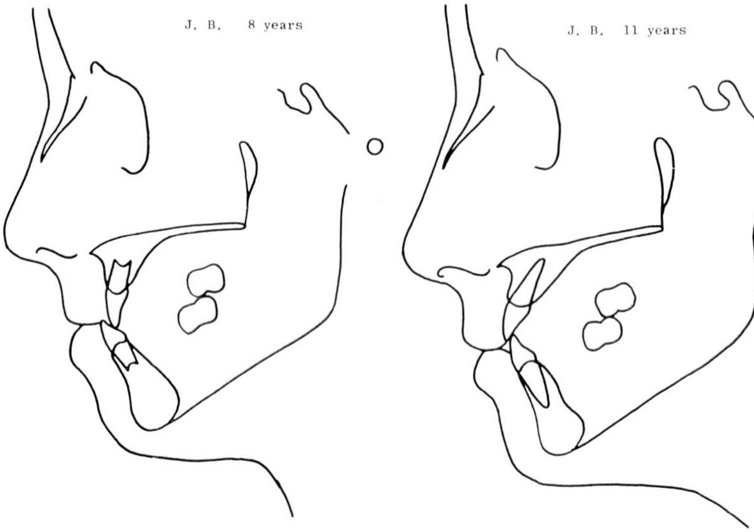

Fig. 230.—Class III malocclusion, mild Skeletal 3 dental base relationship. Upper incisors moved over the bite with removable apparatus as they erupted. Slight overbite is being maintained. Normal size tongue. Note some improvement in profile.

bite goes a long way towards correcting the abnormality. Crowding in both arches can be dealt with later (*Fig.* 231).

Treatment should be confined to the pseudo-Class III and to those cases where the discrepancy in dental base relationship is not too marked. There are limits to which upper incisors can be proclined to maintain an overbite in the face of their soft-tissue environment. *Care must be taken not to put them into a position where they are constantly subjected to conflicting forces from the lower incisors and from the lips and tongue.*

The Mechanics of Treatment.—Treatment can be carried out using all three types of anchorage. There are specific indications for the use of each type.

Extra-oral Anchorage.—The use of traction to the chin from a headgear or cervical strap has been advocated for many years. Even when applied in infancy, there is no proof that the light forces involved change the direction or inhibit the growth of the mandible.

Dramatic changes found in treatment of the deciduous dentition are attributable to the pressure exerted on the lower incisors through the

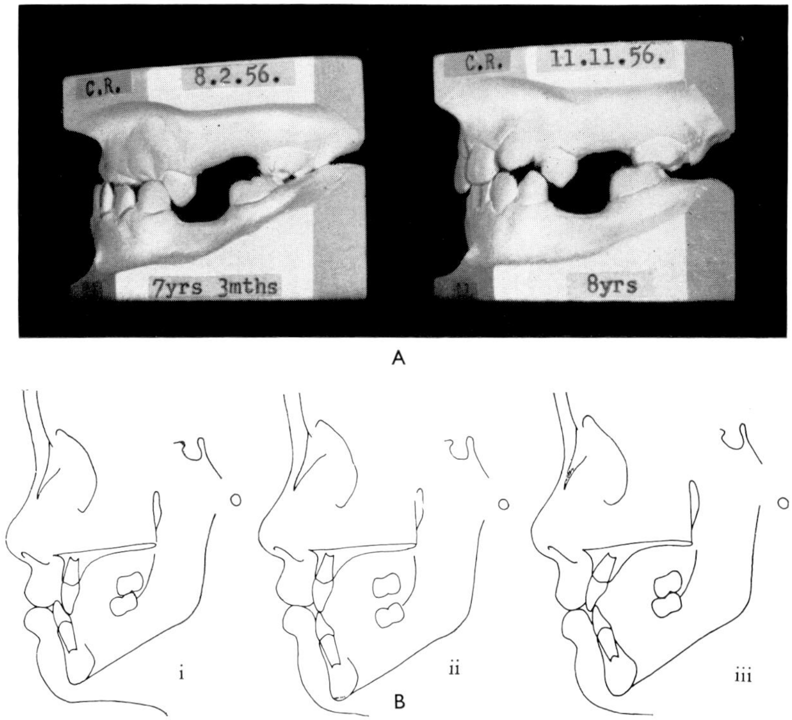

Fig. 231.—A, Overclosure treated by simple removable appliance. Models show that extractions will be required in both arches. B, (i) Tracings of lateral radiographs showing initial overclosure; (ii) Possibility of biting edge-to-edge on incisors; (iii) Upper incisors moved over the bite.

lower lip and the elimination of mandibular displacement which can occur in the deciduous dentition. Spontaneous correction of a Class III malocclusion in the deciduous dentition can occur when it is due to a mandibular displacement (*Fig.* 232). Treatment at this age has no real value when the skeletal relationship is Class III. Follow-up treatment is frequently required when the permanent incisors erupt.

The headgear and chin cap may be of value as an adjunct to other treatment by applying pressure to the lower incisor segment in cases where extraction of lower deciduous canines and later lower premolars are to be carried out.

Intermaxillary Anchorage.—Intermaxillary traction with a full multibanded appliance is required in some cases. The simple labio-lingual type of treatment is not advocated as it will tend to cause

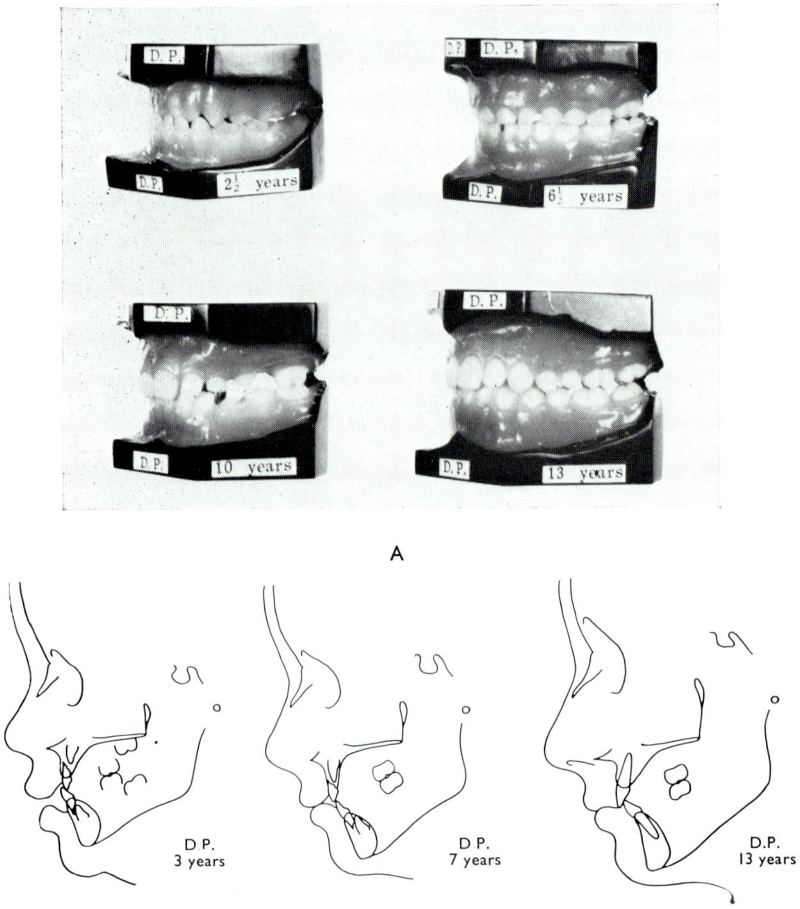

Fig. 232.—A, Models of patient showing Class III relationship in the deciduous dentition which was entirely self-correcting. B, Tracing of same patient showing that this was never a true Skeletal 3 condition. It was a pseudo-Class III in the deciduous dentition.

tilting of the first molar teeth, and does not control the anchorage sufficiently. It also has the disadvantage of moving the upper buccal segments forward and reducing the chance of anterior alinement when the upper arch is small.

However, the use of an inclined plane on the lower incisors is a form of local reciprocal intermaxillary traction which will correct the upper and lower incisor inclinations if there is an excessive incisor overbite of the pseudo-Class III type (*Fig.* 233). It will not work well if there is a reduced overbite. Such an inclined plane may be cast in silver alloy or constructed in acrylic. The inclined plane must be steep and slots cut level with the lower incisal edges to facilitate removal. The appliance

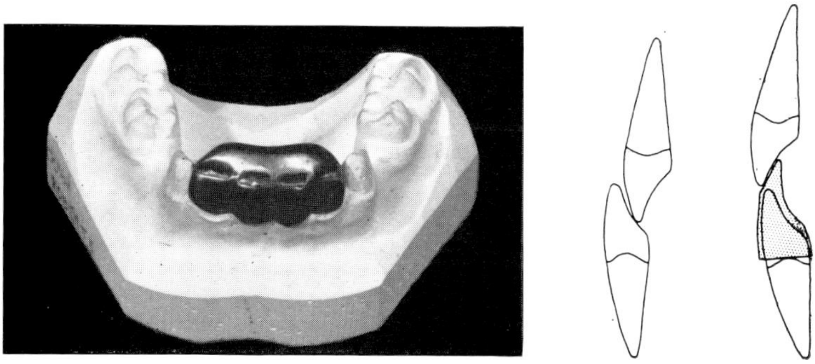

Fig. 233.—Use of a fixed cast inclined plane on lower incisors to correct incisor relationship in cases with overclosure and excessive reverse overbite.

should be effective and removed within three to four weeks. It no longer remains effective when the cheek teeth reach occlusion. A similar use may be made of a lower removable plate with labial bow, where the acrylic inclined plane lips over the lower incisors.

Intramaxillary Anchorage.—Most cases showing pseudo-Class III malocclusions can be treated by removable apparatus. This also applies to many cases where the skeletal discrepancy is not excessive. Upper incisors may be moved forwards over the bite by the use of recurved springs, or screws. The reciprocal distal thrust experienced by the cheek teeth is particularly desirable if early loss in the upper arch has concentrated crowding in the premolar or canine region, as it is desirable to avoid extraction of upper teeth near the front of the arch. *Fig.* 234 illustrates a type of plate with a recurved S-spring in 0·6-mm. wire protected by an adjustable bar of wire so designed that it can continue to protect the spring as it moves forward. The plate should be stabilized with Adams cribs on the first permanent molars and adequate clasps should embrace the first premolar or deciduous canine to prevent the plate dropping anteriorly. *Fig.* 235 illustrates a case treated by this simple technique. *Fig.* 236 illustrates a plate incorporating a screw to move the incisors forward with similar results.

It is not often found necessary to prop open the bite on the cheek teeth but this may be desirable for a short time in some cases where forward movement of incisors is slow.

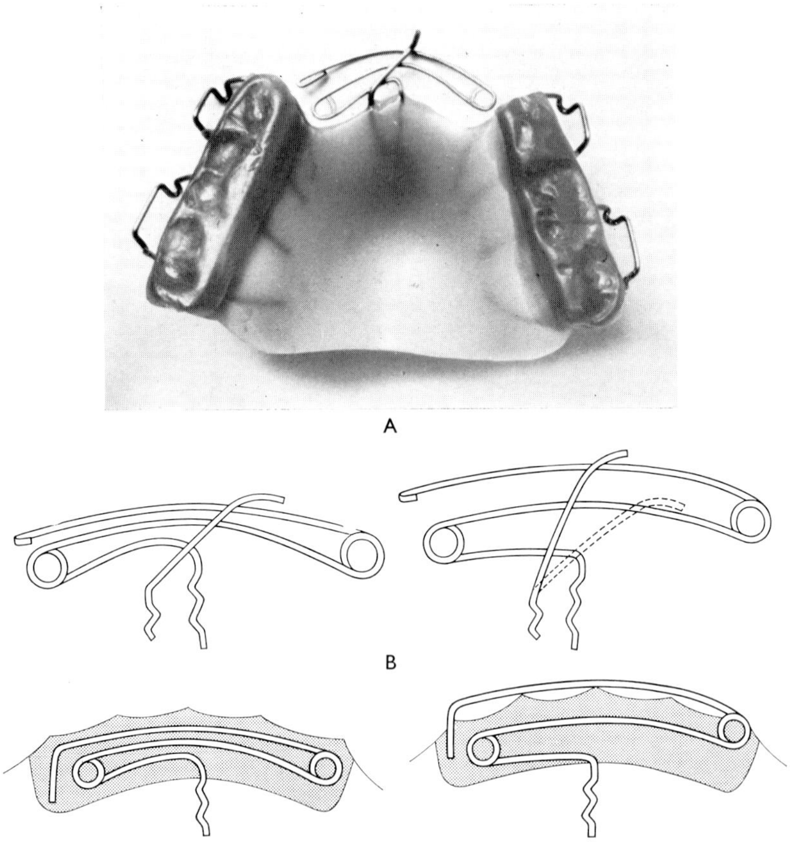

Fig. 234.—A, Appliance with recurved cantilever spring in 0·6-mm. wire to move upper incisors labially. Note adequate stabilization of plate with Adams cribs on $\underline{4|4}$ and $\underline{6|6}$. The overlay is not always required. B, C, show the S-springs in detail. The left-hand illustration shows the spring closed. The right-hand shows how the protecting bar is moved to contain the spring in (B) and the recurved portion of the spring stays under the box in (C).

Intramaxillary forces can sometimes be employed in the lower dental arch in Class III cases to retract the incisor segment following the extraction of lower premolars or even a lower incisor. The feasibility of this depends on the arch size and on the tongue size and behaviour. Where the mandibular dental base is large, the teeth may

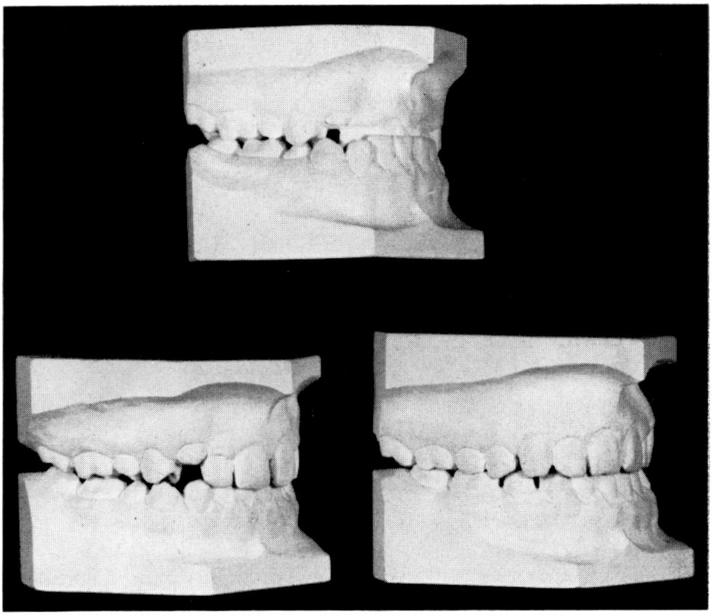

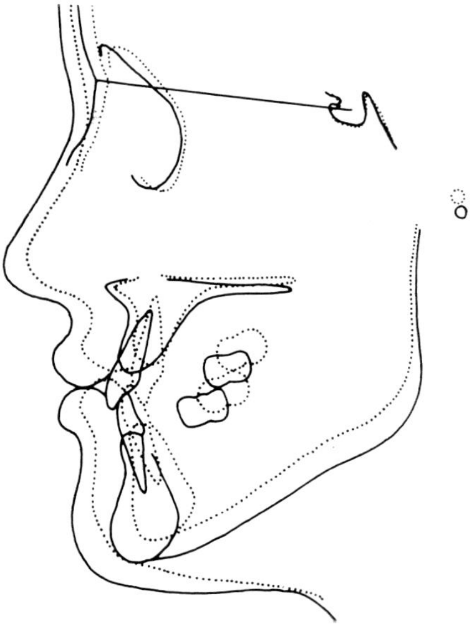

Fig. 235.—Case treated with an appliance, as in *Fig*. 234. Upper incisors moved over the bite. Extraction of $\overline{5|5}$ enabled lower incisor alinement with slight retraction.

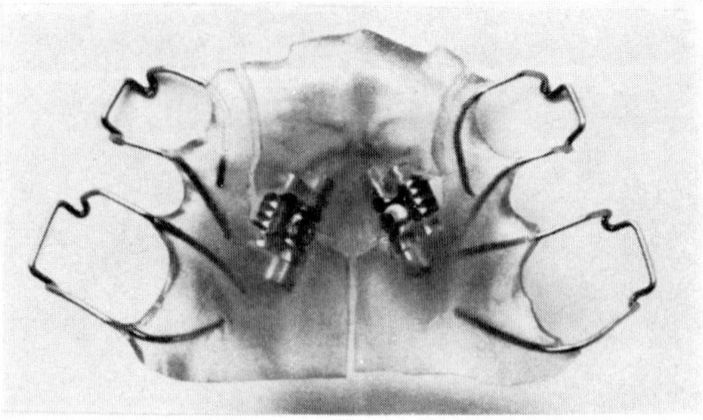

Fig. 236.—Screw plate to effect labial movement of upper incisors and distal movement of upper buccal segments. If used in cases where there is mild crowding in the upper arch, extraction of $\underline{7|7}$ will enable space to be obtained for the accommodation of the remaining upper teeth.

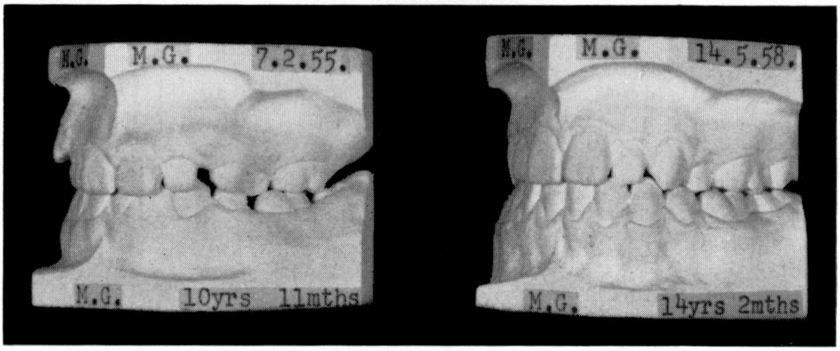

Fig. 237.—Case with Skeletal 3 tendency with crowding in both arches treated by extraction of $\frac{4|4}{5|5}$. Note how the overbite is reducing with growth. Enforced extractions in the upper arch may have increased this tendency.

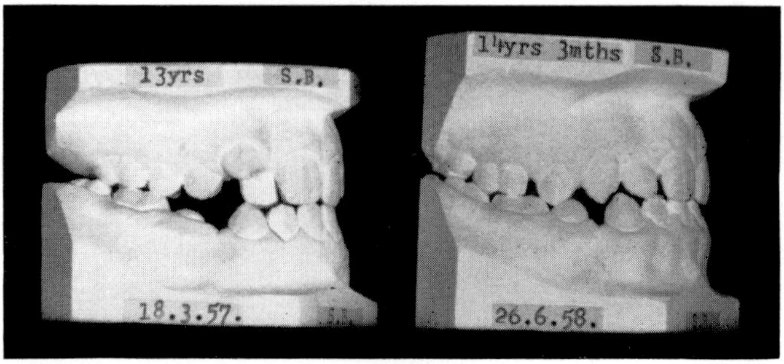

Fig. 238.—Extraction of $\underline{5|5}$ in a Class III malocclusion with a Skeletal 3 relationship may result in reduction of the overbite to the extent that it may become edge-to-edge or the upper incisors fall inside the bite. Where the lower jaw is large and the tongue large, there may be residual spacing when $\overline{4|4}$ are extracted in an attempt to compensate. In this case because there is only a mild Skeletal 3 tendency the treatment has been relatively successful, but $\underline{2|2}$ may fall inside the bite.

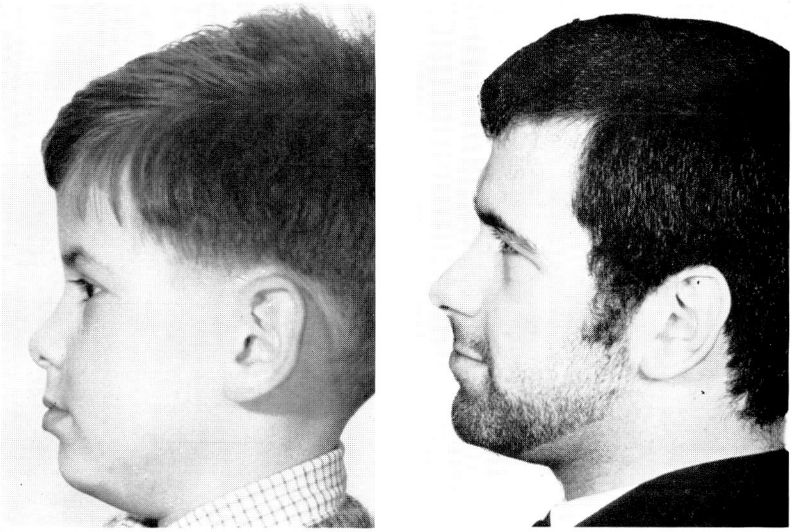

A

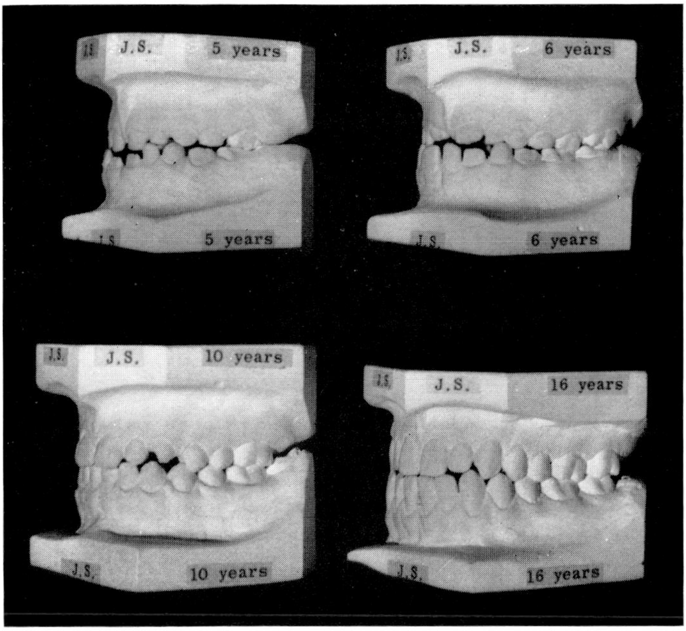

B

Fig. 239 (*continued on p.* 248).

already be spaced; little collapse of the lower arch can be effected to improve the incisor relationship, and any spaces created by extraction

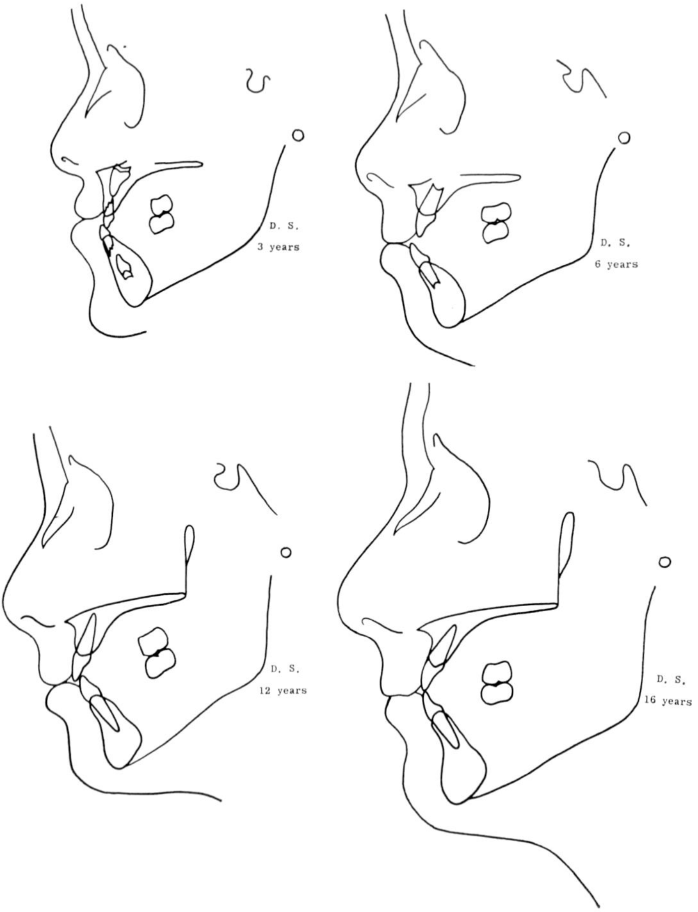

C

Fig. 239.—A, Photographs of patient at 5 years and 21 years whose models and tracings are illustrated below. B, Models of patient where the anterior crossbite was treated between 8 and 10 years, showing the relapse of overbite to edge-to-edge position by 16 years of age. C, Tracings of headplates of patient whose models are shown in B. An incisor overbite had been established by 12 years of age but growth pattern showed steady relapse.

will fail to close. However, where there is some crowding in the lower arch, lingual collapse of the incisor segment can be obtained to a limited extent. There is a strong tendency to relapse in those cases where only a tenuous overbite has been established. A growth spurt in the early teens may cause relapse of what was apparently a good result (*Fig.* 239).

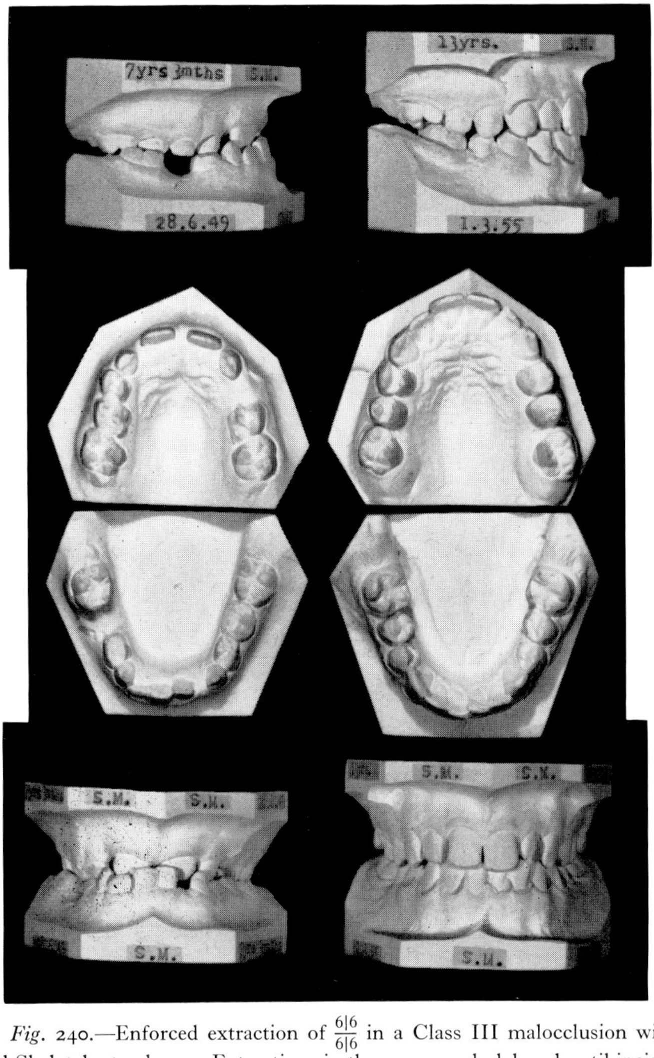

Fig. 240.—Enforced extraction of $\frac{6|6}{6|6}$ in a Class III malocclusion with mild Skeletal 3 tendency. Extractions in the upper arch delayed until incisor overbite corrected. Lower arch was not so large as to leave residual spaces.

The Problem of Crowding.—*As a general principle, upper extractions should be avoided or be carried out as far back as possible.* However, after the correction of the incisor relationship in a Skeletal 1 pseudo-Class III case, crowding exaggerated by early loss of upper and lower cheek teeth may be treated by the extraction of four premolars. Where there is a mild Skeletal 3 tendency with crowding in both arches, upper and lower extractions must be considered. The overbite, however, will tend to reduce (*Figs.* 237–9). Where the discrepancy in the skeletal relationship is so great that an overbite cannot be established, severe crowding in the upper arch may be treated by extraction merely to produce alinement.

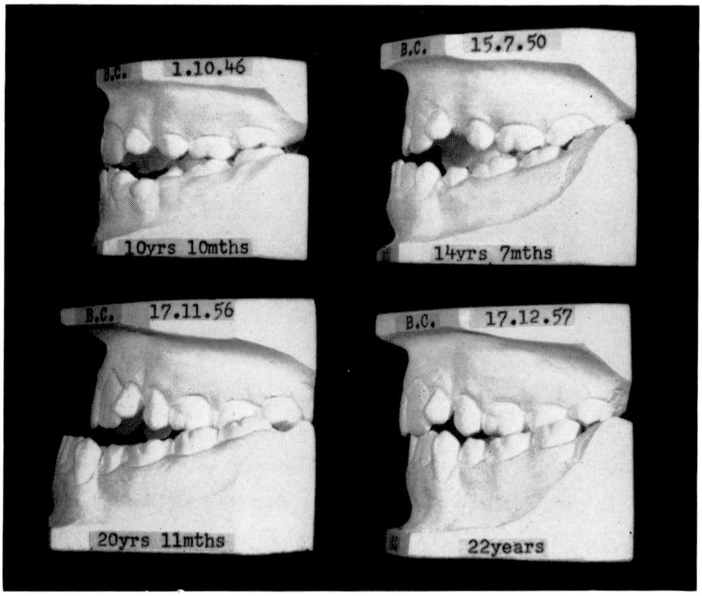

Fig. 241.—Class III malocclusion with Skeletal 3 relationship showing deterioration between 1946 and 1956. Treated surgically by osteotomy of mandibular body. (*By courtesy of Mr. D. M. Macdonald.*) [*Continued opposite.*

Crowding in the lower arch is not so common, but where present extraction of first premolars or even an incisor is permissible to aline the teeth and, if possible, reduce the anteroposterior dimensions of this arch.

Extreme Cases.—Where the discrepancy in dental base relationship is excessive, orthodontic treatment is of no avail. If the condition is really disfiguring, surgical correction may be advised (*Fig.* 240). In such cases orthodontic preparation of the individual arches may well be necessary to produce alinement and to allow a better cuspal interdigitation in the surgically corrected position.

Many of these cases with a marked Skeletal 3 relationship have an open bite, and only the last molar teeth may occlude. This is known as a skeletal open bite and is not due to soft-tissue interference with tooth eruption. There is a very high Frankfort-mandibular-plane as a constant morphological feature. (*See* APPENDIX.)

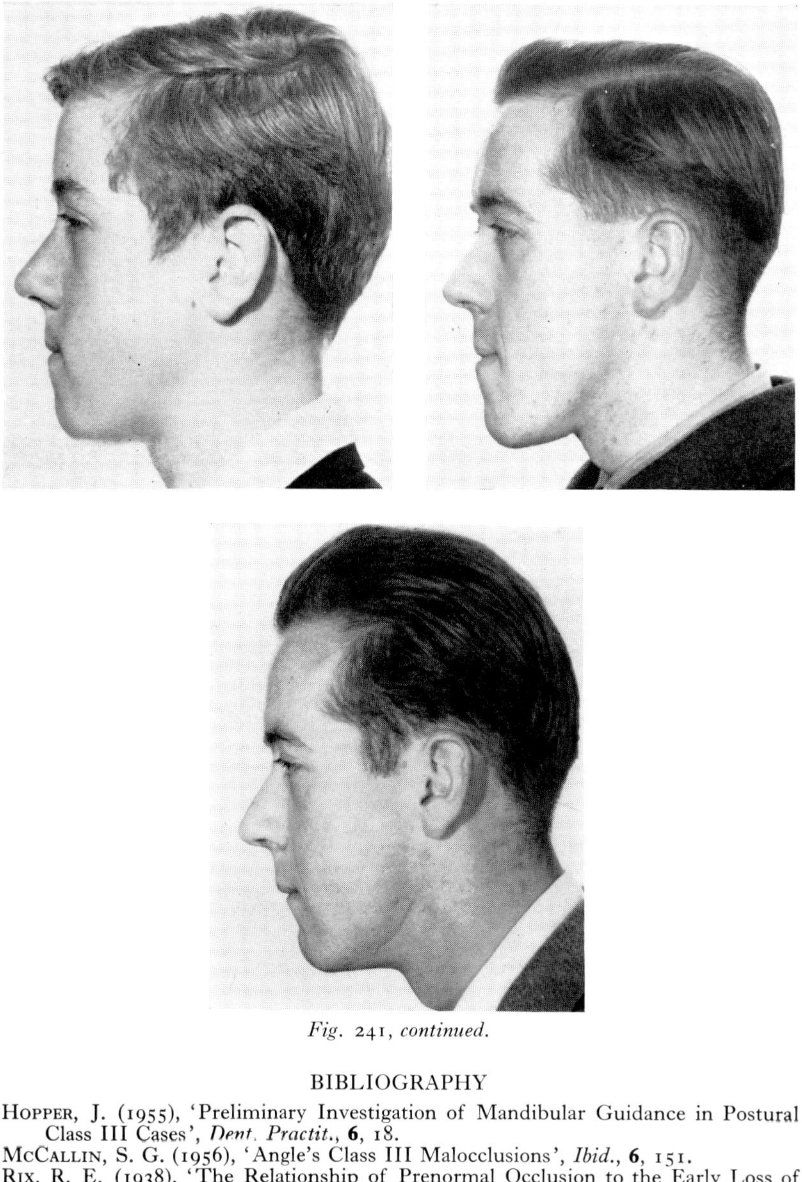

Fig. 241, *continued.*

BIBLIOGRAPHY

HOPPER, J. (1955), 'Preliminary Investigation of Mandibular Guidance in Postural Class III Cases', *Dent. Practit.*, **6**, 18.
McCALLIN, S. G. (1956), 'Angle's Class III Malocclusions', *Ibid.*, **6**, 151.
RIX, R. E. (1938), 'The Relationship of Prenormal Occlusion to the Early Loss of Deciduous Molars', *Proc. R. Soc. Med.*, **31**, 41.

APPENDIX

The contents of this appendix are intended to cover certain aspects of theory and practice which do not appear in the main chapters. They are presented in a shortened form, particularly where there are recent articles on the subject.

The Unerupted Maxillary Canine.—The maxillary canine has farther to erupt from its developmental position than any other tooth. An aberrant path of eruption may be detected during routine examination of the younger patient. Other patients may seek advice in the early teens.

Frequently it is palatally displaced and it may or may not erupt into the palate (*Fig.* 242 A). Alternatively, it may lie high, buccal to the root of the lateral incisor, and it may impact obliquely against the root of the lateral incisor (*Fig.* 242 B) or horizontally against the apex of the central incisor (*Fig.* 242 C).

In assessing its position, the following examination should be made:—

1. Visual examination of the position of the neighbouring teeth and the presence of a buccal or palatal bulge. For example, if the crown of the lateral incisor is displaced labially, the canine may be high and buccal to the apex of the lateral.

2. Palpation of the bone buccally and palatally and comparison of this with the opposite side, if the latter is normal.

3. Radiographic examination. The ordinary oblique occlusal radiograph does not provide enough information about the misplaced canine. However, two occlusal views may be taken by moving the X-ray tube from a position over the pupil of one eye to the other side and repeating the film. These two films can be examined with a stereoscopic viewer which will give depth to the picture (*see Fig.* 248). A true lateral radiograph of the anterior part of the maxilla is helpful to show the depth and tilt of the canine. This may be viewed in conjunction with a true posterior-anterior radiograph which can show the degree of palatal or buccal displacement. A vertex occlusal radiograph may be taken with the tube in the region of the vertex of the skull and angled to expose along the long axis of the incisors (*Fig.* 242 A). There are disadvantages in this technique: a long exposure is required with the ordinary dental apparatus, and the patient may move and spoil a film which is always rather indistinct owing to the density of the bone in

relation to the density of the teeth. It is particularly deceptive where the lateral incisor is lying obliquely.

Having made a radiographic examination the following information should be obtained:—

1. Is the tooth present ? (It is very rarely missing but it may have been extracted.)

2. What is its axial inclination to the horizontal and vertical planes ?

3. Is its apex in the line of the arch and what is the relationship of its apex to that of the first premolar ?

4. Is its crown displaced buccally or palatally, or is it in the alveolus ? How deeply is it placed ?

5. If the deciduous canine is still present, is the crown intact and how much of the root is resorbed ?

6. Is space available in the arch ?

7. Is there any resorption of either the lateral or central incisors due to proximity of the canine ? Such resorption will usually have occurred before the age of 14 years and is unlikely to commence after this age.

Even in favourable situations where the canine could be brought into the arch the overriding factor is whether the patient is prepared to accept treatment and appreciates the time involved. Failures in treatment may occur because of lack of co-operation. This is the main reason for the very cautious approach.

Favourable Circumstances.—In the young adult the unerupted canine that can be brought into the arch has its apex in a normal position but the crown is displaced from the arch buccally or palatally and is quite superficial. It is helpful if the patient is young enough for the canine still to have some eruptive potential. The dentition should be well cared for and space be available or be made available in the arch. Many cases can be helped by removing soft tissue and some bone over the crown of the tooth and packing in such a way as to help to guide the tooth in the direction required. If the canine erupts into the palate it is a relatively simple procedure to move it over the bite, as shown in *Fig.* 243, provided it is not rotated. This appliance does not have to be visible at all and a simple palatal spring in 0·5-mm. wire can be used. Local gingival trimming may be necessary as the mucosa tends to build up as it is moved buccally. In most cases the teeth are rather slow to erupt.

The application of traction to an unerupted canine is rarely needed. However, it can be useful, particularly in cases where there is possible or actual resorption of the roots of incisors. Resorption of the central incisor is prone to occur where there is a missing lateral incisor. (In these cases, surgical removal may be difficult without causing further damage to the central incisor.) *Fig.* 243 shows how such a canine can be guided and allowed to erupt. The incisor remains a useful tooth for many years despite the resorption.

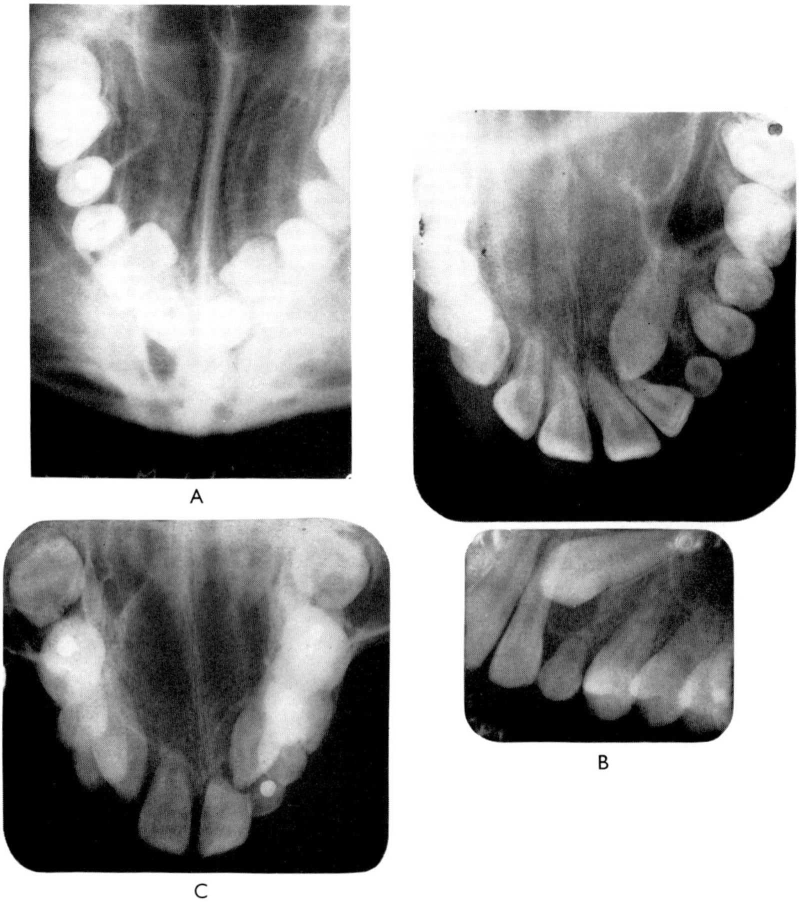

Fig. 242.—A, 'Vertex' occlusal X-ray showing $\underline{3|3}$ displaced palatally. B, Displaced $\underline{|3}$ impacting obliquely against $\underline{|2}$ causing displacement of $\underline{|2}$. C, $\underline{3|3}$ displaced mesially in absence of $\underline{2|2}$, $\underline{|3}$ causing resorption of apex of $\underline{|1}$.

Many methods have been described for the attachment of traction apparatus. The use of a dentine screw accurately placed is one method (*Fig.* 244 B). Traction can be applied from springs on removable or fixed apparatus. Grossly displaced canines which are likely to cause resorption of apices and those showing signs of cystic formation may be surgically removed. It is unusual to find canines moving to cause resorption after the age of 15 years.

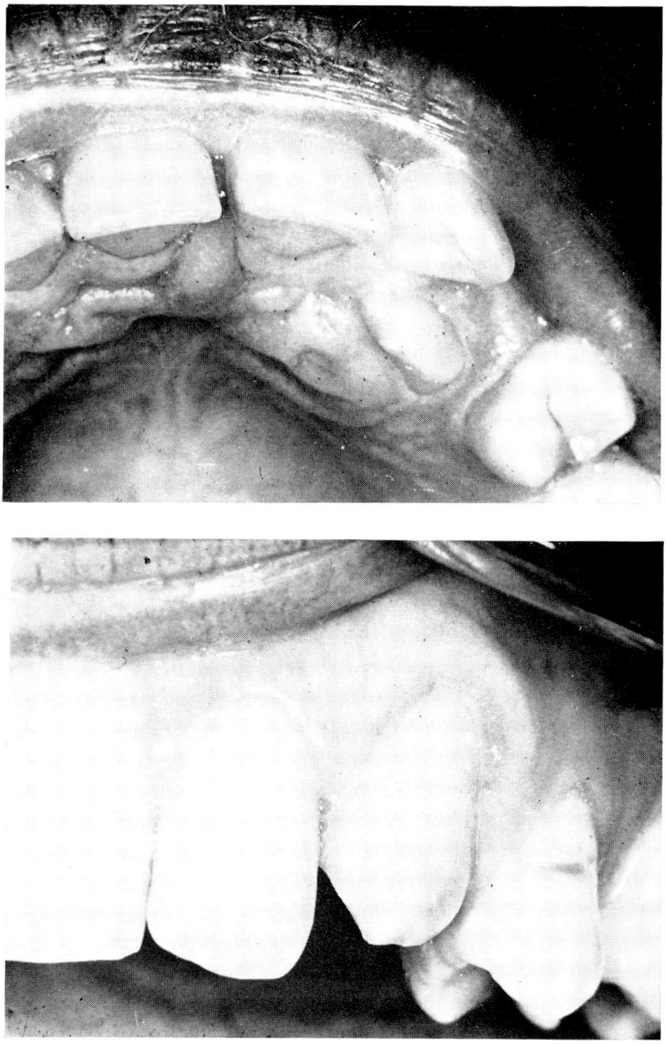

Fig. 243.—Example of delayed eruption of palatally displaced |3 in a young adult. Space was available in upper first premolar region and |45 were retracted and |3 moved over the bite with an appliance similar to that shown in *Fig.* 141.

If for various reasons the lateral incisor has a poor prognosis it may be extracted and the canine allowed to erupt or assisted to erupt into the position of the lateral. In this section the main emphasis will be placed on this situation where the canine cannot be brought into the arch or where it is undesirable to attempt to do so.

Unfavourable Circumstances.—

1. Where there is an excellent occlusion with normal arch relationship and with the deciduous canines retained. The permanent canines may be found lying palatally, almost horizontal, with their crowns

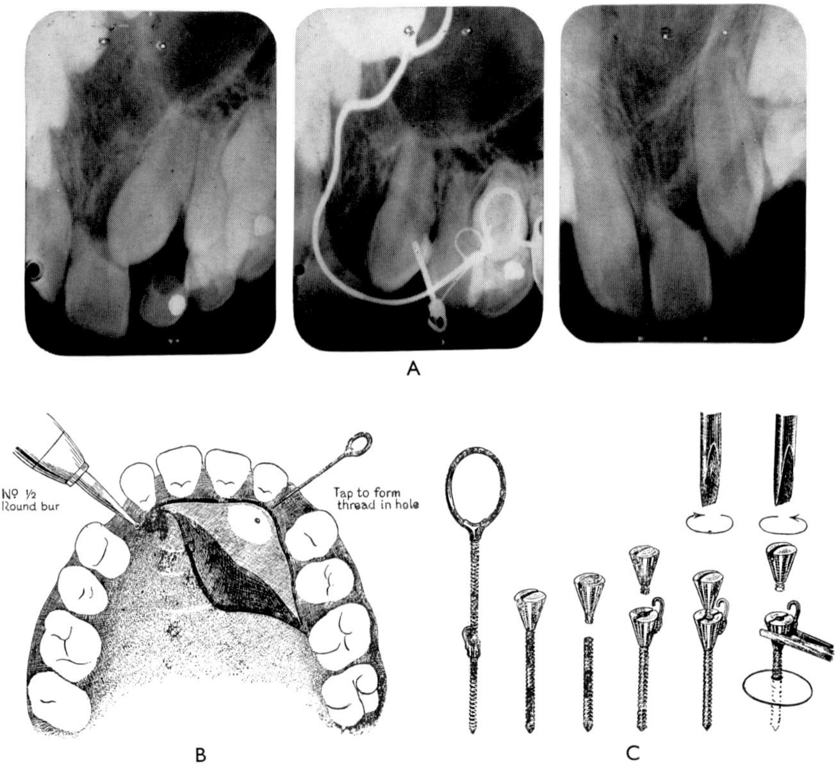

Fig. 244.—A, X-rays to show movement of $\underline{|3}$ by pinning and traction applied from spring. B, Exposure of unerupted canine. C, Dentine screws. (With acknowledgements to M. A. Kettle (1957), *Trans. Brit. Soc. Orthodont.*)

nearly meeting in the midline but causing no resorption of the roots of the incisors.

These canines are best left alone in the young adult; after this age it is rare to find any cystic change or any resorption of the incisors (*Fig.* 245). There is a body of opinion which would favour the surgical removal of canines in any case, even if symptomless, to avoid surgery later.

Their removal is not urgent unless other surgical extractions are indicated, such as the third molars.

The deciduous canines may well remain in place for many years if they are undisturbed and can be quite aesthetically acceptable.

2. In a similar situation to the one above but where the deciduous canines:—

a. Are carious or markedly resorbed and unlikely to be retained for any length of time, *or*

b. Have already been shed (*Fig.* 246), sufficient space may be made available in the canine region by local tooth movement to replace one

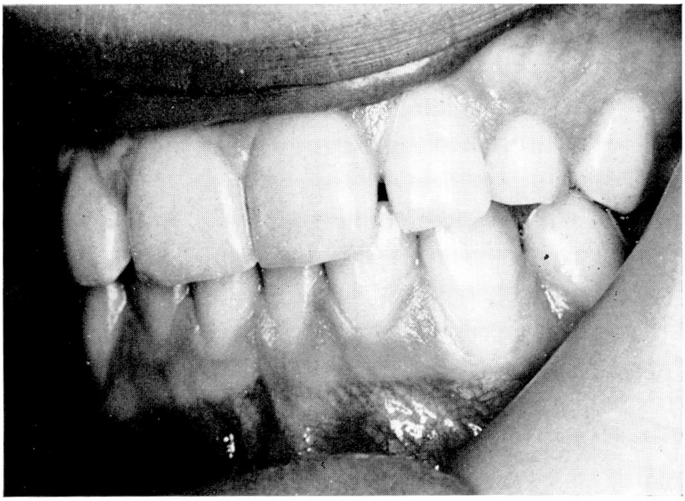

Fig. 245.—Example of excellent arches with good incisor alinement. $\underline{|C}$ retained, unerupted canine in hopeless position.

or both upper canines with a bridge. Where the space is only the width of a deciduous canine, it is better to accept a small pontic rather than extract teeth elsewhere in the arch and open up space still further.

3. In a similar situation to (2), where the spaces are even smaller but aesthetically unacceptable, slight irregularities in the lateral incisor region or in the first premolar region can be corrected, thus reducing the space. In other circumstances extraction of another tooth may be justified and space be made for a reasonable canine bridge.

4. Where there is gross crowding in the arch and no spacing, with the first premolar in contact with the lateral incisor (*Fig.* 247). Providing the premolar is not rotated so as to show its palatal cusp it is quite

aesthetically pleasing. (The canine may or may not be removed surgically).

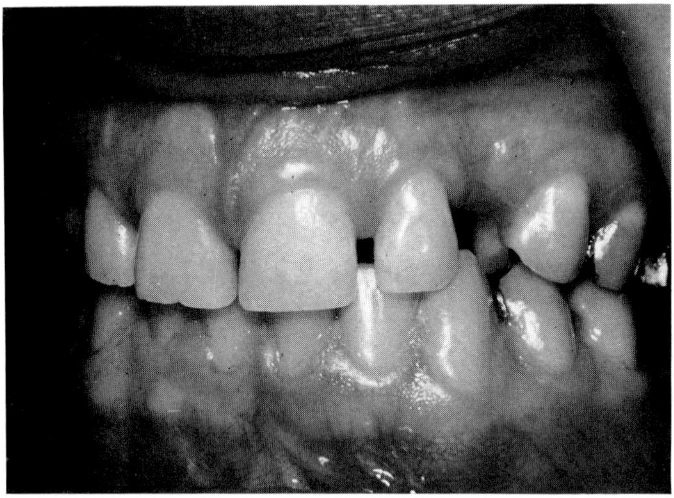

Fig. 246.—Example of good arches, |3 hopelessly displaced, and |C already shed. Mesial movement of |2 with finger spring enabled adequate space to be made for a bridge to replace |3.

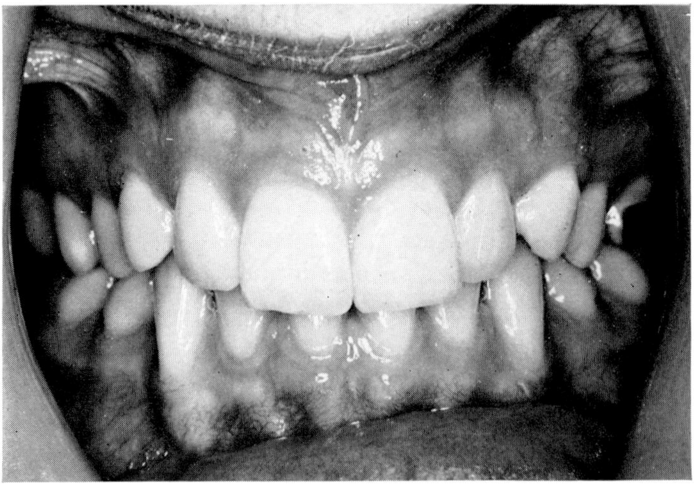

Fig. 247.—Gross crowding, 3|3 hopelessly displaced. 4|4 in contact with 2|2, perfectly acceptable aesthetically.

5. In some cases the position of the canine is closely related to the apex of the lateral incisor but without causing any resorption. If the

lateral incisor is displaced labially it will be necessary to remove the canine surgically before attempting alinement of the displaced incisor.

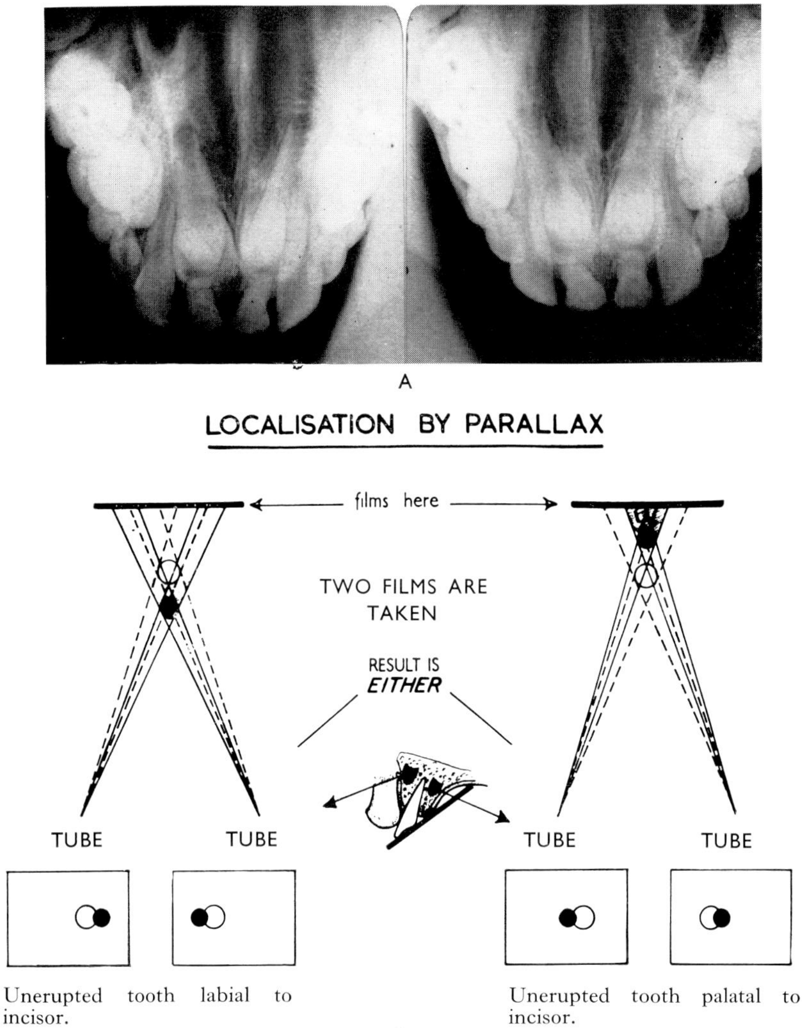

Fig. 248.—Methods of locating unerupted teeth. A, Stereoscopic view of incisor region which can be used with a stereoscope to give depth to the picture. B, Diagram illustrating localization by parallax. The more palatal object moves with the tube.

6. A similar position to that previously described may concern the position of a canine where the first premolar is rotated. If the canine

is preventing de-rotation of the premolar it should be removed surgically and the premolar rotated to a better position to act as an abutment for a bridge to replace the canine.

Removal of Supernumerary Teeth.—In Chapter VI supernumerary teeth have been described as occurring most commonly in the upper incisor region and most frequently palatal to the permanent incisors (*see* pp. 64 and 126).

Localization of the supernumeraries can be achieved partly by examination and palpation of the unerupted incisors and by the same radiographic technique used to locate unerupted canines (*Fig.* 248 A, B). A true lateral radiograph of the incisor region may assist in locating those lying deeply, enabling one to decide whether a buccal rather than a palatal approach should be made. Where they are discovered on routine radiographs but are not likely to cause any ill effects they can be ignored.

These teeth should not be surgically removed before 6 years of age as they sometimes erupt, but they should not be left too long if they are preventing the eruption of upper incisors. Not only must the supernumeraries be removed, but space must be made in the arch for the incisors. This may involve extraction of deciduous canines and later premolars, as the posterior teeth will have drifted around the arch if it is potentially crowded. It is helpful to perform any extractions at the time the supernumeraries are removed if this is being carried out in the theatre under a general anaesthetic.

On rare occasions a dual approach has to be made both buccally and palatally if a supernumerary is located between the apices of displaced upper central incisors. A palatal incision is used to approach supernumeraries overlying the upper central incisors. An adequate flap is necessary to expose the area without danger to the neurovascular bundle entering the incisive canal. Overlying bone may be removed by a bur or chisel, but in many instances it is very thin and can be removed with an excavator. Supernumeraries may often be removed with an apical elevator. One or two sutures are sufficient to hold the flap in place and the healing should be uneventful (*Fig.* 249).

Impacted Teeth.—The presence of impacted teeth is an indication of a discrepancy in the size of the arch compared with the size of teeth, but it may be initiated by an abnormal developmental position of the crypt of the tooth. Impaction of the buried canine has already been discussed. In jaws which are not large enough to accommodate all the teeth in good alinement the impacted third molar is a late manifestation. There may or may not be crowding elsewhere in the arches.

Impacted third molars may well be left to the oral surgeon, but with careful case selection some degree of mesio-angular impaction can be

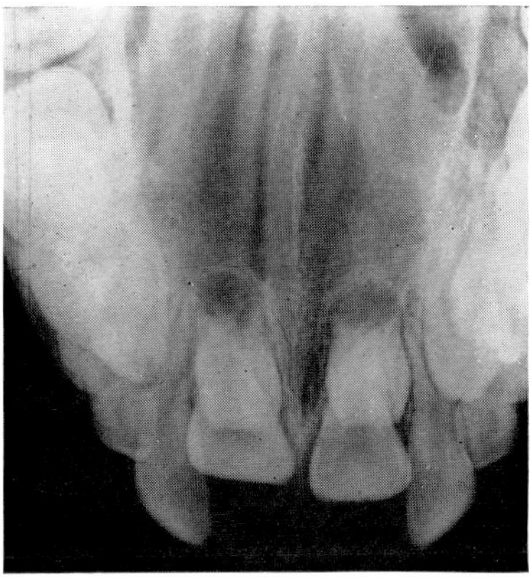

A

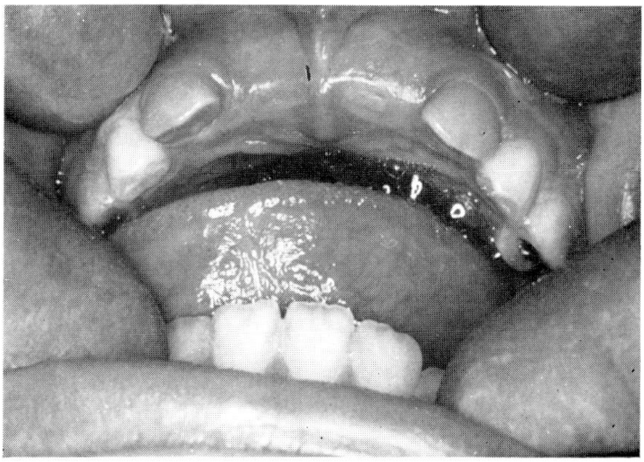

B

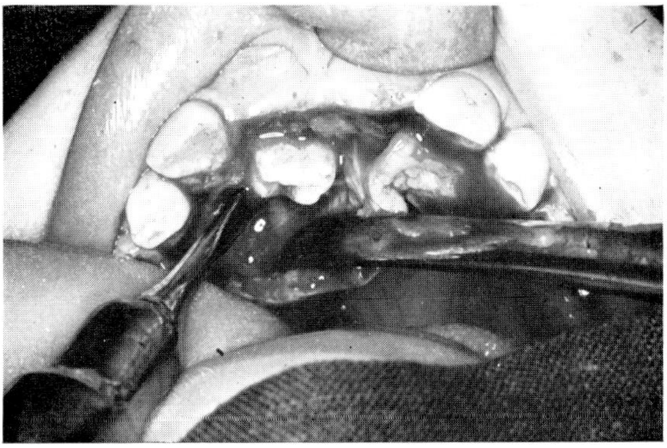

C

Fig. 249 (*continued on p.* 262).

prevented by extraction of the second molars at 14 to 15 years of age. One of the difficulties is to forecast an impaction, and this treatment should only be carried out when the third molars are not likely to be very displaced (*Fig.* 250). Reference has already been made to Cryer's

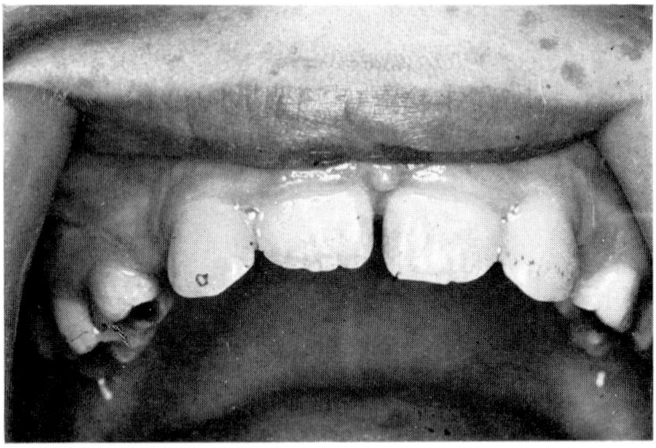

D

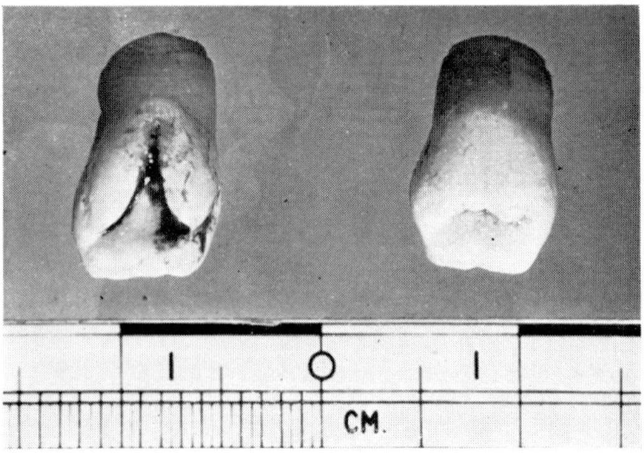

E

Fig. 249.—A, Standard occlusal radiograph showing presence of two supernumeraries palatal to $\underline{1|1}$ (*see also Fig.* 248). B, Intra-oral view showing that $\underline{1|1}$ are unerupted but $\underline{2|2}$ have already erupted. C, Surgical exposure. Palatal flap retracted, supernumeraries being elevated. $\underline{C|C}$ also removed. D, Upper incisors erupting nine months later. No bone was removed over their crowns. Temporary space created by extraction of $\underline{C|C}$ to be followed by extraction of $\underline{4|4}$. E, The two tuberculated supernumeraries after removal.

study and a cautious approach is necessary. If they have an excessive mesio-angular inclination they may move forwards and impact against the first molar when the arches are very small.

The vertical impaction of lower second premolars occurs quite frequently. It has already been shown how they may be disimpacted by extraction of the second molar and may move into the arch by their

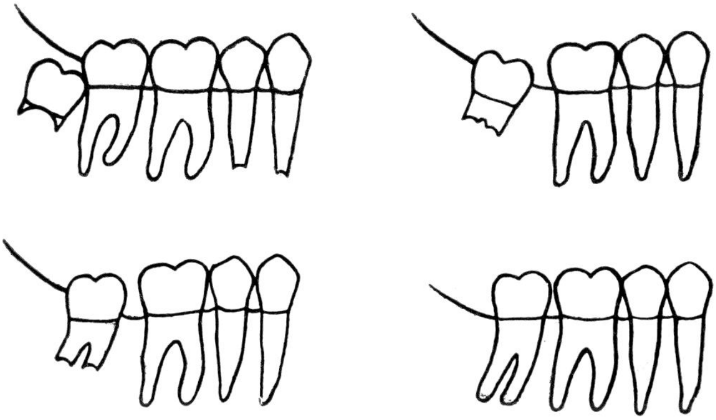

Fig. 250.—Tracing to illustrate the movement of unerupted $\overline{8}|$ following extraction of $\overline{7}|$ at the age of 14 years.

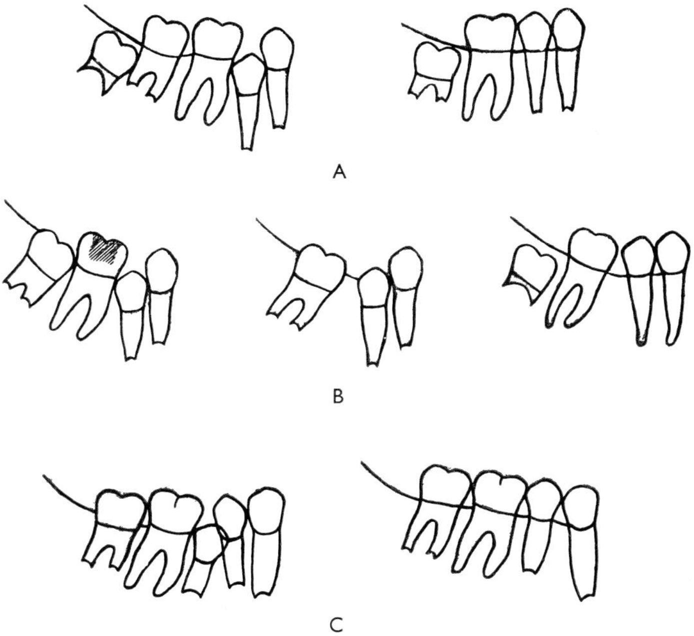

Fig. 251.—A, Tracing from X-ray showing $\overline{5}|$ reaching occlusion without appliance after extraction of $\overline{7}|$ at 13 years of age. B, Enforced extraction of $\overline{6}|$ at 11 years of age, allowing vertically impacted $\overline{5}|$ to erupt. Note that there is a tilt of the $\overline{7}|$ which occurs when the $\overline{6}|$ is extracted late, but this may improve with continued eruption. C, Impacted $\overline{5}|$ allowed to erupt by extraction of $\overline{4}|$.

own eruptive force (*Fig.* 251 A). Where the first permanent molar is carious, its extraction may not produce such a favourable result if left until the second molar has erupted (*Fig.* 251 B). Where the impacted premolar is tilted mesially the first premolar may be extracted where the incisor relationship permits (*Fig.* 251 C). *All these extractions to relieve local impaction must be carried out with reference to the arch form and relationship, and must not be considered as isolated features of the case.*

The upper first molar and the lower first molar may impact against the distal surfaces of the second deciduous molar (*Fig.* 252).

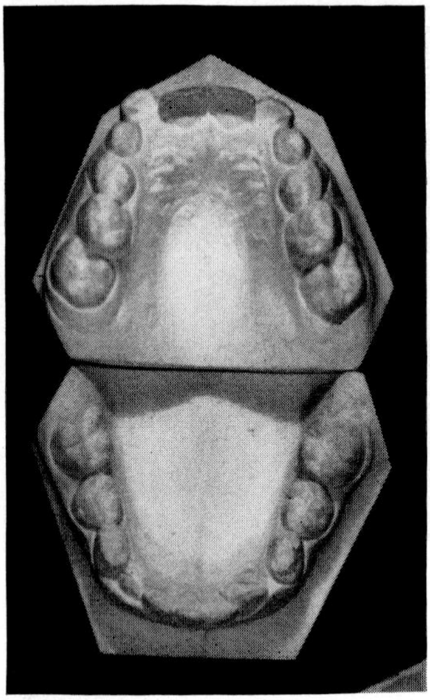

Fig. 252.—Impaction of 6|6.

Occasionally this may happen at a level which allows some resorption of the roots of the deciduous tooth. Unless there are symptoms it is better to leave the deciduous molar in place. As this is a sign of crowding, extractions will be required in the arch, but the first molar should not be allowed to tilt farther forwards. It should be tilted back and a premolar extracted in order to accommodate the canine and one premolar.

Submerged Deciduous Molars.—The relative 'submergence' of one or more deciduous molars is not uncommon. They may even disappear below the level of the alveolar crest. This is thought to be due to a local disturbance in root resorption with an ankylosis of the root to alveolar bone. A recent exhaustive summary of this condition has been made by Dixon.

This interference with eruption while the surrounding teeth are continuing to erupt may only be transient and the deciduous teeth may be shed normally and replaced by the premolars, without interference (*Fig.* 253). Tilting of teeth posterior to this site may cause impaction

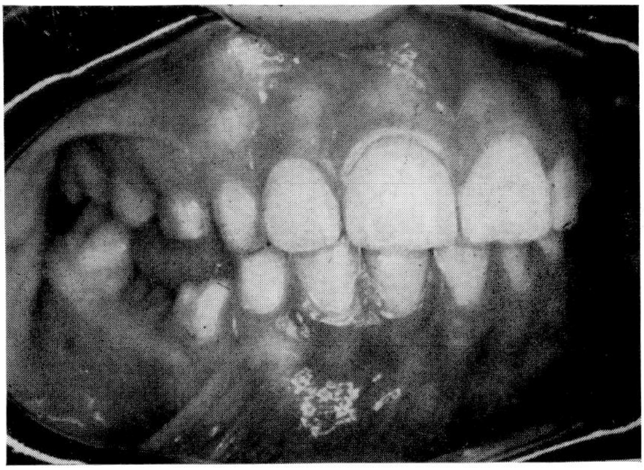

A

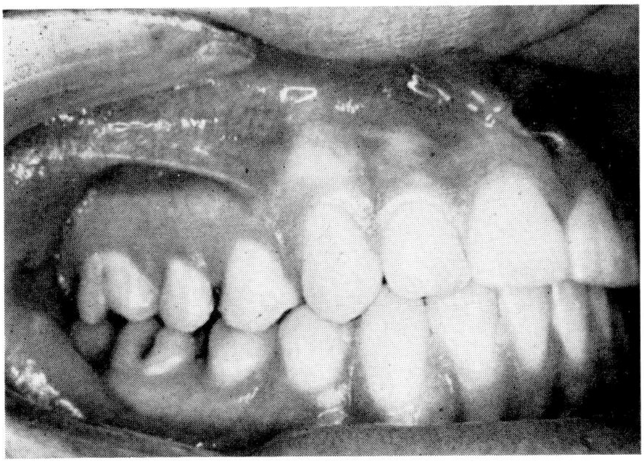

B

Fig. 253.—A, 'Submerging' $\overline{\text{ED}}|$ at the age of 8 years; B, Same patient with premolars in occlusion in the late teens. (*By courtesy of Dr. D. F. Dewel.*)

of the deciduous molar. Teeth that are 'submerging' in this way may be difficult to extract if they are seen in a phase of ankylosis. They should be removed before they become totally 'submerged'.

These phenomena may occur in deciduous molars with or without a successor.

Fraenectomy.—Excision of the superior labial fraenum is rarely performed, as it is not frequently a primary cause of diastema (*see*

18

Chapter IV). However, it is indicated in a few cases where space is available between the central incisors yet the upper lateral incisors lack space and are displaced.

Fraenectomy may also be performed because the fraenum itself is unaesthetic and may bind down the upper lip, preventing the natural

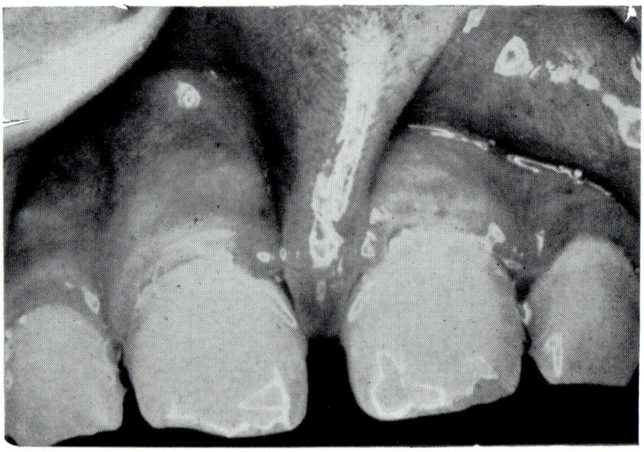

A

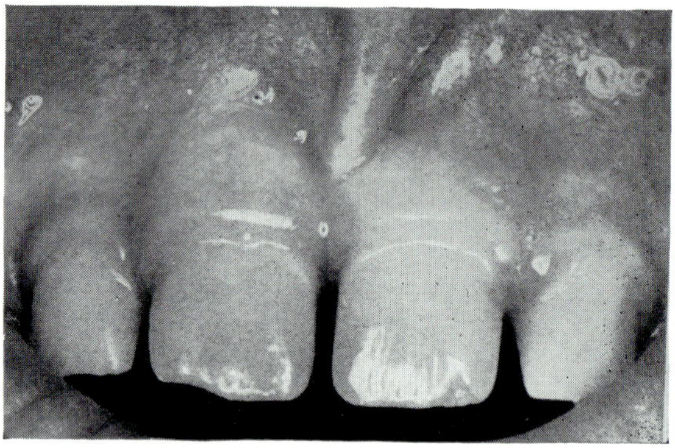

B

Fig. 254.—Large labial fraenum binding down upper lip and causing stagnation. A, Before excision. B, After excision.

cleansing of the labial surfaces of the incisors. It may be thick and fleshy and inserted between the incisors by a dense fibrous band into the mucoperiosteum of the palate (*Fig.* 254).

The procedure is as follows: the thick fibrous band is dissected out from the palate anterior to the incisive papilla and the incision carried forwards on each side between the incisor teeth. A flat plastic instrument can be used as a periosteal elevator to strip it from the bone.

Traction is applied to this tag by grasping it in artery forceps. The aspect of the fraenum attached to the labial gingival surface is cut away by holding the knife obliquely. Finally, it is trimmed from its attachment to the lip with scissors. Sutures, if necessary, should be placed in the opposite direction to the incision. Some writers believe that it is essential to pass a bur or disk into the suture between the incisors as far up as their apices.

PATHOLOGICAL CONDITIONS AFFECTING THE FORM OF THE FACE

Pathological interference with the growth of the facial skeleton has not been given any prominence in this book as the vast majority of malocclusions are the result of inherited variations of the normal. A brief survey is given of some pathological factors which interfere with various aspects of the growth of the jaws and the development of the dentition. They may be grouped as follows. Interference with:—

1. Fusion of primitive processes in foetal life;
2. Interstitial and appositional growth of cartilage;
3. Appositional growth of bones;
4. Growth at sutures of the skull;
5. The soft tissues surrounding and influencing the position of the teeth.

These factors may be inherited, congenital, traumatic, infective, nutritional, or neoplastic in the widest sense of the term.

1. Interference with Fusion of Primitive Processes.—Inherited or congenital factors may interfere with fusion of part of the maxillary process or its palatal processes, producing the various degrees of cleft-lip and cleft palate. In some cases there may be severe derangement of the dentition and deficiency of maxillary growth. The role of the orthodontist in these cases may entail very early repositioning of the segments if necessary to facilitate lip surgery. At a later date, individual teeth or whole segments may need to be moved prior to the insertion of a prosthesis. Valuable work is now being carried out in which segments are placed in improved positions and then maintained with bone grafts. These may not only maintain the arch form but also provide bone through which teeth in the region of the alveolar cleft can erupt prior to their alinement with apparatus. There is extensive and controversial literature on this subject. An orthodontist should be a member of the joint consultative team, but the role of orthodontic treatment is naturally limited where there are major defects in the jaw relationship. It must be remembered that the cleft defect may be superimposed on many variable facial patterns. Where prolonged use of appliances is required, this tends to shorten the life of the teeth, defeating the whole purpose of treatment.

Other major defects in fusion of primitive processes are considered to be sufficiently rare as to be omitted here. Partial aplasia of the mandible, resulting in micrognathia, is extremely rare and many cases described in infancy as micrognathic develop normally.

2. Pathological Factors affecting the Growth of Cartilage.—Achondroplasia is an obscure hereditary condition where there is interference with interstitial growth of cartilage in the skeleton. This results in shortness of the long bones. The cranial base is short, but there is a relative overgrowth of the mandible, as it can continue to grow by apposition of new cartilage cells at the condyle.

Trauma may either cause cessation of condylar growth or in some instances stimulate it. Osteomyelitis due to blood-borne infection in infancy or due to a direct spread from an acute otitis media may cause damage to the condylar cartilage with cessation of growth. This can be unilateral or bilateral and there may be a degree of ankylosis.

Excessive or diminished secretion of the anterior lobe of the pituitary gland may cause excessive or diminished growth which, if operative in the early growth period, may produce a well-proportioned giant or dwarf. In the later stages of growth, increased pituitary secretion may stimulate active sites of cartilage, producing the syndrome known as acromegaly. This particularly affects the extremities and the lower jaw, producing a marked Class III malocclusion.

3. Factors affecting Appositional Growth of Bone and the Normal Remodelling Processes.—Cleidocranial dysostosis is a rare condition which is familial. There is an interference with appositional growth of bone with defects in growth of various parts of the skeleton. Where the facial skeleton is affected, the maxilla fails to grow normally and a relative mandibular protrusion may be found. One of the fairly constant symptoms is that some or all of the teeth fail to erupt at the normal time and supernumerary teeth tend to be present.

Traumatic injuries to the jaws heal with amazing rapidity in the child. Unless the growth sites at the condyles are damaged or there is a gross displacement of fragments, growth will compensate for any slight disturbance of the occlusion.

Severe infective lesions such as the so-called 'osteomyelitis of the newborn', which is a follicular infection, may cause a number of teeth to be exfoliated but may cause very little disturbance in the overall growth pattern of the jaws.

Nutritional abnormalities affecting the growth of bone are now extremely rare in civilized communities. Rickets used to be cited as a cause of certain types of open bite. Owing to the malleability of the bone in rickets there might be an increased tendency to malocclusion in the face of adverse influences, but it is not thought to be clinically important at the present time.

4. **Defects affecting Growth at the Sutures.**—A number of congenital abnormalities appear to be associated with premature closure of the cranial and facial sutures. The maxilla is underdeveloped and the upper dental arch is consequently narrow and small, whereas the mandible is normal in size and there is a relative Class III malocclusion. Many of these patients have only a short expectation of life, and treatment is not considered useful.

5. **Pathological Factors affecting Soft Tissues influencing the Jaws and Dental Arches.**—Lack of tissue in cleft-lip and cleft palate may produce some contraction of the upper arch when surgery has been performed. Congenital enlargement of the tongue will have an effect on the dental arches, producing splaying of the teeth with an open bite. Birth trauma with brain damage may produce spasticity of the tongue musculature with consequent 'wooden tongue', which again fosters an open bite.

Facial paresis in children does not affect the dental arches to any great extent.

Severe burns of the face with marked scarring will produce abnormal pressures on the developing dental arches and sometimes a distortion of jaw growth.

SKELETAL OPEN BITE

Skeletal open bite is the title given to a distinct clinical entity which can occur with a Class I, II, or III occlusal relationship and with a Skeletal 1, 2, or 3 relationship. It is so called to distinguish it from open bites confined to the anterior segments of the arches, which are mainly due to soft-tissue interference. The angle of the mandible is invariably obtuse, carrying the lower teeth downwards away from the maxillary teeth so that only the posterior teeth occlude. It is most commonly noticed on a Skeletal 3 base, and mention has been made of this in Chapter XIII (*see Fig.* 225). The patient does not usually complain of difficulty with feeding, and the marked mandibular prognathism is the main reason for seeking treatment. There is usually excessive depth between the red margin of the lower lip and the point of the chin, and the soft tissues are often of sufficient length to effect a lip seal at rest. This is the particular growth pattern for the individual.

Orthodontic treatment can do little to help these patients. If there is a serious difficulty in feeding or the patient is very concerned about appearance, surgical treatment is the only possibility.

MAJOR SURGERY IN RELATION TO ORTHODONTICS

As has been quite clearly stated, the relationship of the dental bases cannot be materially changed by orthodontic treatment. Various types of osteotomy may be performed where there is a gross disharmony between the jaws.

Quite extensive maxillary osteotomies are being practised, as described by Wasmund and others. The first premolars are extracted as in ordinary orthodontic treatment and the anterior segments of the maxilla repositioned in gross Class II cases. The simple sliding osteotomy originally described by Kostecka involving a cut in the ramus of the mandible has now been superseded by other techniques including those involving the splitting of the ramus, as described by Obgeweser.

Where there is an anterior open bite, ostectomy of the mandible body is still practised in some cases with removal of a segment of bone. These operations are usually not undertaken until growth has ceased, with the exception of the very severe case when a second operation may be justified later.

Owing to the adverse pull of the attached musculature and the influence of the tongue, consideration must be given to muscle stripping and reduction in tongue size in the very severe cases.

Surgical treatment of Skeletal 2 cases showing marked micrognathia are rarely satisfactory because the posterior fragment may slide forwards at the condyle and be splinted in that position, so that the whole mandible goes back into a retruded position after removal of the splints. Another disadvantage is the loss of the suprahyoid incisura, giving the patient a bull-necked appearance. Many surgeons prefer to perform a masking operation in micrognathic cases, placing onlays in the chin region.

These surgical procedures should not be advocated too lightly. Orthodontic preparation of the arches may be required in order to improve the occlusion when the arches are repositioned.

These procedures should not be advocated unless the patient is extremely keen and the whole operation and after-care explained to him. A team approach is essential as preliminary orthodontic preparation of the arches may be required or be undertaken afterwards in order to improve the occlusion by local tooth movements. The reader is referred to modern texts for details of these surgical procedures.

THE AGE FACTOR IN ORTHODONTIC TREATMENT

Although timing of treatment has already received mention in the chapters relating to each type of malocclusion, it is convenient to summarize the subject here. All types of malocclusion can be identified in the complete deciduous dentition, but are not so apparent to the parents. Any treatment during this stage is of little avail and rarely prevents the need for further treatment at a later date, when co-operation may be much greater. A possible exception to this is when there is a deviation in the path of closure from the rest position to occlusion.

During the two years in which the permanent incisors are erupting and finding their position in the dental arches, a number of relatively simple 'interceptive' procedures can be adopted (*see* Chapter VII).

There is still some controversy as to whether treatment of Class II, division 1 cases should be started in the mixed dentition. Many parents are anxious because their children are teased at school, and they also fear that the upper incisors may be injured. However, apart from these factors, case assessment may be clearer if active treatment is delayed until the time of premolar eruption in either a Class II, division 1 or a Class II, division 2 malocclusion. A period of observation during which conservative treatment is completed is often advisable before any orthodontic treatment.

In Class III malocclusions there may be distinct advantages in correcting the permanent incisor relationship at the time of eruption.

Orthodontic procedures for the adult do not differ fundamentally from those used for the younger patient. Theoretically there is no reason why tooth movement should not be possible, but there are many practical reasons which make for difficulties in patients over 16 years of age.

At the present time there is considerable demand for treatment in the late 'teens. This occurs when children emerge from adolescence into the adult world to find there is a premium on appearance. This applies to success at interviews and also in their relationship with the opposite sex. The demand may diminish as dental health education improves and parents come to understand that the ideal age for orthodontic treatment is usually between 10 and 14 years of age.

There will always be some demand for treatment in adult life. Teeth may be lost due to trauma or infection and drifting of neighbouring teeth may make for difficulty in placing a bridge or a prosthetic appliance. The patient may become more aware of increasing irregularities in the anterior region of both arches at the time of eruption of the third molars.

There are certain special problems which must be taken into consideration before attempting orthodontic treatment over the age of 16. The patient may have left school and be studying at a centre of higher education or he may find it difficult to get away from work in a busy office or factory. It is not easy to persuade patients to wear appliances throughout the day and the evenings. Social engagements will tend to take precedence and even if appliances are worn conscientiously at night, this may represent only a small fraction of the twenty-four hours.

People who are much in the public eye may well be torn between a genuine desire to co-operate and the embarrassment of wearing an appliance during the day-time. Many who use telephones or participate in public speaking may find an appliance a severe handicap. Appliances should be modified to suit the particular problem and made as simple as possible. Multibanded techniques will not be popular but some patients will tolerate them if it is explained that procedures can be carried out with more precision and speed.

Another difference in treating adults is that growth of the face and jaws has virtually ceased, which means that the situation is much more static than in the young patient. The orthodontist can never rely on growth producing a change in the basic skeletal relationship of the jaws, even in the growing child, but in the adult there will be little natural help in changing occlusal levels or in space closure by the eruption of posterior teeth with mesial drift.

An important difference in working with adults is that the supporting tissues of the teeth may not be healthy. There may be chronic marginal gingivitis which could be the prelude to more advanced periodontal disease. It is true to say that many children may suffer from marginal gingivitis but this is often reversible. In the young adult, however, it may not be so easily reversed. Where there is an obvious gingival irritation this must be cleared up and a rigid régime of oral hygiene established before any orthodontic treatment is undertaken. In some cases orthodontic treatment may be desirable to correct an irregularity which is preventing adequate cleansing or access for restoration. Reduction of an overjet will facilitate lip seal, especially if there is potential lip competence, and thus the gingival health may be improved.

In the older age range there may be extensive involvement of the periodontal tissues with irregular pocketing. Orthodontic treatment may be desirable to improve alinement before fixation with periodontal splints. This is not a procedure which the authors would advocate in many cases but there is a definite place for it.

Orthodontic treatment for the adult should be limited to the following situations:—

1. Local tooth movements where space is available in one part of the mouth and there is local crowding in another adjacent section of one or both arches.

2. Where space, required for the placing of a bridge or prosthetic appliance, has been partially lost by drifting of teeth. The placing of this appliance will be much more satisfactory if the teeth are better alined.

3. Where there is gross irregularity in one or both arches which could be eliminated by the extraction of the most displaced teeth and simple alinement of adjacent teeth. This would give much better access for restorative work and for scaling and general oral hygiene.

4. Cases with excessive overjet and lack of lip seal, where the upper teeth are splayed forward but there is a Class I arch relationship.

5. Mild abnormalities of arch relationship, both Class II and Class III.

6. Simple tooth movements in one arch or both arches in conjunction with surgical correction of a gross abnormality in jaw relationship.

7. Orthodontic treatment of a minor nature as part of occlusal adjustment may help to relieve pain related to the temporomandibular joint which is primarily associated with muscle spasm.

8. In the younger adult there may be problems of unerupted teeth such as the upper canines. Orthodontic treatment may be required to move them into the arch or make space available for pontics in cases where the displaced teeth have to be surgically removed.

9. To assist in cases of deep overbite where the incisors are causing trauma to the gingivae.

Finally, it is necessary to state quite clearly the contra-indications to orthodontic treatment in the adult. It is wiser not to start on an elaborate and unsuccessful course of treatment in the following cases:—

1. When there is an open bite due to the type of skeletal pattern, with a high Frankfort-mandibular-plane angle, there is a true disparity between the anterior and posterior lower face heights. Even surgical treatment of such an open bite is liable to relapse. Although a severe prognathism may be corrected, the anterior teeth rarely meet properly in occlusion.

2. Unerupted teeth and impacted teeth which are grossly displaced are better left alone or extracted. Heroic efforts to bring them into the arch are rarely justified.

3. Mild incisor crowding with perfect relationship of the buccal segments would be extremely difficult to relieve. The extractions required to relieve the incisor crowding might make for poorer contact relations in the buccal segments.

4. In all cases where there is irregular pocketing and drifting of the teeth unless orthodontic treatment is considered necessary prior to periodontal splinting.

5. There is no advantage in treating a deep overbite where there is no gingival trauma. Such an overbite does not predispose to periodontal disease.

Although the response of the periodontal tissues and the surrounding bone should not differ greatly in the young adult from that of the child, it is definitely less labile and certain adults do show a considerable density of bony pattern which does not make for easy orthodontic tooth movement. Reitan (1966) states as follows: 'A comparison of normal supporting structures in young individuals with those of older individuals reveals that a considerable difference exists with regard to the normal condition of the supporting structures as observed in control material. There are, however, individual variations, especially marked during the transition period of individuals a little above 20 years old, several of whom reveal an inner bone surface partly bordered by osteoid layers. Normal supporting structures of an adult between 30 and 40 years old frequently exhibit a dense alveolar bone tissue with small marrow spaces. Along the inner alveolar bone surface a darkly stained resting line is observed, indicating that only minor tissue changes have taken place over a longer period of time. A continuous movement of teeth whose supporting structures, prior to treatment, are in a resting period will not cause the same reaction as in young individuals.'

There is therefore some variation in the way in which teeth will respond to pressure in the adult and in some instances a cell-free hyalinized area may occur in the periodontal tissues preventing tooth movement, particularly if pressures are excessive.

However, in many of his experiments with adults, Reitan describes an extensive increase in the cellular elements on the pressure side of the periodontal membrane which is quite favourable to tooth movement.

Despite the fact that it is possible to carry out most orthodontic procedures for the young adult, the results will be disappointing unless there is full co-operation. For this reason it is unwise to embark on a scheme of orthodontic treatment of a complex and protracted nature. Considerable experience is required to judge cases which will be successful.

From time to time adult patients will present with acute anxiety states and with a fixation concerning a very mild dental irregularity. They will be very difficult patients and a successful outcome of the orthodontic treatment will be followed by transference of their fixations. It may be in the patient's best interests to obtain a medical opinion before undertaking any treatment.

RETENTION

When upper incisors are moved labially over the lowers and there is a good overbite they are immediately stable in this new position and require no retention. Other relatively local tooth movements, such as the rotation of an incisor tooth, require immediate and prolonged retention even if there is adequate room in the arch, with no displacing forces. Residual disturbances are present in the supporting structures which may bring about rapid reversion to the original position. Teeth which are not rotated, but merely crowded outside or inside the line of the arch, remain stable when they are re-alined, providing adequate space has been acquired.

It has been constantly stressed that lateral expansion of both upper and lower arches merely to accommodate all the teeth moves them out of balance with their soft-tissue environment and is therefore followed by relapse.

Stability of the end-result has to be specially considered in relation to the treatment of Class II, division 1 and Class II, division 2 malocclusions. If teeth are moved into a position out of balance with the soft tissues of the tongue and lips which are acting on them, they will not remain stable even if they are retained for a long time. There are controversial views on the extent to which the soft-tissue activity will adapt to a new tooth position. In a Class II, division 1 case unless the upper incisors are retracted to a position where they can be controlled on their labial aspect by the lower lip, they will not remain stable. However, when such a position is reached, a period of retention is very desirable, with the slow withdrawal of appliances and observation. If there is a persistent tongue-thrust, or an abnormal tongue-resting position or a lower lip scooping under the upper incisal edge to effect a lip seal at rest and in function, the upper and lower incisal contact may not be maintained.

In Class II, division 2 cases the upper incisor position will not be stable if the central incisors have been proclined in the face of pressure from the lower lip. Only minor improvements can be obtained in this direction. Even where adequate space has been created for the retraction of the upper lateral incisors, they still tend to 'creep' forwards.

In general, lower incisors cannot be proclined as they will not remain stable in the face of lower lip activity.

Understanding of the problems of soft tissue posture and behaviour in relation to stability of the incisors makes it feasible in many cases to assess the possibilities of permanent improvement at the time of treatment planning.

The practice of producing a result which requires permanent retention with a night plate is very undesirable from the point of view of oral health.

If residual spacing is present, retention plates must be designed to allow natural mesial movement of teeth distal to the gap.

RADIOGRAPHIC CEPHALOMETRICS

Dr. B. Holly Broadbent's introduction of a technique for examining the skull by serial radiographs taken with standardized head fixation has enabled orthodontists to use this as a research tool to study the growth of the jaws and the development of the dentition (*Fig.* 255). This has extended knowledge beyond the anthropological and craniometric data derived from skull measurements. Serial studies of this kind require a fixed point and plane along which each skull tracing can be superimposed.

Broadbent used a registration point 'R' which is obtained by bisecting a perpendicular dropped from the middle point of the sella turcica to the Bolton plane (*Fig.* 256). Other workers have found this plane difficult to assess in every film and have used the plane from the middle point of the sella turcica to the nasion, the 'S–N' plane, superimposing on the 'S' or 'N' point.

Serial skull tracings have given valuable information on the growth trends of the facial skeleton (*see Fig.* 260). Superimpositions upon various parts of the skull have been used to show the growth at any particular point relative to another.

This method of study has led to the use of cephalometric radiographs for a theoretical appraisal of a case by comparison with the 'normal', which is merely a statistically derived average face taken from the various basic studies, which must be from the same ethnic group.

Cephalometric appraisal has followers, particularly in the United States, and many types of analysis have been developed. It is not within the scope of this book to discuss these in detail, and recent papers and discussions on cephalometrics have failed to reach agreement.

If skull radiographs are to be used in this way, the limitations of orthodontic treatment must be fully appreciated. It is known that the facial skeleton grows according to a predetermined pattern, which is

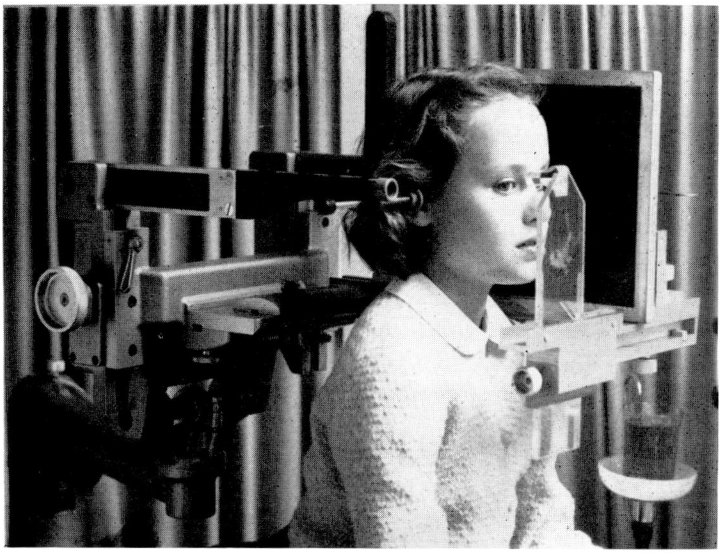

Fig. 255.—Bolton-Broadbent cephalometer for standardized head fixation used in dental research. Apparatus presented to Guy's Hospital Dental School by Charles B. Bolton, F.A.C.D., Cleveland, Ohio.

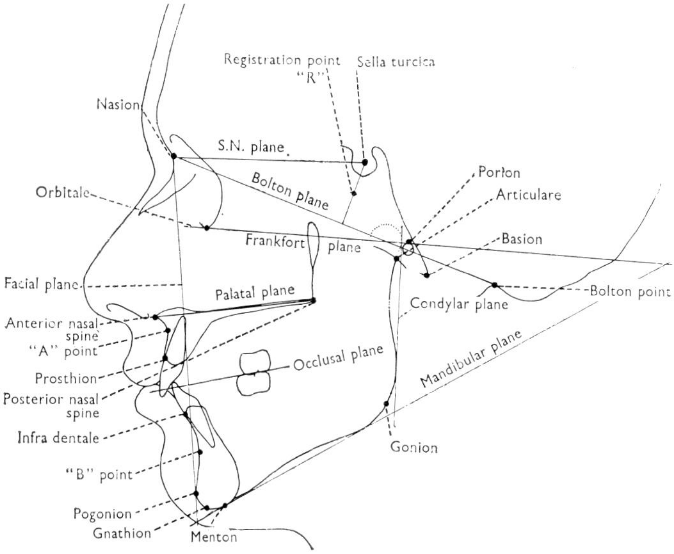

Fig. 256.—Diagram to show landmarks and planes used in cephalometrics.

relatively unchangeable. The cheeks, lips, and tongue place very definite limitations on the amount of change in tooth position on the dental bases.

Among the many methods of assessing the anteroposterior relationship of the dental bases, two deserve mention with their respective advantages and disadvantages:—

1. Down's method assesses the anteroposterior relationship of the 'A' and 'B' points, which are usually quite clearly defined in lateral films. This is achieved by measuring the difference between the angles 'SNA' and 'SNB', and has the advantage of relating these two points to each other and to the cranial base. The average angle for 'SNA' is 80° and for 'SNB' 77°, so that major variations can be appreciated (*Fig.* 257).

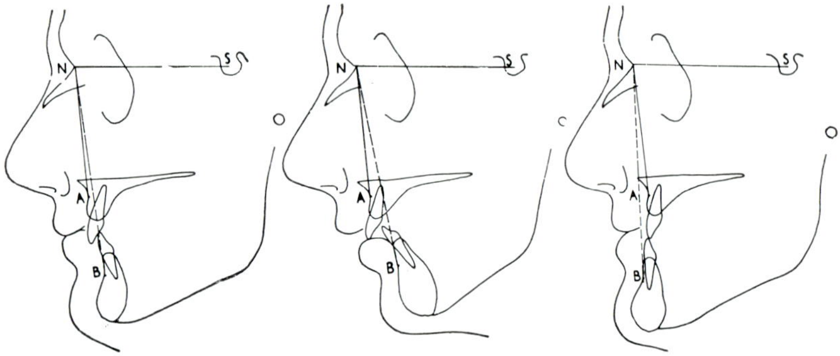

A B C

Fig. 257.—A, *A Skeletal* 1 *Relationship.* The angle SNA is 80° and the angle SNB is 78°. These are the average values found where the dental bases are normally related to each other and to the cranial base. B, *A Type of Skeletal* 2 *Relationship.* In this case the angle SNA is 80° and the angle SNB is 73°. There is a mandibular retrusion with a maxilla normally related to the cranial base. C, *A Type of Skeletal* 3 *Relationship.* The angle SNA is 80° and the angle SNB is 83°. There is a mandibular protrusion in this case with a maxilla normally related to the cranial base.

The real disadvantage is that these points are not truly indicative of the basal bone area. They are points on the alveolar process and do not relate directly to the apical positions of the incisors.

2. Ballard's method is to trace the axial inclination of the upper incisors to the Frankfort plane or to the maxillary plane and to correct this to the theoretical normal angle of 105° to the Frankfort plane or 109° to the maxillary plane; to draw in the lower incisor angle to the mandibular plane and correct this to the theoretical normal of 90° where the Frankfort-mandibular-plane angle is under 25°. Where the Frankfort-mandibular-plane angle exceeds 25° the normal inclination

of the lower incisors will be correspondingly smaller (*Figs.* 258, 259) and therefore the angle of the lower incisors is better corrected in relation to the Frankfort plane, taking as an average the angle 65° as described by Tweed.

If, when the incisors have been placed in their theoretically correct inclinations there is no discrepancy in the anteroposterior relationship of their crowns, a Skeletal 1 relationship is indicated (*Fig.* 259 A). If there is a discrepancy it is indicative of a Skeletal 2 or a Skeletal 3 dental base relationship (*see Fig.* 259 B).

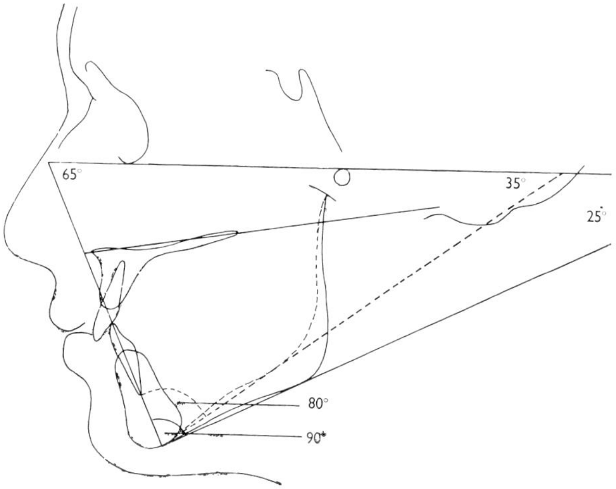

Fig. 258.—Diagram illustrating how the lower incisor-mandibular-plane angle varies inversely with the Frankfort-mandibular-plane angle.

From the clinical point of view there is one disadvantage in this method: it tends to encourage the belief that the axial inclinations of incisors can always be corrected by orthodontic treatment. It must be appreciated that repositioning of teeth will depend on their muscular environment and cannot be expected to comply with a theoretical requirement.

The definitions of some of the principal terms used in cephalometrics are appended.

Anthropological and Cephalometric Landmarks (*Fig.* 256)

Nasion: The anterior point of the suture at the junction of the frontal and nasal bones in the mid-sagittal plane.

Sella Point ('S' point): The mid-point of the sella turcica determined by inspection.

Porion: The uppermost point of the bony external auditory meatus. (Usually located as the upper point on the ear rod on the cephalometer as it is not a clearly distinguishable bony landmark.)

Tragion: The uppermost point of the supratragal notch. The soft-tissue equivalent of the porion.

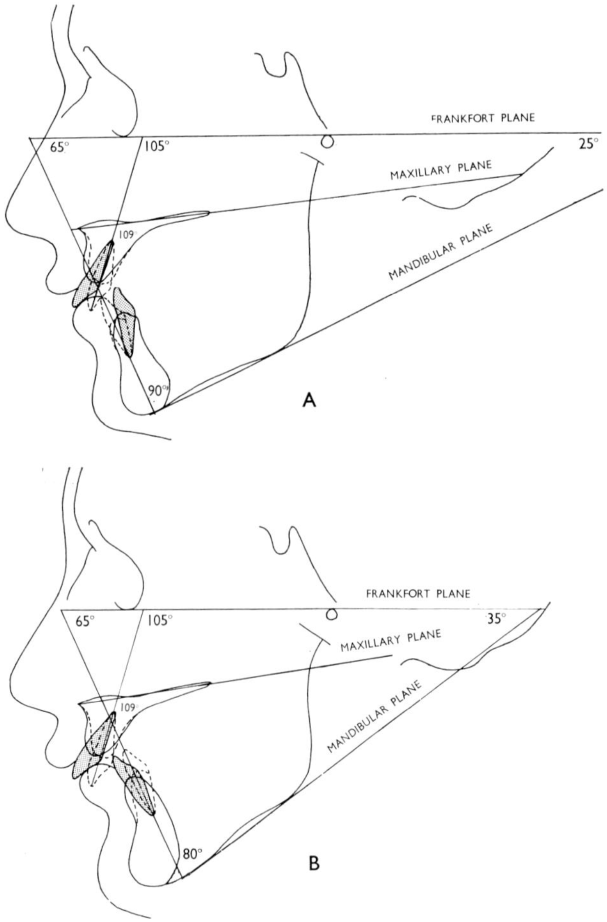

Fig. 259.—Illustrates Ballard's method of correcting lower incisor angle to mandibular plane and upper incisor angle to Frankfort plane, or the maxillary plane, as shown by dotted contour of teeth and then noting whether there is a discrepancy in the incisor relationship indicating the degree of skeletal discrepancy. The actual position of the incisors is indicated by shading. Dotted outlines indicate the theoretically corrected positions. A, Shows Class II, division 1 incisor relationship with normal dental base relationship indicated when incisor inclination is corrected. (Dotted position of incisors.) B, Corrected position of incisors indicates that there is a Skeletal 2 relationship. Corrected lower incisor-mandibular-plane angle is 80° where the Frankfort-mandibular angle is 35°.

Orbitale: The lowest point on the lower margin of the orbit.

Gnathion: The point on the chin determined by bisecting the angle formed by the facial and mandibular planes.

Menton: The lowest point on the symphysial shadow. In some instances the term gnathion and menton have been used synonymously but there are obvious differences between the two.

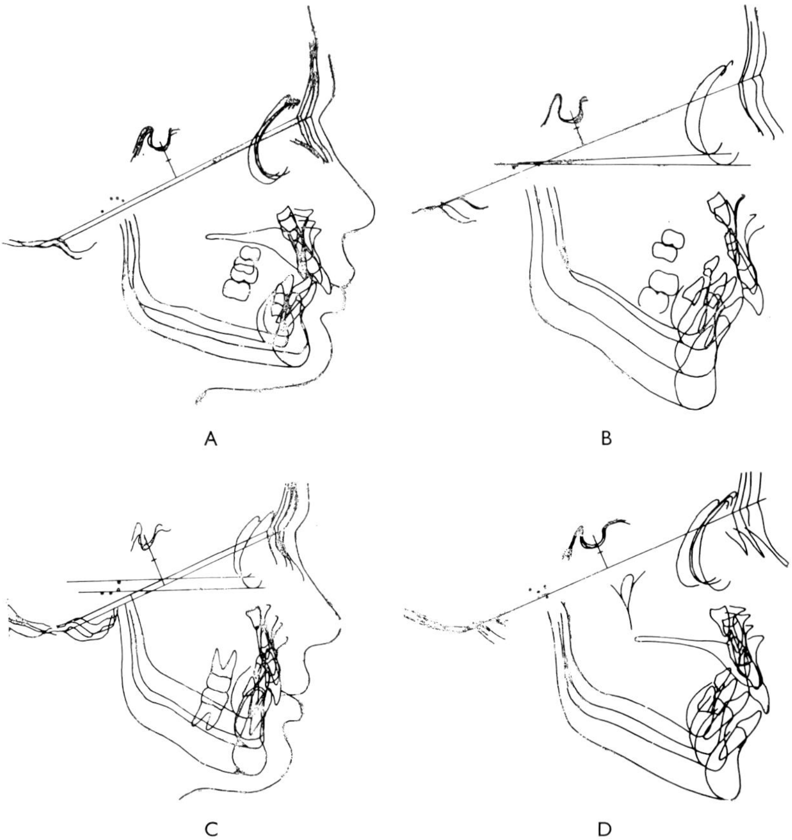

Fig. 260.—Tracings of developing malocclusions from the Bolton study illustrating different growth patterns of the facial skeleton and paths of eruption of the incisor teeth determined by their soft-tissue environment. A and B show variations of growth pattern in a Class II, division 1 malocclusion. A, Shows some downward and forward growth of the mandible. Note proclination of upper incisors as they enter the mouth. B, Shows the mandible growing more downward than forward. Note path of eruption of upper incisors. C and D should be contrasted. C illustrates the development of the dentition with rather a deep overbite of the Class II, division 2 type where the soft tissues are not dispersing the upper and lower incisors and the angle between upper incisors and the Frankfort plane is little more than 90° at any time. D, Shows proclinations of upper and lower incisors becoming more marked as teeth erupt, under the influence of the soft tissues. The tongue is large and the lips flabby.

Pogonion: This point is the most anterior point in the profile of the bony chin.

Gonion: A point midway between the most anterior and posterior points on the angle of the jaw, obtained by bisecting the angle formed by a tangent to the mandibular base and the posterior margin of the ascending ramus.

Anterior Nasal Spine ('ANS'): The tip of the anterior nasal spine seen on the lateral X-ray film.

'*A*' *Point* (Sub-spinale): The deepest midline point between the anterior nasal spine and the prosthion.

Prosthion: The most anterior point on the alveolar process, usually between the upper central incisors.

Infra Dentale: The most anterior point of the alveolar process, situated between the mandibular central incisors.

'*B*' *Point* (Supra mentale): The deepest point in the concavity of the bone between the infra dentale and the pogonion.

Registration Point '*R*': The point used by Broadbent for superimposition, obtained by bisecting a perpendicular drawn from the midpoint of the sella turcica on to the Bolton plane.

Bolton Point: The highest point on the notch immediately posterior to the occipital condyle.

Basion: The lowest point on the anterior margin of the foramen magnum.

Articulare: The point of intersection of the dorsal contours of the condylar process and the external cranial base.

In order to define a plane there must be at least three points of reference and therefore in a tracing of a lateral radiograph it is assumed that planes are represented by lines, as follows:—

Planes.—

Bolton Plane: Represented by a line connecting the nasion with the uppermost point on the post-condylar notch. (The Bolton point.)

Frankfort Horizontal Plane: Represented by a line connecting the lower border of the orbit and the porion (the upper border of the external auditory meatus) or the most superior point of the supratragal notch.

Occlusal Plane: Represented by a line which bisects the incisor overbite and the cuspal height of the first molar teeth.

Mandibular Plane: Represented by a line connecting the two most dependent points of the mandible or a line from menton to gonion.

Facial Plane: Represented by a line drawn from the nasion at a tangent to the pogonion.

Orbital Plane: Represented by a line drawn from the orbitale at right angles to the Frankfort plane.

Palatal or Maxillary Plane: Represented by a line drawn through the anterior and posterior nasal spines.

The use of the cephalometer as a diagnostic or research tool has been criticized owing to the difficulty of locating some of the points of reference with accuracy. However, those who use it as a routine become skilled in the interpretation of these headplates. Its main and most satisfactory role is to allow a general appraisal of facial and dental growth, and if this is linked with further studies of the soft-tissue environment of the teeth, our knowledge of the wide variations of facial form will be greatly enhanced.

Fig. 260 A–D illustrates cases from the files of the Bolton Foundation by kind permission of Dr. B. Holly Broadbent. These make the value of the method abundantly clear.

BIBLIOGRAPHY

BJØRK, A. (1947), 'The Face in Profile', *Svensktandläk Tidskr.*, **40**, No. 5B Suppl. Lund.

— — JENSEN, E., and PALLING, M. (1956), 'Mandibular Growth and Third Molar Impactions', *Trans. europ. orthod. Soc.*, 164.

BROADBENT, B. H. (1931), 'A New X-ray Technique and its Application to Orthodontics', *Angle Orthodont.*, **1**, 45.

BRODIE, A. G. (1938), 'Cephalometric Appraisal of Orthodontic Results', *Ibid.*, **8**, 261.

DOWNS, W. B. (1948), 'Variations in Facial Relationship, Their Significance in Treatment and Prognosis', *Amer. J. Orthodont.*, **34**, 812.

EASTWOOD, A. W. (1952), 'Cephalometric Radiography in Diagnosis and Treatment Analysis', *Dent. Rec.*, **72**, 58.

FLETCHER, G. G. T. (1958), 'Age Factor in Orthodontic Treatment', *Dent. Practit.*, **8**, 31.

GLASS, D. F. (1959), 'Rehabilitation of the Cleft Lip and Palate Child', *Ibid.*, **10**, 47.

HIGLEY, L. B. (1951), 'Application of Cephalometric Appraisal in Orthodontic Diagnosis and Treatment', *Amer. J. Orthodont.*, **37**, 244.

HOVELL, J. (1956), 'The Surgical Correction of Variations in the Facial Skeletal Pattern', *Proc. R. Soc. Med.*, **48**, 546.

— — (1958), 'Some Surgical Procedures related to Orthodontic Treatment', *Dent. Practit.*, **9**, 21.

KETTLE, M. A. (1957), 'Treatment of the Unerupted Maxillary Canine', *Trans. Brit. Soc. Orthodont.*, 74.

KROGMAN, W. M., and SASSOUNI (1957), *Syllabus in Roentgenographic Cephalometry*, P.A. Center for Research in Child Growth. P.A., U.S.A.

PRINGLE, K. E. (1946), 'Variations in Response', *Dent. Rec.*, **66**, 187.

REITAN, K. (1966), 'Tissue Reaction following Orthodontic Tooth Movement', in *Current Orthodontics* (ed. WALTHER, D. P.), p. 457. Bristol: Wright.

TULLEY, W. J. (1952), 'The Age Factor in Orthodontic Treatment', *Dent. Practit.*, **2**, 196.

— — and CRYER, B. S. (1969), *Orthodontic Treatment for the Adult*. Bristol: Wright.

INDEX